MAKING THE DIAGNOSIS

A Video-Enhanced Guide to Identifying
Musculoskeletal Disorders

MAKING THE DIAGNOSIS

A Video-Enhanced Guide to Identifying Musculoskeletal Disorders

Edited by:
Ian J. Dempsey, MD, MBA
Fellow Sports Medicine and Shoulder Surgery
Department of Orthopaedic Surgery
Rush University Medical Center
Chicago, Illinois

Mark D. Miller, MD
S. Ward Casscells Professor
Department of Orthopaedic Surgery
University of Virginia Health System
Charlottesville, Virginia

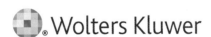

Philadelphia • Baltimore • New York • London
Buenos Aires • Hong Kong • Sydney • Tokyo

Acquisitions Editor: Brian Brown
Development Editor: Sean McGuire
Editorial Coordinator: Alexis Pozonsky
Marketing Manager: Rachel Mante-Leung
Production Project Manager: David Saltzberg
Design Coordinator: Teresa Mallon
Manufacturing Coordinator: Beth Welsh
Prepress Vendor: TNQ Technologies

9 8 7 6 5 4 3 2 1

Printed in China

Library of Congress Cataloging-in-Publication Data

Names: Miller, Mark D., editor. | Dempsey, Ian J., editor.
Title: Making the diagnosis : a video-enhanced guide to identifying musculoskeletal disorders / edited by Ian J. Dempsey, Mark D. Miller.
Description: First edition. | Philadelphia : Wolters Kluwer, [2019] | Includes bibliographical references and index.
Identifiers: LCCN 2018041462 | ISBN 9781496381125 (paperback)
Subjects: | MESH: Musculoskeletal Diseases–diagnostic imaging | Video-Assisted Surgery
Classification: LCC RC925.7 | NLM WE 141 | DDC 616.7/075–dc23
LC record available at https://lccn.loc.gov/2018041462

CCS1218

Dedication

IJD: To my wife, Olivia, for always supporting me and enduring all the long hours spent writing, compiling, and editing this text, and to my family for their love and encouragement in all of my endeavors.

MDM: To my brilliant and beautiful wife, Ann, for allowing me to work on yet another textbook, and to all those who are committed to life-long-learning and improving their clinical acumen in Making the Diagnosis.

Contributors

Bayan Aghadasi, MD
Chief Resident
Department of Orthopaedic Surgery
University of Virginia Health System
Charlottesville, Virginia

Victor Anciano, MD
Resident Physician
Department of Orthopaedic Surgery
University of Virginia Health System
Charlottesville, Virginia

Keith R. Bachmann, MD
Assistant Professor
Department of Orthopaedic Surgery
University of Virginia Health System
Charlottesville, Virginia

Jeffrey D. Boatright, MD, MS
Fellow Hand and Upper Extremity Surgery
Department of Orthopaedic Surgery
University of Virginia Health System
Charlottesville, Virginia

Jourdan M. Cancienne, MD
Fellow Sports Medicine and Shoulder Surgery
Department of Orthopaedic Surgery
Rush University Medical Center
Chicago, Illinois

James B. Carr, II, MD
Resident Physician
Department of Orthopaedic Surgery
University of Virginia Health System
Charlottesville, Virginia

Samuel Evan Carstensen, MD
Resident Physician
Department of Orthopaedic Surgery
University of Virginia Health System
Charlottesville, Virginia

Aaron J. Casp, MD
Resident Physician
Department of Orthopaedic Surgery
University of Virginia Health System
Charlottesville, Virginia

Dennis Chen, MD
Resident Physician
Department of Orthopaedic Surgery
University of Virginia Health System
Charlottesville, Virginia

M. Truitt Cooper, MD
Assistant Professor
Department of Orthopaedic Surgery
University of Virginia Health System
Charlottesville, Virginia

A. Rashard Dacus, MD
Associate Professor
Department of Orthopaedic Surgery
University of Virginia
Charlottesville, Virginia;
Associate Team Physician
James Madison University
Harrisonburg, Virginia

Ian J. Dempsey, MD, MBA
Fellow Sports Medicine and Shoulder Surgery
Department of Orthopaedic Surgery
Rush University Medical Center
Chicago, Illinois

Trent Gause, MD
Resident Physician
Department of Orthopaedic Surgery
University of Virginia Health System
Charlottesville, Virginia

F. Winston Gwathmey, MD
Resident Physician
Department of Orthopaedic Surgery
University of Virginia Health System
Charlottesville, Virginia

Michael M. Hadeed, MD
Resident Physician
Department of Orthopaedic Surgery
University of Virginia Health System
Charlottesville, Virginia

Hamid Hassanzadeh, MD
Assistant Professor
Department of Orthopaedic Surgery
University of Virginia Health System
Charlottesville, Virginia

Timothy Maxwell Hoggard, MD
Resident Physician
Department of Orthopaedic Surgery
University of Virginia Health System
Charlottesville, Virginia

Jason A. Horowitz, MD
Research Assistant
Department of Orthopaedic Surgery
University of Virginia Health System
Charlottesville, Virginia

Daniel E. Hess, MD
Resident Physician
Department of Orthopaedic Surgery
University of Virginia Health System
Charlottesville, Virginia

Michelle E. Kew, MD
Resident Physician
Department of Orthopaedic Surgery
University of Virginia Health System
Charlottesville, Virginia

Kevin L. Laroche, MD
Resident Physician
Department of Orthopaedic Surgery
University of Virginia Health System
Charlottesville, Virginia

Eric S. Larson, MD
Resident Physician
Department of Orthopaedic Surgery
University of Virginia Health System
Charlottesville, Virginia

Harrison S. Mahon, MD
Resident Physician
Department of Orthopaedic Surgery
University of Virginia Health System
Charlottesville, Virginia

Mark D. Miller, MD
S. Ward Casscells Professor
Head, Division of Sports Medicine
Department of Orthopaedic Surgery
University of Virginia Health System;
Team Physician
James Madison University
Charlottesville, Virginia

Mary K. Mulcahey, MD
Associate Professor
Department of Orthopaedic Surgery
Director, Women's Sports Medicine Program
Tulane University School of Medicine
New Orleans, Louisiana

Hakan C. Pehlivan, MD
Resident Physician
Department of Orthopedic Surgery
University of VirginiaHealth System
Charlottesville, Virginia

Felix H. Savoie, MD
Ray J. Haddad Professor and Chairman
Department of Orthopaedics
Tulane University School of Medicine
New Orleans, Louisiana

Nicholas Shen, MD
Research Assistant
Department of Orthopaedic Surgery
University of Virginia Health System
Charlottesville, Virginia

Dimitri S. Tahal, MD
Research Assistant
Department of Orthopaedic Surgery
University of Virginia Health System
Charlottesville, Virginia

Stephen G. Thon, MD
Chief Resident and Clinical instructor
Department of Orthopaedic Surgery
Tulane University School of Medicine
New Orleans, Louisiana

Brian C. Werner, MD
Assistant Professor
Department of Orthopaedic Surgery
University of Virginia Health System
Charlottesville, Virginia

Foreword

It is my distinct pleasure and honor to be invited to write the foreword for Dempsey and Miller, *Making the Diagnosis*. I must say that I am biased as Mark Miller, MD, is a dear friend and Ian Dempsey, a University of Virginia trainee, will soon start his sports medicine fellowship at Rush in August 2018. I have known Mark Miller, MD, for nearly 25 years and have witnessed his ability to identify educational resource needs and to address those deficiencies by spearheading new textbooks—nearly 40 in number at last count. Some of the most impactful textbooks in orthopedic surgery and sports medicine have the DNA of Dr. Miller. The consummate educator, he is renowned for the Miller Review Course and is the editor in chief for *Clinics in Sports Medicine*. He is an educational giant, on whose shoulder so many of us—orthopedic colleagues, academicians, private practitioners, fellows, residents, primary care sports fellows, and students—have benefitted. For those who have edited textbooks, it is not the royalty benefits that drives us, as the "ergs per stitch" ratio pales in comparison to the hours and hours of preparation, editing, and cajoling contributors to meet deadlines.

So, I ask, why another textbook—particularly one entitled *Making the Diagnosis*? From a conceptual sense this text is "spot on". Many of our trainees are woefully educated in the art of history taking and physical examination skills. The 80-hour work week has strained the abilities of our trainees to spend time in the office or clinic at the expense of being exposed to more surgical cases. One may be exceedingly well trained technically but the art of medicine is in the decision-making processes outside of the operating room theatre. I look at my clinical practice as two overlapping bell-shaped distribution curves—normal and abnormal. The extremes are easy to diagnose. So much of what we do is not "black and white"; we live in a gray zone of overlapping normals and abnormals. The ability to ferret out these subtleties can make the difference between well-indicated and poorly indicated surgeries. Although we are trained as surgeons, our goals should not be to figure out which surgery a patient needs, but rather when performing a meticulous history and careful examination arrive at a correct diagnosis that allows us to put into place a treatment plan. A carefully crafted physical therapy recommendation for someone with core weakness, patellar pain and instability, activity modification for an overuse condition, an evaluation for osteopenia for a young woman with oligomenorrhea and multiple stress fractures, a rheumatologic referral for a patient with polyarticular joint complaints, and appropriate surgical recommendations only when the patient has a clear-cut diagnosis that can be benefitted from a surgical intervention.

Making the Diagnosis is a step in the right direction. This is a "no nonsense" textbook that covers broadly key areas of orthopedic surgery. Multiple anatomic sections are covered quite thoroughly: the knee, hip, elbow, hand and wrist, foot and ankle, the pediatric patient, and the spine. Each section is subdivided into specific pathologic conditions. For example, the knee section is divided into the major pathologies we encounter: the anterior cruciate ligament (ACL) injuries, posterior cruciate ligament (PCL) injuries, posterolateral corner injuries, medial-sided injuries, meniscal injuries, patellar instability, and osteochondral injuries. As one dissects the anatomy of each topic in a bullet-formatted presentation the classic history, appropriate physical examination tests, and pertinent imaging studies are presented, along with evaluation flowcharts, appropriate images (physical examination, radiographic, MRI [magnetic resonance imaging],

CT [computed tomography], and intraoperative findings). Each chapter is accompanied by key references and original videos.

    I look forward to seeing this textbook in its final form. I believe there will be a major role in one's library for this contribution. Congratulations to the authors for having the vision, tenacity, and passion to produce this outstanding contribution to the orthopedic community.

Bernard R. Bach, Jr., MD
The Claude Lambert–Helen Thomson Professor of Orthopedics
Director (*Emeritus*) Rush Sports Medicine division and Sports Medicine Fellowship
Midwest Orthopedics at RUSH
Department of Orthopedic Surgery
Rush University Medical Center
Assistant Team Physician, Chicago Bulls and White Sox
Chicago, Illinois

Preface

Making the correct diagnosis requires a mastery of multiple clinical variables. One of the most important of these is the physical examination, which, unfortunately, is sometimes overlooked in this era of advanced technology. This is further complicated by the fact that there is often a plethora of physical examination maneuvers described for each diagnosis. To make things even more complicated, these examinations have often been incorrectly performed, modified, or simply misunderstood over the years. We are unaware of a definitive resource that accurately describes each key musculoskeletal examination, including the original description, until now. We reviewed the original sources to document the authors' unedited descriptions of key examinations in musculoskeletal medicine. We then produced new illustrations, clinical photographs, and videos to further elucidate the key features of each examination.

Although physical examination is a critical component of making the diagnosis, it is only one part of the story. Every clinical encounter begins with a history, as well as a general and focused physical examination. This, combined with appropriate imaging, culminates in an accurate diagnosis. Therefore, each anatomically based chapter in this book takes this approach. Key elements in the patient's history include his or her age, activity level, chronicity of his or her complaints, mechanism of injury, associate symptoms, past injuries, and prior treatment to include surgery. Physical examination includes overall components (observation, palpation, range of motion, strength testing, neurovascular testing, and general examination features) and then proceeds to a focused examination. For those less familiar with musculoskeletal medicine, we have included algorithms in each chapter to help the clinician focus on the appropriate areas. Finally, we have outlined what imaging should be obtained, how and when to order it, and how to interpret the results.

Our goal was to create a stand-alone reference for all providers from the beginning medical student, technician, physician assistant, or resident to the most senior orthopedic surgeon who may need a quick refresher on the particulars of an examination that he does not routinely perform. We hope that it will be used to solve arguments in clinic and conference regarding the exact maneuvers involved for a particular examination. However, perhaps most importantly, we hope it improves the care that we offer our patients, leading to their correct diagnoses and, ultimately, their best treatment and outcome.

Ian J. Dempsey
Mark D. Miller

Acknowledgments

We gratefully acknowledge and appreciate the excellent work done on this textbook by the section editors; the faculty, fellows, and residents of the Department of Orthopaedic Surgery at the University of Virginia; and Dr Eric Vess who provided invaluable technical assistance for the video accompanying this text. Finally, we wish to acknowledge and thank the excellent team from Wolters Kluwer to include Lexi Pozonsky, Sean McGuire, and Brian Brown.

Contents

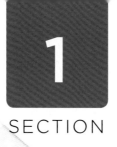

1

SECTION

The Knee

Section Editor
Mark D. Miller

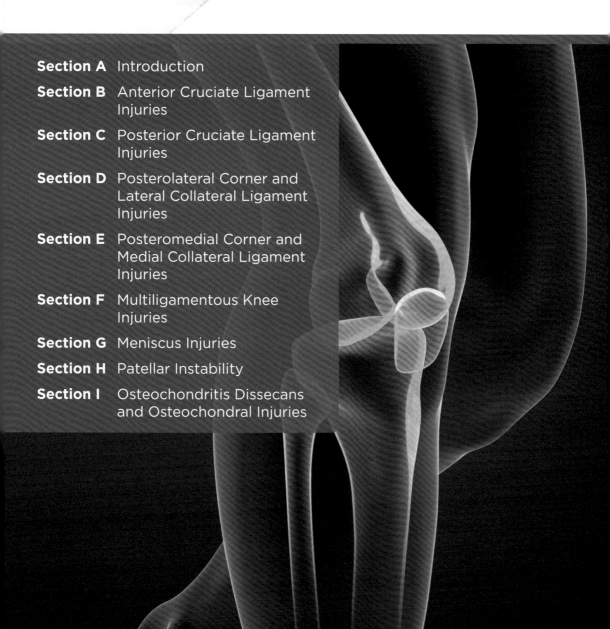

QUICK REFERENCE FLOW CHARTS

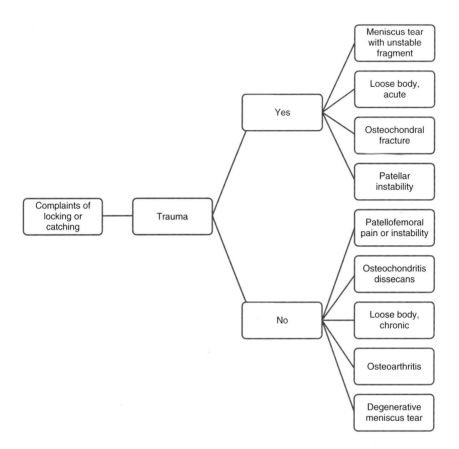

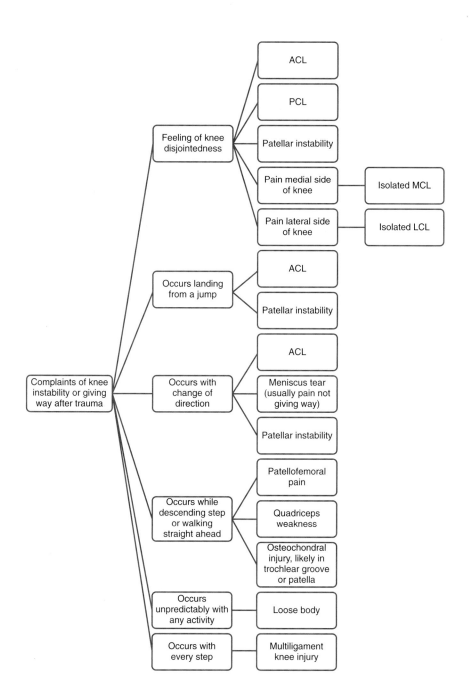

4

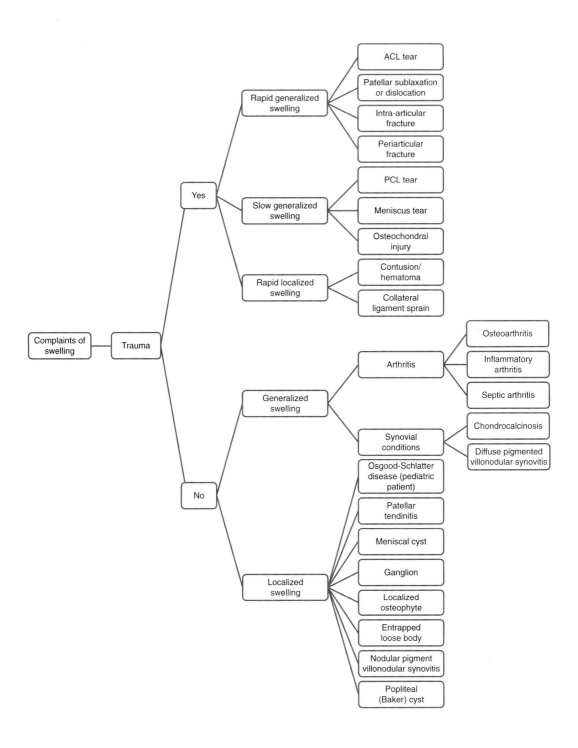

SECTION A
Introduction

Ian J. Dempsey and Mark D. Miller

HISTORY

It is important to consider the following parameters when a patient presents to the clinic with a knee complaint:

- Patient age
  - Younger patients are more likely to have a ligament or acute meniscal injury
  - Older patients are more likely to have osteoarthritis and/or chronic meniscal injuries
- Chronicity of symptoms
  - Acute injuries may involve ligament tears, fractures, dislocations, and meniscal tears
  - Chronic injuries may represent untreated or unrecognized ligament injures (+/− recurrence), osteoarthritis, and chronic/complex/degenerative meniscal tears
- Mechanism of injury (if any)
  - Noncontact pivoting or landing injury with a "pop" and immediate swelling may represent an ACL tear or an acute patellar dislocation
  - Blow to the proximal tibia (MVA dashboard injury or fall on the front of the leg with the foot plantar flexed) may represent a PCL injury
  - Blow to the patella (direct blow or fall on the front of the leg with the foot dorsiflexed) may represent a patellar injury
  - Twisting injury may represent a meniscal tear or a "corner" injury
  - Blow to the outside (lateral side) of the knee may represent an MCL injury
  - Blow to the inside (medial side) of the knee is less common but may represent an LCL injury
  - Pain with climbing stairs or sitting for long periods may be associated with patellofemoral syndrome or arthritis
- Associated swelling (effusion)
  - The following conditions can be associated with acute or subacute swelling:
    - ACL tear
    - Patellar dislocation
    - PCL tear
    - Peripheral meniscal tear
    - Acute osteochondral fracture
- Mechanical symptoms (locking, catching)
  - Commonly associated with meniscal tears, loose bodies, or osteochondral injury/ osteoarthritis
- History of knee injury
  - One must be concerned about reinjury
- History of knee surgery
  - One must critically analyze the prior surgery to determine if there may have been any technical errors
  - Obtain prior operative reports and images; patient reports are often incomplete or inaccurate

- Prior treatment
- Current medications
- One-finger test: Ask patients to point, with 1 finger, to the area where it hurts (they often cannot do so, but it can be helpful)

PHYSICAL EXAMINATION

Observation

- Observe the patients' posture, how they get onto the examination table, and how they describe their pain
- Look at the patient's alignment (Figure 1A.1)
- Evaluation of gait pattern and standing attitude of the entire lower limb as it relates to the knee
  - Antalgic gait: Patients may walk with limp on the affected extremity
  - Trendelenburg gait: Patients may lean to one side because of hip pain
  - Quadriceps avoidance gait: Patients may lean forward and have a short stance phase with ACL deficiency
  - Varus recurvatum gait: Patients' affected knee hyperextends with relative varus during the stance phase of the affected limb with PCL deficiency

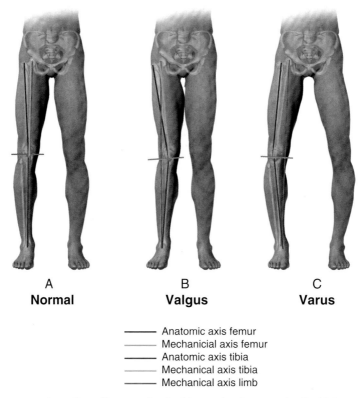

A	B	C
Normal	**Valgus**	**Varus**

──────── Anatomic axis femur
──────── Mechanicial axis femur
──────── Anatomic axis tibia
──────── Mechanical axis tibia
──────── Mechanical axis limb

Figure 1A.1. Lower extremity alignment. A, Normal alignment. B, Valgus alignment. C, Varus alignment. (From Moore KL, Agur AMR, Dalley AF. *Essential Clinical Anatomy*. 5th ed. International edition. Philadelphia: Wolters Kluwer Health; 2015.)

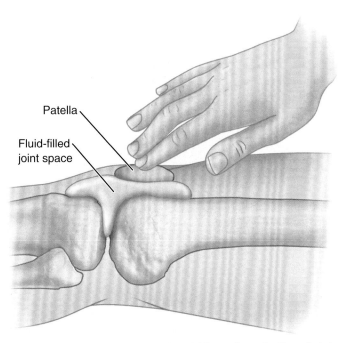

Patella

Fluid-filled joint space

Figure 1A.2. Ballotable patella test. The leg should be relaxed. The clinician gently pushes the patella downward into the groove. If a joint effusion is present, the patella rebounds and floats back up. (From Anderson MK, Barnum M. *Foundations of Athletic Training: Prevention, Assessment, and Management*. Philadelphia: Wolters Kluwer Health; 2017.)

Palpation

- Effusion
  - If an effusion is present, the patella may be ballotable, graded 1 to 4 (Figure 1A.2)
  - Check for swelling in the suprapatellar pouch
  - If a tense effusion is present, any palpation of knee will be painful
  - If a mild effusion is present, there may not be a specific palpable area of tenderness
- Tenderness
  - Joint line tenderness may signify a meniscal tear
  - Medial tenderness may represent an MCL or proximal medial patellofemoral ligament (MPFL) injury
  - Deep tenderness may represent a bone bruise or osteochondral injury

Range of Motion (Figure 1A.3)

- Normal range of motion is typically full extension (0°) or up to 10° of hyperextension (we prefer to designate this as "HE" rather than "+" or "−" because that can be confusing)
- Loss of extension (compared with the opposite side) may represent a "locked knee" (typically from a displaced meniscal tear or loose body). Chronic loss of extension is more ominous and difficult to treat. Full extension must be obtained before reconstructive surgery
- Loss of flexion may be associated with an effusion or poor quad tone

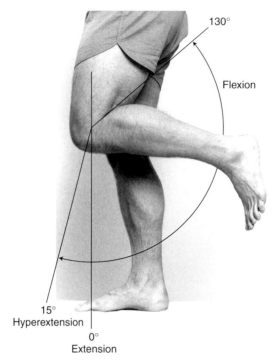

Figure 1A.3. Knee range of motion. (From Jones RM. *Patient Assessment in Pharmacy Practice*. Philadelphia: Wolters Kluwer Health; 2016.)

Muscular Strength

- Normally graded 0 to 5 as follows:
  - Grade 0: no contraction or muscle movement
  - Grade 1: trace contraction
  - Grade 2: movement at the joint with gravity eliminated
  - Grade 3: movement against gravity only
  - Grade 4: movement against external resistance but weak
  - Grade 5: normal strength
- Extensor weakness may represent an injury to the extensor mechanism
  - Patellar fracture
  - Patella tendon rupture (typically seen in patients <40 years of age)
  - Quadriceps tendon rupture (typically seen in patients >40 years of age)
- Flexor weakness may represent a hamstring injury
- Foot and toe loss of extension may represent a common peroneal nerve injury (commonly associated with knee multiple ligament injuries from a knee dislocation)

Sensation (Figure 1A.4A and 1A.4B)

- Can be viewed as dermatomes L2-S1 or as peripheral nerves listed below:
  - Saphenous
  - Sural
  - Superficial peroneal
  - Deep peroneal
  - Tibial

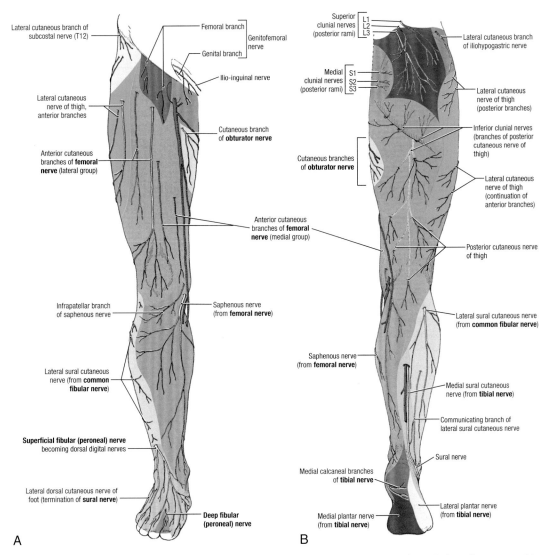

Figure 1A.4. Sensation of the lower extremity as dermatomes and peripheral nerves (A, anterior view and B, posterior view). (From Agur AMR, Dalley AF. *Grant's Atlas of Anatomy*. Philadelphia: Wolters Kluwer Health; 2017.)

KEY EXAMINATION MANEUVERS

- **Anterior Cruciate Ligament Injuries**
  - Anterior drawer test
  - Lachman test
  - KT-1000 arthrometer
  - Classic pivot shift test or MacIntosh test
  - Jerk test
  - Flexion rotation drawer test
  - Losee test
  - Lever sign or Lelli test

- **Posterior Cruciate Ligament Injuries**
  - Posterior sag sign
  - Posterior drawer test

- Godfrey test
- Reverse or posterior Lachman test
- Reverse pivot shift
- Quadriceps active drawer test
- Dynamic posterior shift test

- **Posterolateral Corner and Lateral Collateral Ligament Injuries**
  - External rotation asymmetry or dial test (30° and 90°)
  - Posterolateral drawer test
  - External rotation recurvatum test
  - Varus stress test

- **Posteromedial Corner and Medial Collateral Ligament Injuries**
  - Slocum test
  - Valgus stress test

- **Meniscus Injuries**
  - **Direct Palpation Maneuvers**
    - Bragard test
    - McMurray test
    - Steinmann second test
  - **Rotation Maneuvers**
    - Apley test and grind test
    - Bohler sign
    - Helfet test
    - Steinmann first test
    - Merke test
    - Payr test
    - Duck walk or Childress test
    - Thessaly test

- **Patellar Instability**
  - Fairbank apprehension and modified apprehension test
  - Bassett sign
  - Lateral and medial patellar glide test
  - Patellar tilt test
  - Gravity subluxation test
  - J-sign
  - Q-angle
  - Patella position
  - Vastus medialis obliquus strength

- **Osteochondritis Dissecans and Osteochondral Injuries**
  - Wilson test
  - Passive and active patellar grind test

IMAGING

Plain Radiographs

- AP view (Figure 1A.5A)
- Lateral view (Figure 1A.5B)
  - Condyle overlap
  - Patellar height
- Patellar views
  - Sunrise (Figure 1A.5C)
  - Merchant
  - Laurin

- Flexion weight-bearing PA (Rosenberg view)
- Stress radiographs
  - Physeal injuries
  - Collateral ligament injuries
  - PCL stress radiographs

Magnetic Resonance Imaging

Classic findings (described in detail in the appropriate sections):

- Bone bruise pattern
- Direct and indirect ACL signs
- Double PCL sign
- Double anterior horn sign
- PCL injury

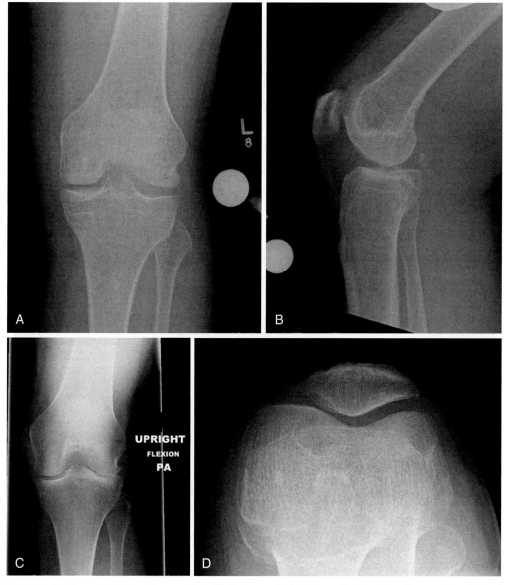

Figure 1A.5. Normal AP radiograph of left knee (A). Normal lateral radiograph of the left knee (B). Normal Flexion weight-bearing PA (Rosenberg view) (C). Normal sunrise view of the left knee (D).

Computed Tomography

- Helpful in revision ACL to evaluate tunnel osteolysis
- TT-TG for patellar instability

Ultrasound—Knee Arthroscopy (Figure 1A.6)

- Portals
- Accessory portals
- Visualization

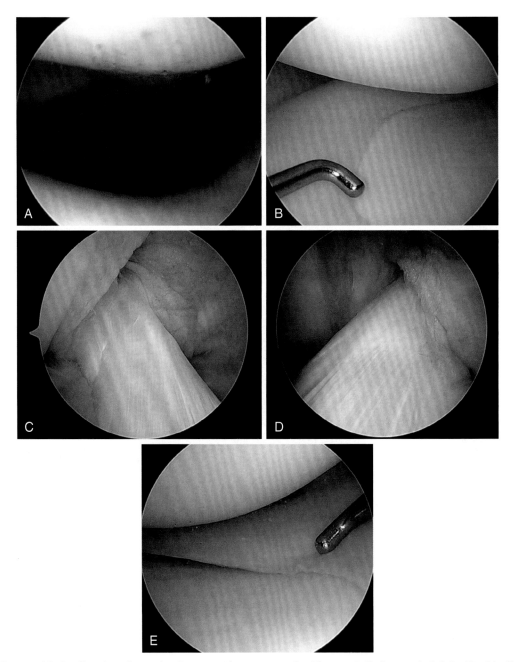

Figure 1A.6. Classic views in knee arthroscopy. A, The patellofemoral joint. B, Medial compartment containing medial femoral condyle, medial meniscus, and medial tibial plateau. C, ACL viewed from the anterolateral portal. D, ACL viewed from the anteromedial portal. E, Lateral compartment containing lateral femoral condyle, lateral meniscus, and lateral tibial plateau.

SECTION B
Anterior Cruciate Ligament Injuries

Ian J. Dempsey and Mark D. Miller

HISTORY

- Classically a noncontact mechanism of injury
  - Example: cutting maneuvers during athletic play such as soccer or football
- Many patients hear an audible "pop" during the injury
- Immediate swelling and effusion formation
- Feeling of instability in the knee, "my knee gives out," "I can't trust my knee"

PHYSICAL EXAMINATION

KEY EXAMINATION MANEUVERS

- **Anterior Drawer Test** 📹 (Sensitivity: 0.38-0.41 [acute] or 0.53-95 [chronic], Specificity: 0.81-0.97 [both acute and chronic]) (Figure 1B.1)
  - First described in the literature in 1875 by George Noulis
  - The test was further popularized by Marshall and Warren in 1975
  - **Maneuver:**
    - The patient lies supine with the involved knee bent to 90° in neutral rotation
    - The examiner sits so that his/her thigh restrains the foot
    - The examiner then grasps the tibia and pulls anteriorly assessing the amount of anterior translation relative to the femur
  - **Limitations of Maneuver:**
    - Many patients have considerable laxity in the 90° flexed position; this makes it difficult to distinguish normal form abnormal
    - It may also be difficult to flex the knee to 90° if the patient has an effusion present
    - If the patient has difficulty relaxing, the hamstrings may disallow anterior tibial translation

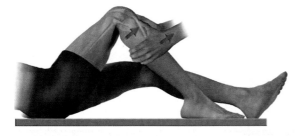

Figure 1B.1. The anterior drawer test. (From Chila AG, American Osteopathic Association. *Foundations of Osteopathic Medicine.* Philadelphia: Wolters Kluwer Health/Lippincott Williams & Wilkins; 2011.)

Lachman Test ▶ (Sensitivity: 0.81-0.99, Specificity: 0.81-0.95) (Figure 1B.2)
- First described by Torg and his mentor Lachman
- There have been no significant modifications
- Considered the "gold standard"
- **Maneuver**:
  - Best completed with the knee flexed to 20° to 30° on a pillow
  - The examiner stands at the side of the supine patient
  - Grasp the lower leg with a thumb over the tibial tubercle and the hand wrapped around the calf
  - The other hand grasps the thigh with the thumb over the quadriceps tendon and fingers wrapped around the posterior thigh
  - The examiner then pulls forward on the tibia feeling for a firm endpoint
  - In the presence of an ACL tear, there is increased anterior translation of the tibia best appreciated at Gerdy tubercle on the lateral side of the knee

KT-1000 Arthrometer by Medmetric ▶ (Figure 1B.3)
- Given the subjective nature of many tests to assess for ACL injuries, Markolf et al[9] in 1978 began developing an instrument to quantitatively assess the anterior translation of the tibia in the ACL-deficient knee
- Multiple devices were tested including the KT-1000, Stryker knee laxity tester, and Genucom knee analysis
- The KT-1000 has been validated through multiple studies and used in orthopedic research[1]
- **Maneuver:**
  - To use the device, both knees are positioned with the same degree of flexion of the knees and ankles by way of thigh and foot rests
  - The foot rest partially constrains external rotation of the tibia
  - The arthrometer is placed on the anterior aspect of the leg and held with 2 straps with 2 sensor pads in contact with the patella and tibial tubercle
  - To test for ACL deficiency, an anterior force is applied through a force-sensing handle, which is located 10 cm distal to the joint line; this is typically 89 newtons of force
  - Data received are plotted as force versus tibial displacement, which may be read to the nearest newton of force and 0.1 mm of displacement
  - Daniel et al created a compliance, which was calculated as the increase in anterior displacement between 67 and 89 newtons of anterior force[4]
  - Individuals with intact ACLs had no more than a 0.5 mm compliance index difference between the 2 intact sides, whereas an individual with a deficient ACL demonstrated more than a 0.5 mm difference
  - Bach et al had similar results who also noted[2]:
    - ACL competent knees should have maximal translation of 11.0 mm or less with 89 newtons of force and maximum manual force
    - Translation of 11.0 mm or more with either force should be considered diagnostic for ACL deficiency
    - If the side-to-side difference exceeded greater than 3.0 mm with 89 newtons of force, the examiner should suspect an ACL deficiency

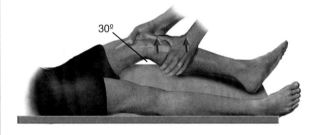

30°

Figure 1B.2. Lachman test. (From Chila AG, American Osteopathic Association. *Foundations of Osteopathic Medicine.* Philadelphia: Wolters Kluwer Health/Lippincott Williams & Wilkins; 2011.)

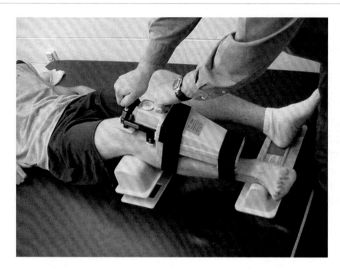

Figure 1B.3. General set-up for KT-1000. Note the foot rest disallows excessive tibial external rotation. (From Fu F, ed. *Master Techniques in Orthopaedic Surgery: Sports Medicine*. Philadelphia: Wolters Kluwer Health/Lippincott Williams & Wilkins; 2011.)

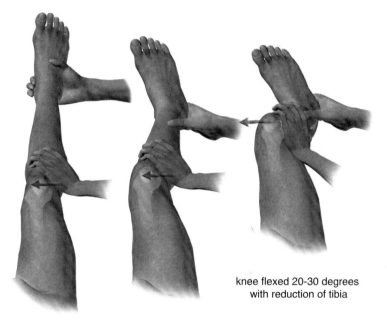

knee flexed 20-30 degrees
with reduction of tibia

Figure 1B.4. Classic pivot shift test. (From Fu F, ed. *Master Techniques in Orthopaedic Surgery: Sports Medicine*. Philadelphia: Wolters Kluwer Health/Lippincott Williams & Wilkins; 2011.)

- **Classic Pivot Shift Test or MacIntosh Test** 🔵 (Sensitivity 0.35-0.98, Specificity 0.98) (Figure 1B.4)
  - First described by Galway and McIntosh[5] in 1972
  - The initial description was performed with the lower limb internally rotated
  - The **modern pivot shift test** 🔵 is commonly performed with the lower limb neutral or even externally rotated
  - There is a grading scheme described by Jakob et al[6] in 1987 but can be somewhat subjective
    - Grade I: positive in medial rotation
    - Grade II: positive in medial and neutral rotation
    - Grade III: positive in medial, neutral, and lateral rotation
  - Bach et al[3] in 1988 expanded on this grading system finding that external rotation most reliably recreated the pivot shift test; they also used a grading system that is also somewhat subjective but evolved into

- Grade I: demonstrating a "gentle sliding reduction"
- Grade II: demonstrating a "palpable clunk"
- Grade III: demonstrating a "palpable clunk with locking"

• Currently, investigators are developing instruments to measure rotational forces that can be used during the pivot shift test to make it a more quantifiable test but nothing is yet on the market

• **Maneuver:**
  - The examiner holds the foot and extends the leg in the air, causing the femur to fall posterior relative to the tibia if the ACL is deficient
  - A hand is then placed on the proximal and lateral aspect of the tibia applying a gentle valgus force
  - The knee is gently flexed; at 20° to 30° of flexion, the anteriorly subluxed tibia reduced to the posterior femur, which is demonstrated by a visible jump or shift
  - The best place to watch this is laterally around Gerdy tubercle

• **Limitations of Maneuver:**
  - Pivot shift may not be accurate if the knee cannot reach full extension

● **Jerk Test** 🔘 (Figure 1B.5)

• Variant of classic pivot shift test described by Hughston

• **Maneuver:**
  - This the reverse of the pivot shift test
  - The examiner begins with the knee flexed and the tibia reduced and watches the tibia sublux, as the knee is passively extended

• **Limitations of Maneuver:**
  - The patient must stay completely relaxed throughout the whole examination

● **Flexion-Rotation Drawer Test** 🔘 (Figure 1B.6)

• Gentler version of the pivot shift test

• **Maneuver:**
  - The examiner grasps the patient's leg at the ankle with both hands
  - An internal rotation, valgus, and flexion force is applied at the ankle
  - This typically produces a less violent reduction than the classic pivot shift

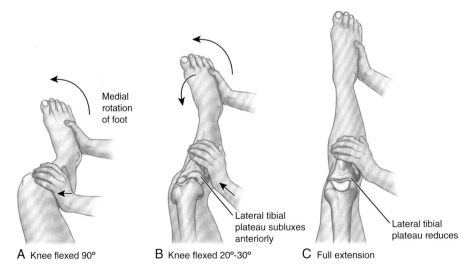

A Knee flexed 90°   **B** Knee flexed 20°-30°   **C** Full extension

Figure 1B.5. Jerk test. A, While the knee is flexed to 90°, the examiner places one hand behind the head of the fibula to produce internal tibial rotation. B, When the knee reaches 20°-30°, the lateral tibial plateau subluxes anteriorly. C, When the knee moves into full extension, the lateral tibial plateau reduces.

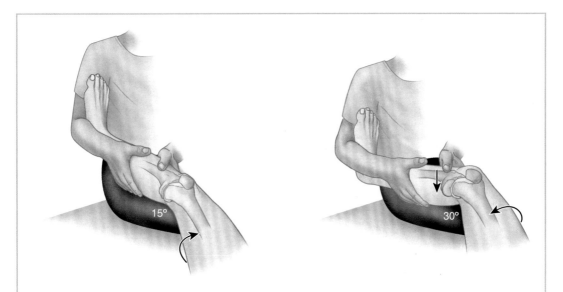

Figure 1B.6. Flexion-rotation drawer test. (From Anderson MK, Parr GP. *Foundations of Athletic Training: Prevention, Assessment, and Management.* Baltimore: Wolters Kluwer Health/Lippincott Williams & Wilkins; 2013.)

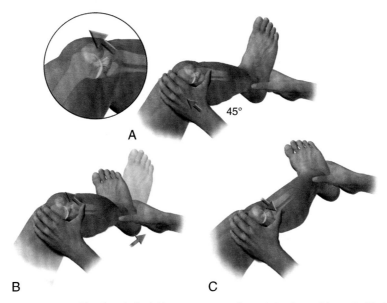

Figure 1B.7. Losee test. The leg is held in an externally rotated position at 45 degrees with a valgus force applied (A). The leg is gradually extended to 30 relaxing the hamstring with an internal rotation force and an anterior direct force on the fibular head (B). The test is positive if the lateral tibial plateau is felt to sublux anteriorly, and then clunks into a reduced position at full extension (C).

- **LoseeTest**[8] 🔘 (Figure 1B.7)
    - Another technique demonstrating the pivot shift phenomenon first described by Losee
    - **Maneuver**:
        - The examiner stands facing the supine patient at the side of the examination table
        - To examine the right knee, the examiner's right hand is placed to support the right foot and ankle in an externally rotated position braced against the examiner's abdomen
        - The knee is then pushed from 45° to 30° of flexion to relax the hamstrings

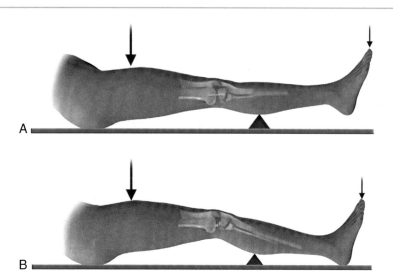

Figure 1B.8. The lever sign or Lelli test. A, With the fist acting as a fulcrum under the calf and a second hand pushing down on the quadriceps (large arrow), the ACL is able to counteract the downward force of the weight of the foot (small arrow). B, With the fist acting as a fulcrum under the calf and a second hand pushing down on the quadriceps (large arrow), the deficient ACL is unable to counteract the downward force of the weight of the foot (small arrow).

- The examiner's left hand is placed on the knee over the patella and the thumb behind the fibular head applying a valgus stress
- As the knee is slowly extended, the fibular head is pushed forward
- The test is positive if the lateral tibial plateau is felt to sublux anteriorly, as the knee approaches full extension

- **The Lever Sign or Lelli Test** (Figure 1B.8)
  - First put into practice by Dr Lelli et al in 2014[8]
  - **Maneuver**:
    - The examiner stands at the side of the patient and places a closed fist under the proximal third of the calf causing slight knee flexion
    - With the other hand, a moderate downward force is applied to the distal third of the quadriceps, with the leg acting as a lever over the examiner's fist (the fulcrum)
    - The downward force applied on the quadriceps in an ACL intact knee offsets the force of gravity on the heel
    - This causes the knee to rotate into full extension, and the heel rises off of the examination table
    - The test is positive if the heel does not rise off the examination table; this occurs because in the ACL-deficient knee, the tibial plateau slides anterior relative to the femoral condyle and the pull of gravity continues to keep the heel on the examination table

IMAGING

Plain Radiographs

- Flexion weight-bearing posteroanterior radiographs: allow assessment of arthritis and offer a good view of the notch
  - Segond fracture/lateral capsular sign: avulsion fracture of the lateral capsule (anterolateral ligament) off the lateral tibial plateau should raise suspicion for an ACL injury (Figure 1B.9)

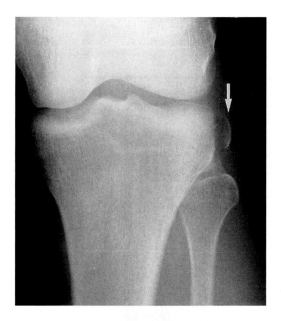

Figure 1B.9. AP radiograph of the right knee demonstrating an avulsion fracture of the lateral capsule (white arrow) commonly known as a Segond fracture. (From Greenspan A, Beltran J. *Orthopedic Imaging: A Practical Approach.* Wolters Kluwer Health/Lippincott Williams & Wilkins; 2015.)

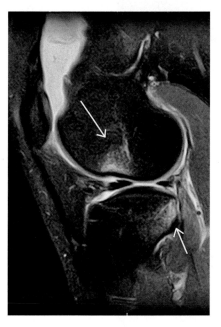

Figure 1B.10. Sagittal section of T2-weighted MRI of the knee demonstrating classic "bone bruise" (white arrows) of the midlateral femoral condyle and posterior lateral tibial plateau.

- Lateral radiographs: done in full extension if possible
  - Effusion can be assessed on the lateral radiograph
- Patellar "sunrise" view: allows evaluation of patellofemoral arthrosis
- Long-leg cassette views from hip to ankle are important if there is any question regarding mechanical alignment
- Stress radiographs: assess tibial translation relative to femur; good to have a comparison view of the unaffected side

Magnetic Resonance Imaging

- Evaluation of associated injuries, including other ligaments, patellar dislocation, menisci, and articular cartilage
- The typical pattern for trabecular microfracture (bone bruise), associated with 50% to 60% of ACL injuries, involves the far lateral aspect of the midlateral femoral condyle and posterior lateral tibia (Figure 1B.10)

Classic Arthroscopic Findings (Figures 1B.11-1B.17)

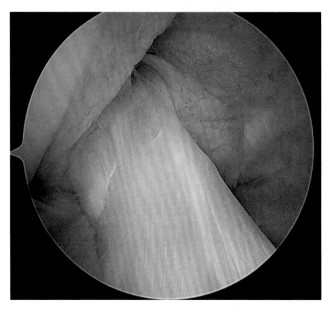

Figure 1B.11. Arthroscopic image of an intact ACL of the right knee.

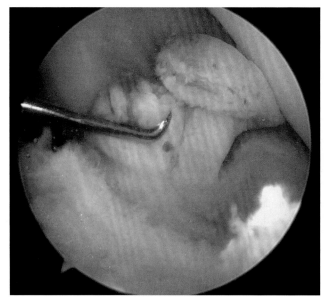

Figure 1B.12. Complete tear of the ACL of the left knee with arthroscopic probe demonstrating incompetence of ACL.

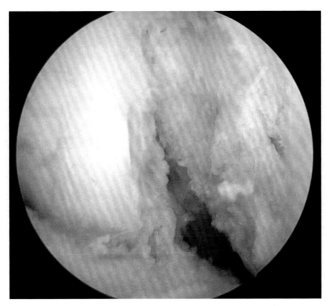

Figure 1B.13. Arthroscopic image demonstrating femoral insertion of ACL after ACL remnant has been removed.

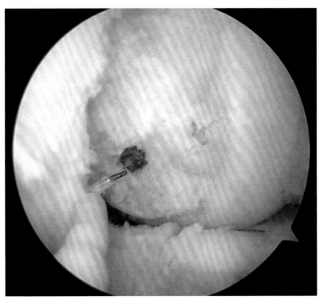

Figure 1B.14. Arthroscopic image marking femoral tunnel placement for single bundle ACL reconstruction.

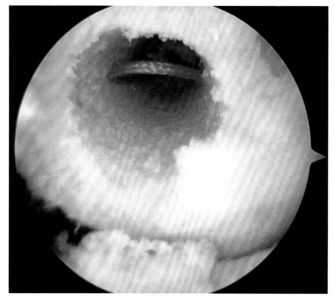

Figure 1B.15. Arthroscopic image of femoral tunnel with suture to guide passage of graft.

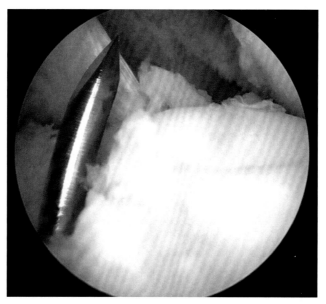

Figure 1B.16. Arthroscopic image of guide wire placed for tibial tunnel placement of ACL reconstruction.

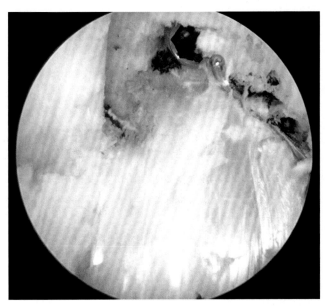

Figure 1B.17. Arthroscopic image demonstrating final placement of ACL graft. Purple marking pen was used to mark appropriate placement of graft with interference screw fixation.

REFERENCES

1. Anderson AF, Lipscomb AB. Preoperative instrumented testing of anterior and posterior knee laxity. *Am J Sports Med.* 1989;17(3):387-392.
2. Bach Jr BR, Warren RF, Flynn WM, et al. Arthrometric evaluation of knees that have a torn anterior cruciate ligament. *J Bone Joint Surg Am.* 1990;72(9):1299-1306.
3. Bach BR, Warren RF, Wickiewicz TL. The pivot shift phenomenon: results and description of a modified clinical test for anterior cruciate ligament insufficiency. *Am J Sports Med.* 1988; 16(6):571-576.
4. Daniel DM, Malcom LL, Losse G, et al. Instrumented measurement of anterior laxity of the knee. *J Bone Joint Surg Am.* 1985;67(5):720-726.
5. Galway RD, Beaupre A, MacIntosh DL. Pivot shift: a clinical sign of symptomatic anterior cruciate insufficiency. *J Bone Joint Surg Br.* 1972;54(4):763-764.
6. Jakob RP, Staubli H, Deland JT. Grading the pivot shift. Objective tests with implications for treatment. *Bone Joint J.* 1987;69(2):294-299.
7. Losee RE, Johnson TR, Southwick WO. Anterior subluxation of the lateral tibial plateau. A diagnostic test and operative repair. *J Bone Joint Surg Am.* 1978;60(8):1015-1030.
8. Lelli A, Di Turi RP, Spenciner DB, et al. The "Lever Sign": a new clinical test for the diagnosis of anterior cruciate ligament rupture. *Knee Surg Sports Traumatol Arthrosc.* 2014:1-4.
9. Markolf KL, Graff-Radford A, Amstutz HC. In vivo knee stability. A quantitative assessment using an instrumented clinical testing apparatus. *J Bone Joint Surg Am.* 1978;60(5):664-674.
10. Malanga GA, Andrus S, Nadler SF, McLean J. Physical examination of the knee: a review of the original test description and scientific validity of common orthopedic tests. Arch Phys Med Rehabil. 2003;84(4):592-603.
11. Marshall JL, Wang JB, Furman W, et al. The anterior drawer sign: what is it? *J Sports Med.* 1974;3(4):152-158.
12. van Eck CF, van den Bekerom MP, Fu FH, et al. Methods to diagnose acute anterior cruciate ligament rupture: a meta-analysis of physical examinations with and without anaesthesia. *Knee Surg Sports Traumatol Arthrosc.* 2013;21(8):1895-1903.

SECTION C
Posterior Cruciate Ligament Injuries

Ian J. Dempsey and Mark D. Miller

HISTORY

- Commonly from a direct blow to the proximal tibia with a flexed knee
  - Example: dashboard injury
- Noncontact fall onto a hyperflexed knee with a plantar flexed foot
- Hyperextension movement about the knee
- Patients will often have vague symptoms of unsteadiness or discomfort compared with the classic "pop" felt during an ACL injury

PHYSICAL EXAMINATION

KEY EXAMINATION MANEUVERS

- **Posterior Sag Sign** 🔵 (Sensitivity: 0.46-1.00, Specificity: 1.00) (Figure 1C.1)
  - First described by Robson in 1903[10], but unknown who coined the term
  - Biomechanical testing and sectioning of the PCL by Grood et al[3] and Ogata et al[7] produced the greatest posterior laxity when the knee is flexed between 70° and 90°. This is why many of the maneuvers to test the PCL occur in this position
  - **Maneuver**:
    - The patient lies supine with hips and knees flexed to 90°; this also demonstrates the "dropback phenomenon," as gravity causes the tibia sag posteriorly
    - The examiner supports the ankles and observes a posterior shift of the tibia compared with the contralateral uninvolved tibia
    - This is best noted by observing the prominence of the tibial tubercle
    - Normally the anterior cortex of the proximal tibia sits about 10 mm anterior to the distal of the femoral condyles when the knee is flexed to 90°
      - There is a grading system associated with every 5 mm of posterior dropback of the tibia relative to the femoral condyles
        - Grade 1: 5 mm
        - Grade 2: 0 mm, the tibia is flush with the femoral condyles
        - Grade 3: −5 mm, the tibia is posterior to the femoral condyles
        - Grade 4: −10 mm

- **Posterior Drawer Test** 🔵 (Sensitivity: 0.22-1.00, Specificity: 0.98) (Figure 1C.2)
  - First observed by Noulis in 1875
  - The maneuver was first described by Hughston et al in 1976[4,5] and again by Clancy et al[1] in 1983.
  - Clancy et al noted that the posterior drawer test was decreased with the knee internally rotated likely due to the fact that the meniscofemoral ligaments of Humphrey or Wrisberg were still competent resisting posterior translation of the tibia

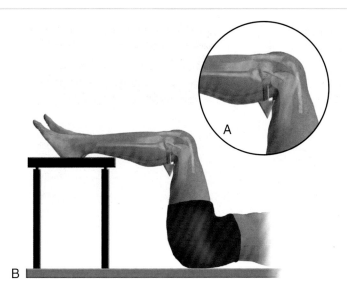

Figure 1C.1. Posterior sag sign with the leg flexed (A) and propped on the bench (B). (From Hertling D, Kessler RM. *Management of Common Musculoskeletal Disorders: Physical Therapy Principles and Methods*. Philadelphia: Lippincott Williams & Wilkins; 2006.)

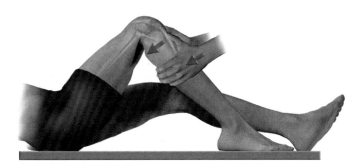

Figure 1C.2. Posterior drawer test. (From Chila AG, American Osteopathic Association. *Foundations of Osteopathic Medicine*. Philadelphia: Wolters Kluwer Health/Lippincott Williams & Wilkins; 2011.)

- **Maneuver:**
  - The patient lies supine with the involved knee bent to 90° in neutral rotation
  - The examiner sits so that his/her thigh restrains the foot
  - The examiner then grasps the tibia and pushes posteriorly assessing the amount of posterior tibial translation relative to the femur
- **Limitations of Maneuver:**
  - The patient must be relaxed
  - Unlike the anterior drawer test, there is typically a firm endpoint felt once the posterior laxity has been stretched tensioning the posterior capsule even in complete PCL tears

- **Godfrey Test** (Figure 1C.3)
  - First described by Joseph Godfrey in 1973[11]
  - Also demonstrates the dropback phenomenon

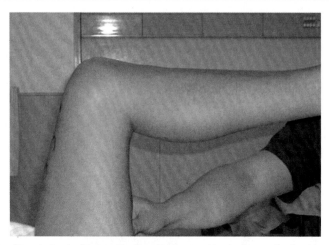

Figure 1C.3. Godfrey's test. (From Fu F, ed. *Master Techniques in Orthopaedic Surgery: Sports Medicine*. Philadelphia: Wolters Kluwer Health/Lippincott Williams & Wilkins; 2011.)

- **Maneuver**:
  - The examiner holds the patient's legs so that the hip and knees are both flexed to 90°
  - In this position, gravity causes the tibia to sublux posterior relative to the femoral condyles
- **Reverse or Posterior Lachman Test** (Sensitivity: 0.63, Specificity: 0.89) (Figure 1C.4)
  - Not truly considered a test but first described by Trillat et al in 1971[9]
  - **Maneuver**:
    - Best completed with the patient prone; the patient's knee is flexed 20° to 30°
    - The examiner stands at the side of the prone patient
    - Grasp the lower leg with the fingers over the tibial tubercle and the hand wrapped around the calf
    - The other hand grasps the thigh with the thumb over the posterior thigh
    - The examiner then pulls back on the tibia feeling for a firm endpoint
    - In the presence of a PCL tear, there is a soft or absent endpoint
    - This may also be completed with the patient in a supine position with the knee flexed 20° to 30° on a pillow much like the Lachman test
- **Reverse Pivot Shift** 🔵 (Sensitivity: 0.19-0.26, Specificity: 0.95) (Figure 1C.5)
  - First described by Jakob et al[6]
  - **Maneuver**:
    - The patient is supine
    - The examiner rests the patient's foot on his pelvis with the foot in external rotation
    - The examiner supports the lateral side of the calf and bends the knee to 70° to 80°
    - In patients with posterolateral rotatory instability, external rotation in this position causes the lateral tibial plateau to sublux posteriorly relative to the lateral femoral condyle
    - This is felt as a posterior sag of the proximal tibia
    - The examiner then allows the knee to extend leaning into the foot to transmit an axial and valgus load on the knee
    - As the knee approaches 20° of flexion, the lateral tibial plateau reduces from its posteriorly subluxed position

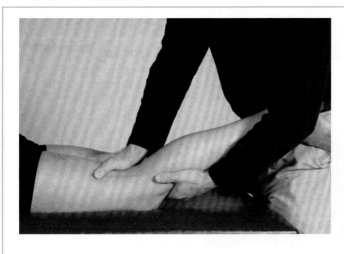

Figure 1C.4. Reverse or posterior Lachman test. (From Anderson MK, Barnum M. *Foundations of Athletic Training: Prevention, Assessment, and Management*; 2017.)

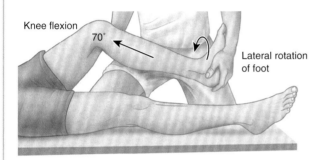

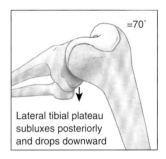

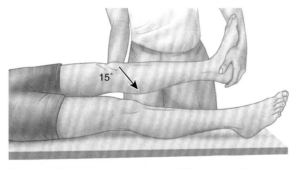

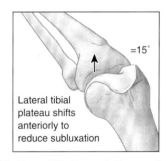

Figure 1C.5. Reverse pivot shift test. (From Anderson MK, Parr GP. *Foundations of Athletic Training: Prevention, Assessment, and Management*. Baltimore: Wolters Kluwer Health/Lippincott Williams & Wilkins; 2013.)

- **Quadriceps Active Drawer Test** (Sensitivity: 0.53-0.98, Specificity: 0.96-1.00) (Figure 1C.6)
  - Initially called the Muller test but later termed the quadriceps active drawer test by Daniel et al in 1988[2]
  - Helpful test when the dropback phenomenon is not well observed

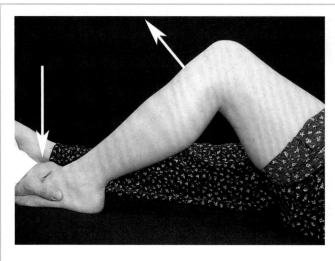

Figure 1C.6. Quadriceps active drawer test. (From Stuart LW, John MF. *Lovell and Winter's Pediatric Orthopaedics*. Vol 1. Wolters Kluwer Health/Lippincott Williams & Wilkins; 2014.)

- **Maneuver**:
  - The patient is supine with the knee flexed to 90°
  - An isometric contraction of the quadriceps is created by asking the patient to slide the ipsilateral foot up the examination table while the examiner secures the leg in place and resists the movement
  - In the setting of a PCL tear, the posteriorly subluxed tibia will shift anteriorly into a reduced position
  - Compare with the uninjured side, as some patients have a small amount of translation of the tibia normally
- **Limitations of Maneuver:**
  - Need to make sure quadriceps is actively firing by either visualization or palpation

- **Dynamic Posterior Shift Test** (Sensitivity: 0.58, Specificity: 0.95) (Figure 1C.7)
  - First described by Shelbourne et al[8] in 1989.
  - Adjunctive test that may be abnormal in posterior or posterolateral laxity
  - **Maneuver**:
    - The examiner places the patient's leg so that the hip and knee are both flexed to 90°
    - In this position, the hamstrings may tighten and sublux the tibia posteriorly
    - The examiner then passively extends the patient's knee while keeping the hip flexed at 90°
    - The passive extension causes the subluxed tibia to reduced sometimes with a noticeable shift

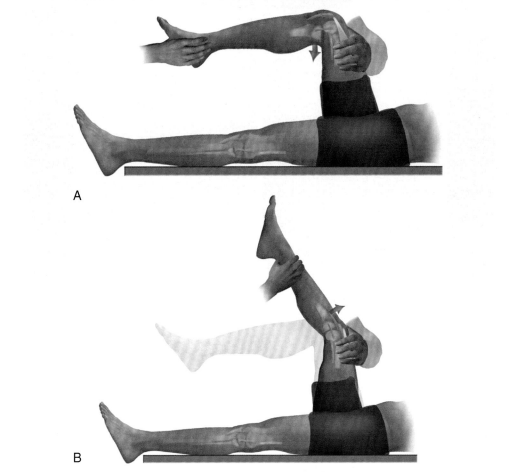

Figure 1C.7. Dynamic posterior shift test. The knee and hip are held at 90 degrees with the hamstrings tight pulling the tibia posteriorly (red arrow, A). Passive extension at the knee causes the subluxed tibia to reduce (red arrow, B).

IMAGING

Plain Radiographs

- Flexion weight-bearing posteroanterior radiographs allow assessment of arthritis and offer a good view of the notch
  - Chronic PCL injuries may be associated with medial compartment and patellofemoral arthrosis
  - A reduced knee on radiography does not mean the joint was not previously dislocated
- Lateral view is required to look for relationship between the tibia and femur
- Radiographs can also demonstrate avulsions on either the femoral or tibial side
- Patellar "sunrise" views allows evaluation of patellofemoral arthrosis, also associated with chronic PCL injuries
- Long-leg cassette views from hip to ankle are important if there is a question about mechanical alignment
- Telos stress radiographs: 15 dekanewtons (D_AN) of stress is applied to each tibia, and radiographs are taken. The normal side is compared with the injured side (Figure 1C.8)

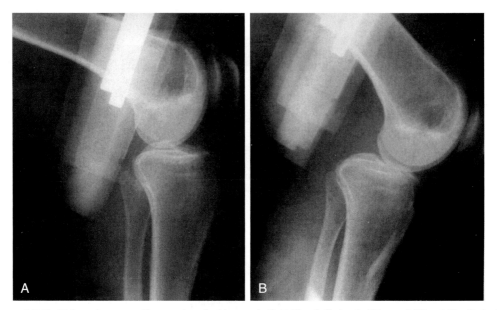

Figure 1C.8. Telos stress radiographs. A, Normal. B, PCL-deficient. (From Miller MD, Cole BJ, Cosgarea A, et al. *Operative Techniques: Sports Knee Surgery*. Philadelphia, PA: Saunders Elsevier; 2008, with permission.)

Magnetic Resonance Imaging

- Helpful for evaluation of associated injuries
  - Other ligaments (PCL)
  - Extensor injury
  - Menisci
  - Articular cartilage
  - Bony edema:
    - With ACL intact: medial compartment edema likely PCL + PLC injury
    - With ACL intact: lateral compartment edema PCL + MCL injury

Classic Arthroscopic Findings (Figures 1C.9-1C.21)

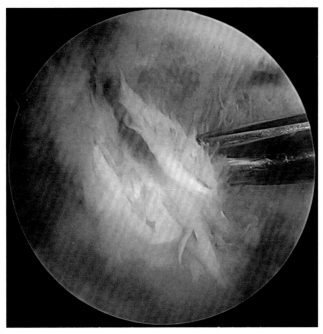

Figure 1C.9. Arthroscopic image demonstrating peel off lesion noted on femoral attachment of PCL of the right knee with PCL scarred into ACL (also torn).

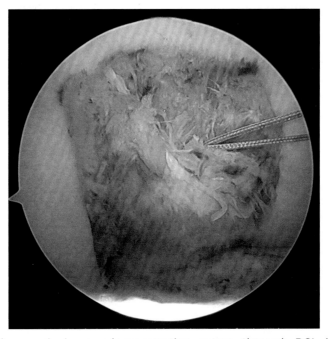

Figure 1C.10. Arthroscopic image demonstrating suture through PCL in preparation of making drill holes to pass PCL.

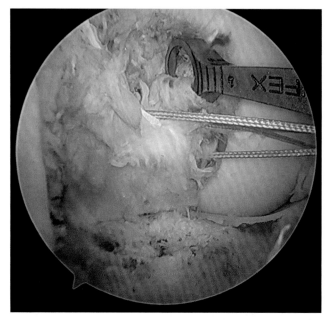

Figure 1C.11. Arthroscopic image demonstrating arthroscopic to create drill holes through femoral attachment of PCL.

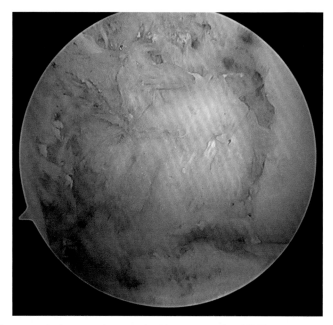

Figure 1C.12. Arthroscopic image demonstrating a repaired PCL.

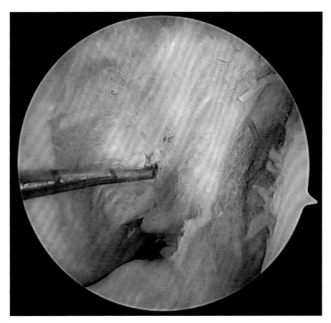

Figure 1C.13. Arthroscopic image demonstrating complete rupture of PCL off femoral insertion.

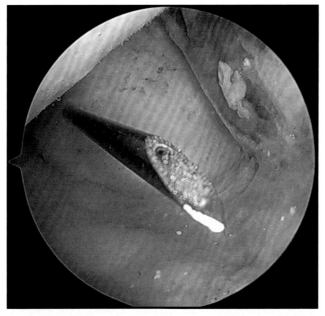

Figure 1C.14. Arthroscopic image demonstrating a spinal needle used to aid in the creation of a posteromedial portal to aid in debridement of PCL stump and facilitate tunnel creation and graft passage.

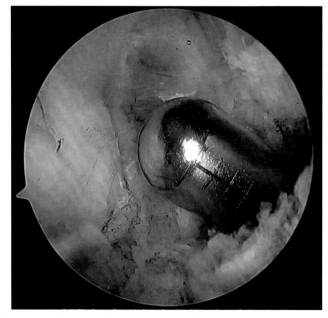

Figure 1C.15. Arthroscopic image demonstrating debriding PCL stump at the femoral and tibial insertion.

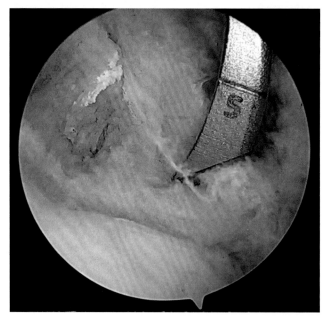

Figure 1C.16. Arthroscopic image demonstrating outside-in guide passing the guide wire for transtibial PCL reconstruction on the tibial side.

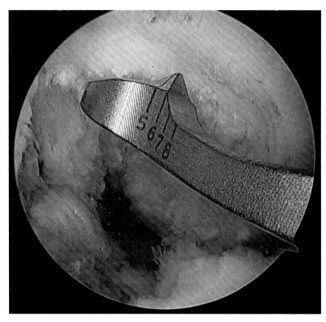

Figure 1C.17. Arthroscopic image demonstrating outside-in guide passing the guide wire for transtibial PCL reconstruction on the femoral side.

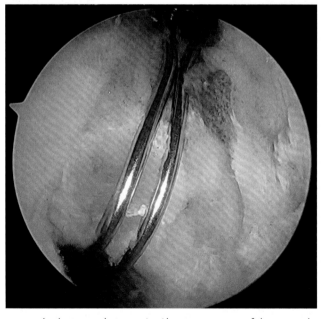

Figure 1C.18. Arthroscopic image demonstrating passage of luque wire to assist in graft passage.

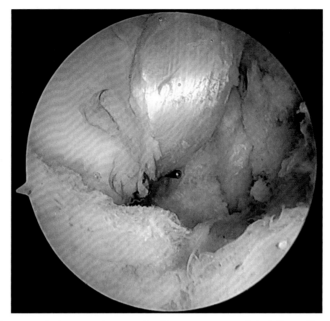

Figure 1C.19. Arthroscopic image demonstrating passage of Achilles allograft.

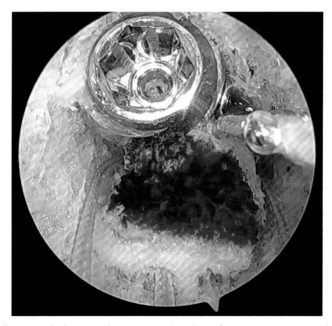

Figure 1C.20. Arthroscopic image demonstrating interference screw on the femoral side of transtibial PCL reconstruction. Purple marking pen was used to mark end of the graft.

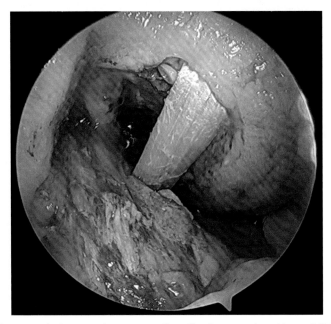

Figure 1C.21. Arthroscopic image demonstrating final reconstruction of PCL.

REFERENCES

1. Clancy WG, Shelbourne KD, Zoellner GB, et al. Treatment of knee joint instability secondary to rupture of the posterior cruciate ligament. Report of a new procedure. *J Bone Joint Surg Am.* 1983;65(3):310-322.
2. Daniel DM, Stone ML, Barnett P, et al. Use of the quadriceps active test to diagnose posterior cruciate-ligament disruption and measure posterior laxity of the knee. *J Bone Joint Surg Am.* 1988;70(3):386-391.
3. Grood ES, Stowers SF, Noyes FR. Limits of movement in the human knee. Effect of sectioning the posterior cruciate ligament and posterolateral structures. *J Bone Joint Surg Am.* 1988;70(1):88-97.
4. Hughston JC, Andrews JR, Cross MJ, et al. Classification of knee ligament instabilities. Part I. The medial compartment and cruciate ligaments. *J Bone Joint Surg Am.* 1976;58(2):159-172.
5. Hughston JC, Andrews JR, Cross MJ, et al. Classification of knee ligament instabilities. Part II. The lateral compartment. *J Bone Joint Surg Am.* 1976;58(2):173-179.
6. Jakob RP, Hassler H, Staeubli H. Observations on rotatory instability of the lateral compartment of the knee: experimental studies on the functional anatomy and the pathomechanism of the true and the reversed pivot shift sign. *Acta Orthop Scand.* 1981;52(suppl 91):1-34.
7. Ogata K, McCarthy JA, Dunlap J, et al. Pathomechanics of posterior sag of the tibia in posterior cruciate deficient knees an experimental study. *Am J Sports Med.* 1988;16(6):630-636.
8. Shelbourne DK, Benedict F, McCarroll JR, et al. Dynamic posterior shift test an adjuvant in evaluation of posterior tibial subluxation. *Am J Sports Med.* 1989;17(2):275-277.
9. Trillat A, Dejour H, Bousquet G. *Lere Jounies Luonnaises de Chirurgie du Genou.* Lyon: Bernadet; 1971.
10. Mayo Robson AW. Ruptured crucial ligaments and their repair by operation. *Ann Surg.* 1903;37: 716-718.
11. Godfrey JD. Ligamentous injuries of the knee. *Curr Pract Orthop Surg.* 1973;5:56-92.

SECTION D
Posterolateral Corner and Lateral Collateral Ligament Injuries

Ian J. Dempsey and Mark D. Miller

HISTORY

- Usually presents as a result of acute trauma from motor vehicle collisions or sports injuries
- Blunt trauma to the anteromedial aspect of the tibia with a posterolaterally directed force with knee extension and external tibial rotation with a fixed foot in a common mechanism
- Rare to be an isolated injury, commonly occur with ACL and/or PCL injuries

PHYSICAL EXAMINATION

KEY EXAMINATION MANEUVERS

- **External Rotation Asymmetry or Dial Test (30° and 90°)** 🎬 🎬 (Figure 1D.1)
  - First described by Hughston and Norwood in 1980[7]
  - **Maneuver**:
    - Classically the maneuver is completed in a supine position (Figure 1D.1) but can also be completed in a prone position
    - The patient is asked to flex the knees to 30° and 90° while keeping the knees and ankles together
    - The examiner then passively externally rotates the feet at 30° and 90°
    - The test is considered positive if there is greater than 15° of asymmetry between the feet
    - If asymmetry is only present at 30° of knee flexion, this is consistent with an isolated PLC injury
    - If asymmetry is present at both 30° and 90° of knee flexion, this consistent with a combined PLC and PCL injury

- **Posterolateral Drawer Test** (Figure 1D.2)
  - First described by Hughston and Norwood in 1976
  - **Maneuver**:
    - Similar to the posterior drawer test
    - The patient lies supine with the involved knee bent to 90°
    - The examiner then grasps the tibia and pushes posteriorly assessing the amount of posterior translation relative to the femur
    - This is performed with the foot externally rotated, neutral, and internally rotated
    - The test is positive with increased posterior excursion with the foot externally rotated

- **External Rotation Recurvatum Test** (Figure 1D.3)
  - First described by Hughston and Norwood in 1976

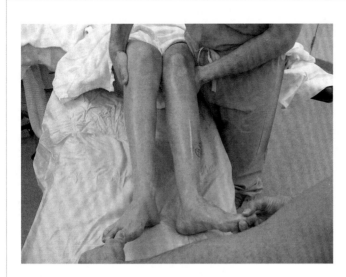

Figure 1D.1. External rotation asymmetry or dial test at 30 degrees in the supine position. (From Johnson D, Amendola NA, Barber F. *Operative Arthroscopy.* Philadelphia: Wolters Kluwer; 2015.)

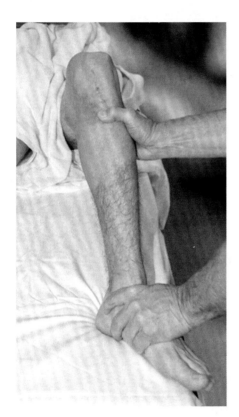

Figure 1D.2. Posterolateral drawer test. (From Johnson DL. *Reconstructive Knee Surgery.* Philadelphia: Wolters Kluwer Health; 2017.)

- **Maneuver**:
  - The patient lies supine with the legs extended
  - The examiner stands at the edge of the examination table and grasps the great toes in each hand and lifts them straight up off the examination table
  - The test is positive if the knee falls into recurvatum (hyperextension) and varus compared with the uninjured side

- **Varus Stress Test** (Sensitivity 0.25, Specificity not reported) (Figure 1D.4)
  - First described as adduction and rocking in 1938 by Palmer[8]
  - Later modified to varus stress by Hughston et al,[2] but concepts further refined by Marshall et al[5]
  - **Maneuver**:
    - The patient lies supine on the examination table
    - The examiner places one hand on the lateral side of the ankle and other on the medial side of the knee
    - A force going lateral to medial is placed on the ankle while a force going medial to lateral is placed on the knee

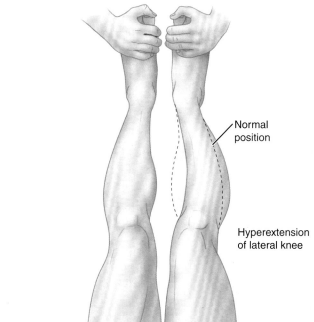

Normal position

Hyperextension of lateral knee

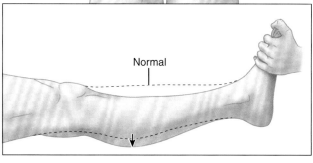

Normal

Figure 1D.3. External rotation recurvatum test. (From Anderson MK, Barnum M. *Foundations of Athletic Training: Prevention, Assessment, and Management*. Philadelphia: Wolters Kluwer Health; 2017.)

- This is performed in both full extension and at approximately 30° of knee flexion
- A positive test results in no to minimal discernible endpoint with the force applied
- A positive test at 30° is concerning for an isolated LCL injury
- A positive test in full extension is concerning for a combined LCL and ACL and/or PCL injury

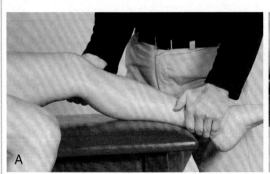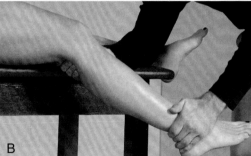

Figure 1D.4. Varus Stress Test at 0° (A) and 30° (B), The test is repeated with the knee fully extended. (From Anderson MK, Barnum M. *Foundations of Athletic Training: Prevention, Assessment, and Management*. Philadelphia: Wolters Kluwer Health; 2017.)

IMAGING

Plain Radiographs

- Usually negative, although fibular head avulsion involving PLC structures may be seen (Figure 1D.5)
- Critical to assess overall limb alignment in chronic cases. Genu varum may develop in chronic PLC-deficient knees

Stress Radiographs

- Helpful when MRI findings are not conclusive or in chronic injuries
- Greater than 4 mm of lateral compartment opening compared with the contralateral side with varus stress indicates LCL/PLC injury (Figure 1D.6)

Magnetic Resonance Imaging

- With significant LCL/PLC injuries, there is often substantial edema in the soft tissue on the lateral side of the knee (Figure 1D.7)
- Injuries to individual structures that make up the posterolateral corner can be detected on high-quality scans and may aid in planning of primary repairs

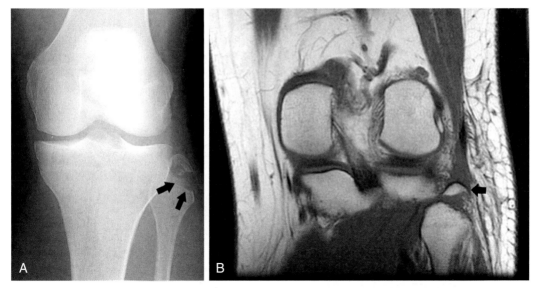

Figure 1D.5. Radiograph (A) and MRI (B) of a fibular head avulsion (black arrows) seen in a PLC injury. This is also called an "Arcuate sign". (From Pope TL, Harris JH, Harris JH. *Harris & Harris' Radiology of Emergency Medicine.* Wolters Kluwer/Lippincott Williams & Wilkins; 2013.)

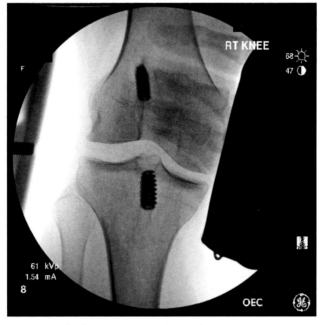

Figure 1D.6. Stress radiograph demonstrating lateral compartment opening concerning for PLC/LCL injury. (From Wiesel SW, ed. *Operative Techniques in Orthopaedic Surgery.* Vol 4. Wolters Kluwer/Lippincott Williams & Wilkins; 2016.)

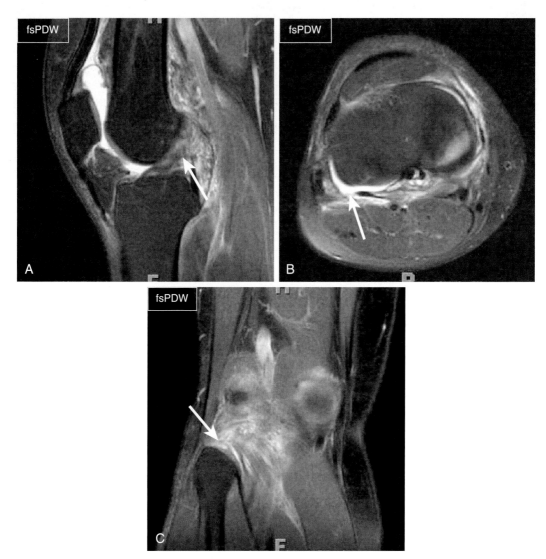

Figure 1D.7. Posterolateral corner injury with associated anterior cruciate ligament tear. Sagittal (A), axial (B), and coronal (C) images display complete tear of the anterior cruciate ligament (arrow in A), along with arcuate ligament tear, and popliteofibular ligament tear (arrows in B and C), in keeping with posterolateral corner injury. (From Chhabra A, Soldatos T. *Musculoskeletal MRI Structured Evaluation: How to Practically Fill the Reporting Checklist*. Wolters Kluwer/Lippincott Williams & Wilkins; 2015.)

Classic Arthroscopic Findings (Figure 1D.8)

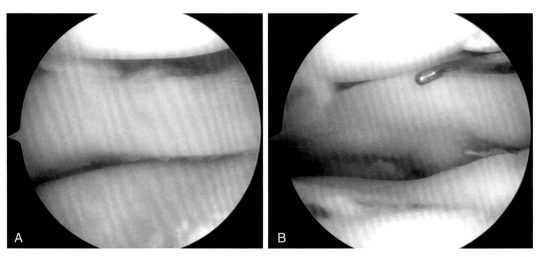

Figure 1D.8. Athroscopic appearance of lateral compartment of knee demonstrating widening (A) and undersurface tearing of the lateral meniscus (B). The meniscus is more adherent to the femoral side of the lateral compartment consistent with a tibial sided injury of the PLC.

REFERENCES

1. Gollehon DL, Torzilli PA, Warren RF. The role of the posterolateral and cruciate ligaments in the stability of the human knee: a biomechanical study. *J Bone Joint Surg Am*. 1987;69:233-242.
2. Hughston JC, Andrews JR, Cross MJ, et al. Classification of knee ligament instabilities. Part II. The lateral compartment. *J Bone Joint Surg Am*. 1976;58(2):173-179.
3. LaPrade RF, Heikes C, Bakker AJ, Jakobsen RB. The reproducibility and repeatability of varus stress radiographs in the assessment of isolated fibular collateral ligament and grade-III posterolateral knee injuries. An in vitro biomechanical study. *J Bone Joint Surg Am*. 2008;90(10):2069-2076.
4. Lunden JB, Bzdusek PJ, Monson JK, Malcomson KW, Laprade RF. Current concepts in the recognition and treatment of posterolateral corner injuries of the knee. *J Orthop Sports Phys Ther*. 2010;40(8):502-516.
5. Marshall JL, Baugher WH. Stability examination of the knee: a simple anatomic approach. *Clin Orthop Relat Res*. 1980;146:78-83.
6. Seebacher JR, Inglis AE, Marshall JL, Warren RF. The structures of the posterolateral aspect of the knee. *J Bone Joint Surg Am*. 1982;64:53.
7. Hughston JC, Norwood LA Jr. The posterolateral drawer test and external rotational recurvatum test for posterolateral rotatory instability of the knee. *Clin Orthop Relat Res*. 1980;147:82-87.
8. Palmer I. On injuries to the ligaments of the knee joint. A clinical study. *Acta Chir Scand Suppl*. 1938;53:282.

SECTION E
Posteromedial Corner and Medial Collateral Ligament Injuries

Ian J. Dempsey and Mark D. Miller

HISTORY

- Most commonly injured ligament of the knee
- Commonly occurs from contact injuries such as sliding into a base during baseball or being tackled during football
- Can also occur as a noncontact injury such as landing awkwardly on the ground after a jump
- Can occur in conjunction with ACL and meniscal injuries

PHYSICAL EXAMINATION

KEY EXAMINATION MANEUVERS

- **Slocum Test** (Figure 1E.1)
  - First described by Slocum[4] in 1968
  - Can be used to assess anteromedial and anterolateral rotatory instability
  - **Maneuver**:
    - Similar to the anterior drawer test
    - The patient lies supine with the involved knee bent to 90°
    - The leg is assessed in 2 positions:
      - With the tibia internally rotated 30° to assess for posterolateral corner injuries
      - The examiner then grasps the tibia and pulls anteriorly assessing the amount of anterior translation relative to the femur in this position

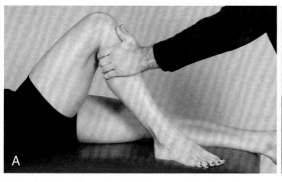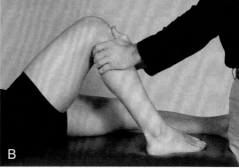

Figure 1E.1. Slocum test. A, An anterior drawer force is applied for anteromedial rotatory instability with the tibia externally rotated at 15°. B, Anterolateral rotatory instability is tested with the tibia internally rotated at 30°. (From Anderson MK, Barnum M. *Foundations of Athletic Training: Prevention, Assessment, and Management.* Wolters Kluwer Health; 2017.)

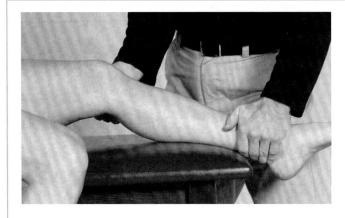

Figure 1E.2. Valgus stress test at 30°. The test is repeated with the knee fully extended. (From Anderson MK, Barnum M. *Foundations of Athletic Training: Prevention, Assessment, and Management.* Wolters Kluwer Health; 2017.)

- If there is considerable laxity, this points to a posterolateral corner injury (see section D for further tests)
- In this setting the test for anteromedial instability may be of less value
- Next the tibia is externally rotated 15°
- The examiner then grasps the tibia and pulls anteriorly, assessing the amount of anterior translation relative to the femur in this position
- Increased anterior excursion in this position is concerning for injury to the posteromedial capsule and possibly medial collateral ligament
- The tibia will appear to roll out during the maneuver

- **Valgus Stress Test** (Sensitivity 0.86-0.96, Specificity not reported) (Figure 1E.2)
  - First described as abduction and rocking in 1938 by Palmer
  - Nomenclature further refined by the Committee on the Medical Aspects of Sports's Standard[1] within the American Medical Association (AMA) who created a severity system
  - Later modified to valgus stress by Hughston et al[2] who also added a laxity system for grading
  - These clinical examination findings were also further refined by Marshall et al[3]
  - AMA grading system:
    - Grade I: 0 to 5 mm opening with up to 2 mm being physiologic
    - Grade II: 6 to 10 mm opening
    - Grade III: >10 mm opening with valgus stress at 30° of flexion
  - Hughston Grading System (Figure 1E.3):
    - Grade I: no clinical instability, tear of a few fibers of the MCL resulting in localized tenderness
    - Grade II: no clinical instability, disruption of more fibers of the MCL with generalized tenderness
    - Grade III: complete disruption of the MCL with varying instability with valgus stress at 30° of flexion
      - 1+ (3-5 mm of opening)
      - 2+ (6-10 mm of opening)
      - 3+ (>10 mm of opening)
- **Maneuver:**
  - The patient lies supine on the examination table
  - The examiner places one hand on the medial side of the ankle and the other hand on the lateral side of the knee
  - A force going medial to lateral is placed on the ankle while a force going lateral to medial is placed on the knee
  - This is performed in both full extension and at approximately 30° of knee flexion
  - A positive test results in no to minimal discernible endpoint with the force applied
  - A positive test at 30° is concerning for an isolated MCL injury
  - A positive test in full extension is concerning for a combined MCL and ACL and/ or PCL injury

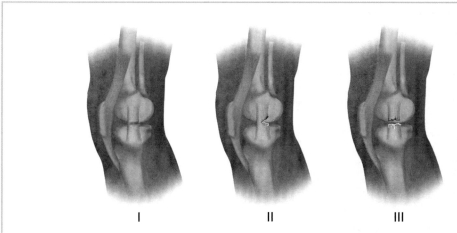

I   II   III

Figure 1E.3. Hughston classification of MCL injuries. (From Frassica FJ. *The 5-Minute Orthopaedic Consult*. Philadelphia: Lippincott Williams & Wilkins; 2007.)

IMAGING

Plain Radiographs

- Usually normal
- A Pellegrini-Stieda lesion: indicative of a chronic femoral-sided MCL injury with residual ossification adjacent to the medial epicondyle (Figure 1E.4)

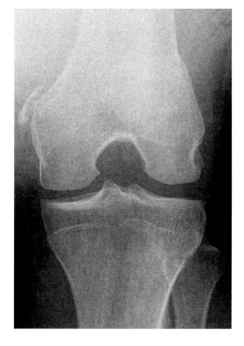

Figure 1E.4. Pellegrini-Stieda lesion. (From Miller MD, ed. *Operative Techniques in Sports Medicine Surgery: Free Fully Searchable Text and Image Bank Online*. Philadelphia: Lippincott Williams & Wilkins; 2011.)

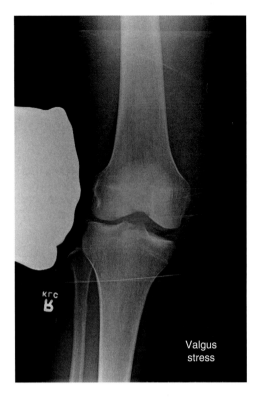

Figure 1E.5. Stress radiograph demonstrating medial compartment opening concerning for MCL injury. (From Johnson D, Amendola NA, Barber F. *Operative Arthroscopy.* Philadelphia: Wolters Kluwer; 2015.)

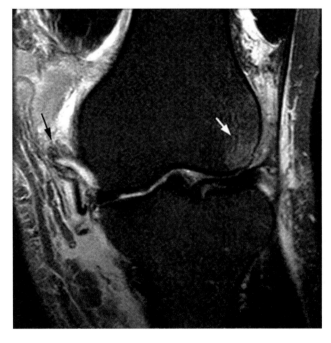

Figure 1E.6. MRI demonstrating a torn MCL (black arrow) and associated lateral condyle bone bruise (white arrow).

Stress Radiographs

- Compare with the uninjured side and consider operative intervention with >4 mm asymmetry (Figure 1E.5)

Magnetic Resonance Imaging

- Used to determine location of MCL tear as both the deep and superficial MCL can tear in different locations (Figure 1E.6)

- Can also determine if tissue is interposed between the tear like the pes tendons
- Bone bruising shows contrecoup bone contusion in the lateral compartment
- Allows for evaluation of concomitant ligament and meniscal injuries

Classic Arthroscopic Findings (Figure 1E.7)

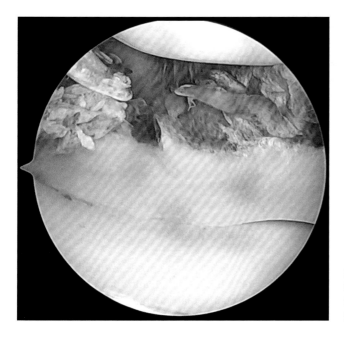

Figure 1E.7. Arthroscopic view of the medial knee with a significant femoral-sided MCL injury with MCL flipped into medial joint space.

REFERENCES

1. Committee on the Medical Aspects of Sports, American Medical Association. *Standard Nomenclature of Athletic Injuries.* American Medical Association; 1968:99-101.
2. Hughston JC, Andrews JR, Cross MJ, et al. Classification of knee ligament instabilities. Part I. The medial compartment and cruciate ligaments. *J Bone Joint Surg Am.* 1976;58(2):159-172.
3. Marshall JL, Baugher WH. Stability examination of the knee: a simple anatomic approach. *Clin Orthop Relat Res.* 1980;146:78-83.
4. Slocum DB, Larson RL. Rotatory instability of the knee. Its pathogenesis and a clinical test to demonstrate its presence. *J Bone Joint Surg Am.* 1968;50:211-225.

SECTION F
Multiligamentous Knee Injuries

Ian J. Dempsey and Mark D. Miller

HISTORY

- Devastating and potentially limb threatening injury, as it is often associated with a knee dislocation
- Typically seen in high-energy, low-energy, and ultralow-energy mechanisms
- High-energy mechanism is usually from an MVC or a fall from height
- Low-energy mechanism is usually from athletic play most commonly being tackled during football
- Ultralow-energy mechanism is usually from a ground-level fall in the morbid obese and super obese
- In 1963 Kennedy et al[3] classified knee dislocations in terms of the position of the tibia relative to the femur, which included anterior, posterior, lateral, medial, and rotatory
  - Rotatory was further subdivided into anteromedial, anterolateral, posteromedial, and posterolateral, with posterolateral being the most frequently described
- In 1997 Eastlack and Schenck[2,4] reported on knee dislocations, which ultimately led to the anatomic knee dislocation classification by Schenck:
  - KD I: knee dislocation with one cruciate intact and both collaterals intact, either ACL or PCL
  - KD II: knee dislocation with both cruciates torn but both collaterals intact
  - KD III: knee dislocation with both cruciates torn and one collateral torn
    - Additional modifier "M" or "L" is added
    - "M" designates an MCL injury
    - "L" designates a PLC injury
  - KD IV: knee dislocation with all 4 ligaments torn
  - KD V: knee dislocation with fracture dislocation of either the femoral or tibial side
    - Additional modifiers "C" and "N" are added
    - "C" designates an arterial injury
    - "N" designates a neural injury, either tibial or peroneal

PHYSICAL EXAMINATION

- The patient will typically present to a clinic with the knee reduced in an immobilization device
- In some situations, an external fixator device is required to keep the knee in a reduced position, making the patient unable to undergo any ligamentous examination

KEY EXAMINATION MANEUVERS

Refer to the previous sections for tests related to ACL (section B), PCL (section C), PLC (section D), and MCL (section E) injuries

IMAGING/DIAGNOSTIC TESTING

Ankle-Brachial Index

- Required in situations where a knee dislocation is occurred
- Should be performed after the knee is reduced
- The systolic pressure of the ankle is divided by the systolic pressure of the brachium to obtain a ratio
- A ratio of less than 0.9 requires further investigation by duplex arteriography or CT angiogram

Plain Radiographs

- In the setting of a knee dislocation, radiographs can be used to determine direction of dislocation, typically an anterior dislocation (Figures 1F.1 and 1F.2)
- Can be used to determine if there is a concomitant tibial plateau fracture, which may require a CT to determine its 3D characteristics
- Used for postoperative follow-up and assess hardware placement (Figures 1F.3 and 1F.4)

Stress Radiographs

- Compare with the uninjured side, including varus, valgus, anterior, and posterior stress testing

Magnetic Resonance Imaging

- Used to confirm which ligaments are injured and the extent of ligamentous injury
- Sometimes difficult to determine and why stress radiographs are an important adjunct
- Also helpful to determine if there are associated osteochondral lesions or meniscal pathology

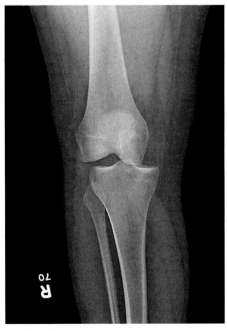

Figure 1F.1. AP radiograph of a right knee dislocation with medial displacement of the tibia. (From Court-Brown CM, Heckman JD, McQueen MM, et al. *Rockwood and Green's Fractures in Adults*. Philadelphia: Wolters Kluwer Health; 2015.)

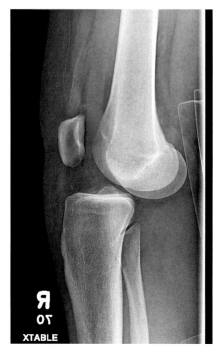

Figure 1F.2. Lateral radiograph of a right knee dislocation with anterior displacement of the tibia demonstrating an anterior knee dislocation. (From Court-Brown CM, Heckman JD, McQueen MM, et al. *Rockwood and Green's Fractures in Adults*. Philadelphia: Wolters Kluwer Health; 2015.)

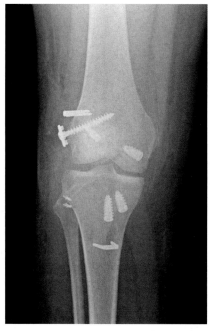

Figure 1F.3. AP radiograph of the right knee after reconstruction of combined ACL, PCL, and PLC injuries.

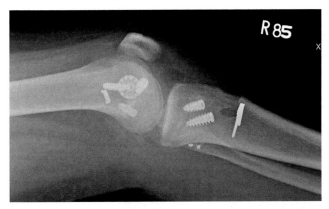

Figure 1F.4. Lateral radiograph of the right knee after reconstruction of combined ACL, PCL, and PLC injuries.

Classic Arthroscopic Findings (Figures 1F.5-1F.7)

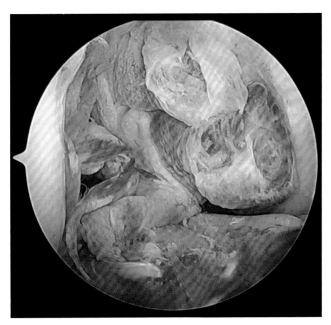

Figure 1F.5. Arthroscopic view of the femoral notch demonstrating disruption of both the ACL and PCL.

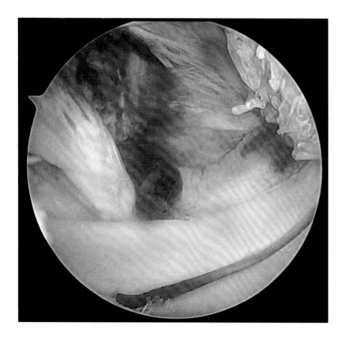

Figure 1F.6. Arthroscopic view of the lateral side of the knee demonstrating avulsion of the popliteus tendon.

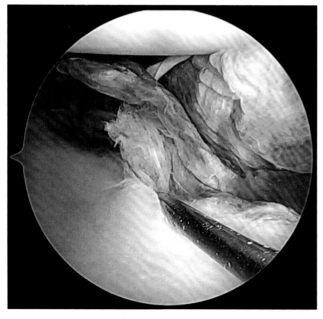

Figure 1F.7. Arthroscopic view of the medial side of the knee demonstrating medial meniscus tearing and intrasubstance tearing of the deep MCL with intra-articular displacement.

REFERENCES

1. Butler DL, Noyes FR, Grood ES. Ligamentous restraints to anterior-posterior drawer in the human knee. *J Bone Joint Surg Am*. 1980;62(2):259-270.
2. Eastlack RK, Schenck Jr RC, Guarducci C. The dislocated knee: classification, treatment, and outcome. *US Army Med Dept J*. 1997;11:2-9.
3. Kennedy JC. Complete dislocation of the knee joint. *J Bone Joint Surg Am*. 1963;45:889-904.
4. Schenck Jr RC. Classification of knee dislocations. In: *The Multiple Ligament Injured Knee*. New York: Springer; 2004:37-49.

SECTION G
Meniscus Injuries

Ian J. Dempsey and Mark D. Miller

HISTORY

- Commonly occur from twisting injury at the knee
- Medial meniscus tears are more common than lateral meniscus
- Can occur concomitantly with ACL injuries where the lateral meniscus is typically torn acutely
- Medial meniscus tears can occur secondarily in an ACL-deficient knee, as it blocks anterior tibial translation

PHYSICAL EXAMINATION

- Most meniscal injury examination maneuvers require direct palpation of the femorotibial joint or a rotational force to elicit pain, thus resulting in a positive test
- Pay close attention to overall range of motion of the knee
- A block to extension may be due to a displaced or bucket handle meniscus tear

KEY EXAMINATION MANEUVERS

Direct Palpation Maneuvers

- **Bragard Test** 🔘 (Figure 1G.1)
  - First described by Bragard in 1929[8]
  - Also used to assist in the diagnosis of lumbar spine pathology
  - **Maneuver**:
    - The patient is supine and the examiner takes the affected leg and extends the knee fully while holding the foot
    - The foot is then externally rotated; pain with palpation at the medial joint line is a positive test for a medial meniscus tear
    - The foot is then internally rotated; pain with palpation at the lateral joint line is a positive test for a lateral meniscus tear
    - Note that pain radiating from the back down into the leg may also occur, which may be related to lumbar spine pathology and not a meniscus tear. See the straight leg raise maneuver in section 7E.

- **McMurray Test** 🔘 (Sensitivity 0.16-0.58, Specificity 0.77-0.95) (Figure 1G.2)
  - First described by McMurray[5] in 1928 to test the medial meniscus
  - The test has been modified by Fouche to test for lateral and posterior meniscus injuries
  - Additionally what is considered a positive test has been slightly modified
  - **Maneuver**:
    - The patient is supine and the examiner flexes the knee to 90°

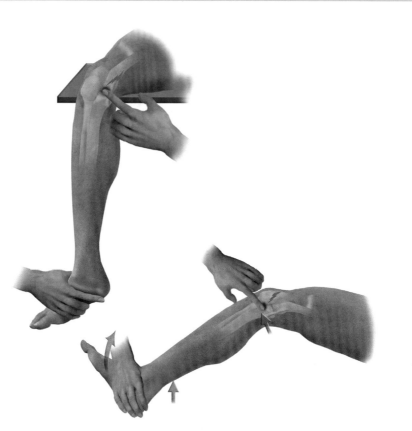

Figure 1G.1. Bragard test. (From Chila AG, American Osteopathic Association. *Foundations of Osteopathic Medicine.* Philadelphia: Wolters Kluwer Health/Lippincott Williams & Wilkins; 2011.)

- To test for a medial meniscus tear, the examiner holds the patient's hindfoot and externally rotates the foot while placing a varus stress on the knee with the other hand compressing the medial compartment
- The knee is then passively extended while the medial joint line is palpated with the index finger of the hand that is grasping the knee
- In the original description, a positive test occurs if there is pain at the medial joint line and a click is felt by the examiner at the medial joint line
- More commonly medial joint line pain is elicited without a click, but this still may indicate a medial meniscus tear
- To test for a lateral meniscus tear, by Fouche modification, the examiner holds the hindfoot and internally rotates the foot while placing a valgus stress on the knee with the other hand compressing the lateral compartment
- The knee is then passively extended while the lateral joint line is palpated with the index finger of the hand that is grasping the knee
- Like the medial side, pain and a palpable click is a positive test, but pain alone on the lateral side is also considered positive
- Note that pain from osteoarthritis may also occur with this test
- Note that starting with the leg extended and reversing the steps essentially constitute Steinmann I meniscal signs

- **Steinmann Second Test** (Figure 1G.3)
  - First mentioned in the early 1980s but likely developed in the 1960s
  - **Maneuver:**
    - The patient may lay supine or sit at the edge of the bed allowing for the knee to flex and extend from 0° to 90° of flexion

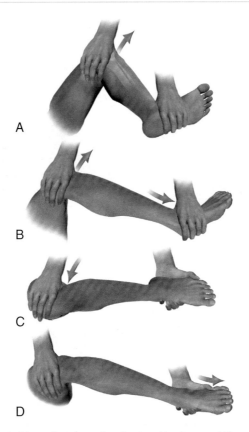

Figure 1G.2. McMurray's Test. One hand palpates the knee at the medial and lateral joint line. The other hand holds the foot to control external and internal rotation of the foot and tibia. To test the medial meniscal test (A and B), the foot and tibia are externally rotated, the 2 hands place the tibia into valgus, and while holding this position, the leg is slowly extended. For the Fouche variation for lateral and posterior meniscus injuries (C and D), the foot and tibia are internally rotated, the 2 hands place the tibia into varus, and while holding this position, the leg is slowly extended. Pain with a palpable "click" constitutes a positive test. Note that starting with the leg extended and reversing the steps essentially constitute Steinmann I meniscal signs. (From Chila AG, American Osteopathic Association. *Foundations of Osteopathic Medicine.* Philadelphia: Wolters Kluwer Health/Lippincott Williams & Wilkins; 2011.)

- Joint line tenderness, either medial or lateral, is noted and moves posteriorly with knee flexion and anteriorly with knee extension
- This is consistent with a meniscus tear that is slightly mobile during knee range of motion, causing the pain to travel compared with stationary pain that you would see in articular cartilage injuries

Rotation Maneuvers

- **Apley Test and Grind Test** 🔵 (Sensitivity 0.13-0.16, Specificity 0.8-0.9) (Figures 1G.4 and 1G.5)
  - First described by Apley[1]
  - The Apley grind test is a modification that was created at the same time
  - **Maneuver:**
    - The patient lies prone on the examination table with the knee flexed to 90°
    - The examiner holds the foot in his hand and uses the other hand to hold the thigh to the examination table
    - A distraction force is applied in the Apley test, and a compressive force is applied in the Apley grind test to the knee

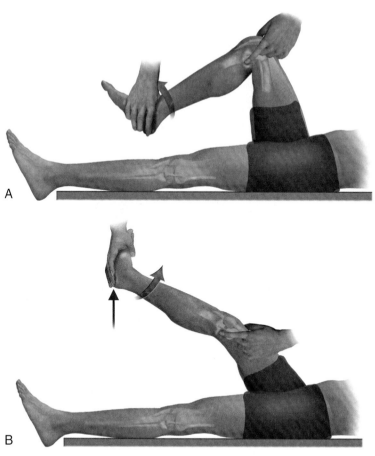

Figure 1G.3. Steinmann second test. Tenderness move anterior with extension (red and black arrow).

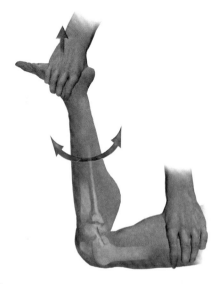

Figure 1G.4. Apley test.

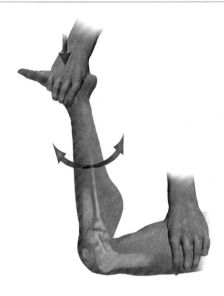

Figure 1G.5. Apley grind test. (From Boulware DW, Heudebert GR. *Lippincott's Primary Care Rheumatology.* Philadelphia: Wolters Kluwer Health/Lippincott Williams & Wilkins; 2012.)

- After the force is applied, the leg is rotated internally and externally at the knee
- If there is pain only with distraction and rotation, it is thought there is a capsular or ligamentous injury without meniscal involvement
- If there is pain only with compression and rotation, it is thought there is a meniscal injury

● **Bohler Sign** (Figure 1G.6)
- **Maneuver:**
  - The patient is supine on the examination table with the leg in extension
  - The examiner grabs the ankle with one hand and applies a valgus force to the knee compressing the lateral compartment
  - The other hand is used to palpate the lateral joint line
  - Pain during palpation and the force may be consistent with a lateral meniscus tear
  - Applying a varus force with palpation of the medial joint line may be consistent with a medial meniscus tear
  - Pain from joint space widening due to either a valgus or varus load is likely due to a ligamentous knee injury and should be noted

● **Helfet Test** (Figure 1G.7)
- First described by Helfet[3] in 1963
- This test is useful with a locked knee where there is a mechanical block to motion
- **Maneuver**:
  - This maneuver relies on an understanding of the **Q-angle**
  - The **Q-angle** is also utilized in patellar instability
  - The **Q-angle** is created by a vertical line drawn from the tibial tuberosity up through the middle of the patella and a second line that connects the anterior superior iliac spine with the midpoint of the patella
  - A normal Q-angle is typically 10 to 15 for men and 15 to 20 for women
  - It is normally measured in extension
  - During the maneuver, the tibial tubercle cannot externally rotate with knee extension
  - The Q-angle is unable to increase back to its normal value

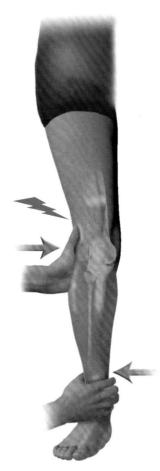

Figure 1G.6. Bohler test.

- **Steinmann First Test** 🔵 (Figure 1G.8)
  - First mentioned in the 1980s but likely developed in the 1960s
  - **Maneuver**:
    - The patient is sitting with the knee flexed to 90°
    - Sudden external rotation of the foot by the examiner elicits medial joint line pain consistent with a medial meniscus tear
    - Sudden internal rotation of the foot by the examiner elicits lateral joint line pain consistent with a lateral meniscus tear

- **Merke Test** (Figure 1G.9)
  - First referred to as Merke sign or test in 1964 by Springorum[7]
  - This is similar to Steinmann first test
  - **Maneuver**:
    - Instead of sitting, the patient is standing bearing weight through the affected extremity
    - Internal rotation of the body and thigh causes relative external rotation of the tibia, causing medial joint line pain consistent with a medial meniscus tear
    - External rotation of the body and thigh causes relative internal rotation of the tibia causing lateral joint line pain consistent with a lateral meniscus tear

- **Payr Test** 🔵 (Figure 1G.10)
  - First mentioned in the 1917s by Payr[6]

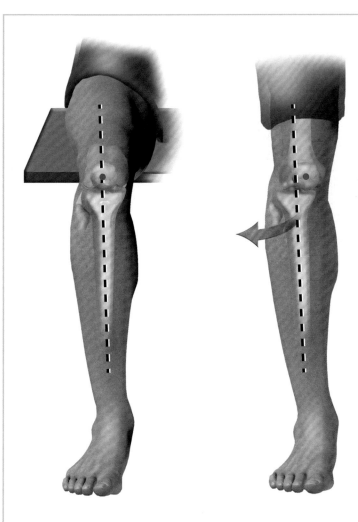

Figure 1G.7. Helfet test.

- **Maneuver**:
  - The patient sits with legs crossed or the so-called Turkish sitting position
  - The examiner places a downward force of the affected knee
  - If medial joint line pain is elicited, this is consistent with a medial meniscus tear
  - There is no variation to detect lateral meniscus tears
- **Duck Walk or Childress Test** (Figure 1G.11)
  - First described by Childress[2] in 1957
  - **Maneuver**:
    - The patient performs a deep squat and attempts to "duck walk" across the room
    - This walking causes increased compressive force on the posterior horns of the menisci
    - Joint line tenderness on the medial side may be consistent with a tear of the posterior horn of the medial meniscus
    - Joint line tenderness on the lateral side may be consistent with a tear of the posterior horn of the lateral meniscus
- **Thessaly Test** (Figure 1G.12A-C)
  - First described by Karachalios[4] in 2005
  - Named after the county in Greece where the test was developed

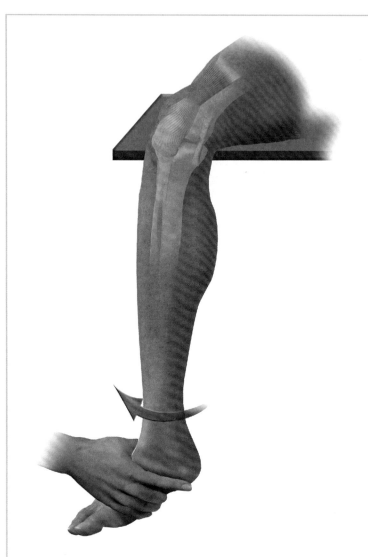

Figure 1G.8. Steinmann first test.

- **Maneuver**:
  - The test is performed with the patient standing flat-footed on the affected leg holding the unaffected leg in the air
  - The examiner holds the patient's arms for balance
  - The examination is performed at 5° and 20° of flexion
  - At 5° of flexion, the patient is asked to rotate the knee and body internally and externally 3 times keeping the knee at 5°
  - The test is then repeated at 20° of flexion of the same knee
  - The test is positive if the patient endorses pain at either joint line during the maneuver

Internal body rotation   External body rotation

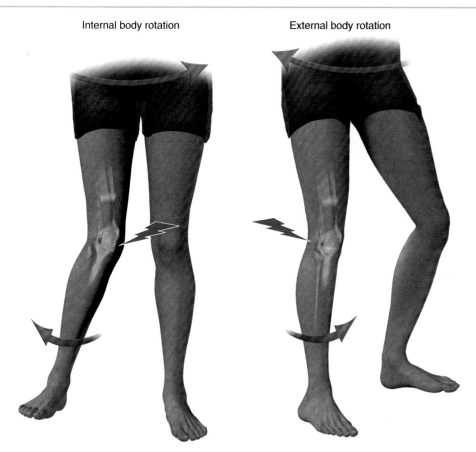

Figure 1G.9. Merke test.

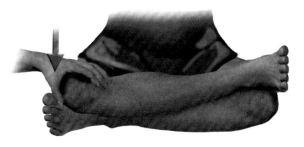

Figure 1G.10. Payr test. (From Palmer ML, Epler MF. *Fundamentals of Musculoskeletal Assessment Techniques*. 2nd ed. Philadelphia: Lippincott; 1998.)

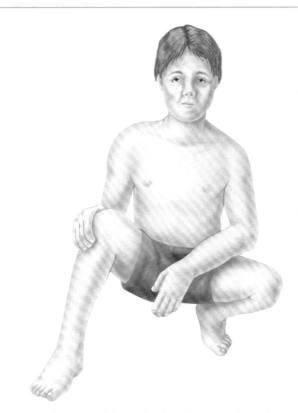

Figure 1G.11. Duck walk or Childress test. (From Bickley LS, Szilagyi P. *Bates' Guide to Physical Examination and History Taking.* 8th ed. Philadelphia: Lippincott Williams & Wilkins; 2003.)

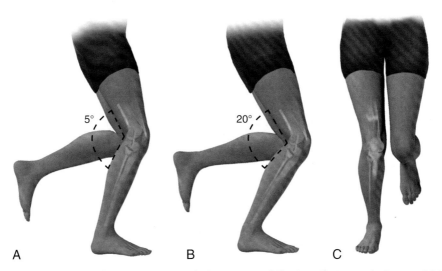

A   B   C

Figure 1G.12. Thessaly test. A, Lateral view at 5° of flexion. B, Lateral view at 20° of flexion. C, Frontal view at 20° of flexion.

IMAGING

Plain Radiographs

- Usually normal

Stress Radiographs

- Not typically used for isolated meniscus injuries

Magnetic Resonance Imaging

- Used to determine location and characteristics of meniscus tear in addition to possible concomitant pathology
- Be wary of the double anterior horn sign and double PCL sign, which is consistent with a flipped bucket handle tear of the meniscus (Figures 1G.13 and 1G.14)

Classic Arthroscopic Findings

- Anatomic representation of typical meniscus tears (Figure 1G.15)
- Arthroscopic findings (Figure 1G.16)

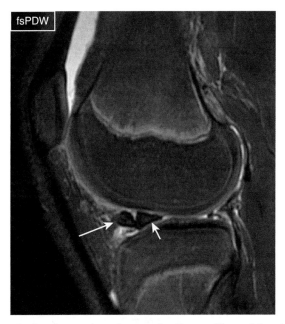

Figure 1G.13. Double anterior horn sign demonstrating a flipped bucket handle tear (short arrow) of the lateral meniscus behind the native anterior horn of the lateral meniscus (long arrow). (From Chhabra A, Soldatos T. *Musculoskeletal MRI Structured Evaluation: How to Practically Fill the Reporting Checklist*. Philadelphia: Wolters Kluwer/Lippincott Williams & Wilkins; 2015.)

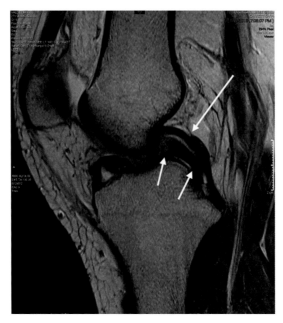

Figure 1G.14. MRI demonstrating double PCL sign that demonstrates a flipped medial meniscus tear (short arrows) with an intact PCL (long arrow). (From Chew FS, Ovid Technologies Inc. *Skeletal Radiology the Bare Bones*. Philadelphia: Wolters Kluwer Health/ Lippincott Williams & Wilkins; 2010.)

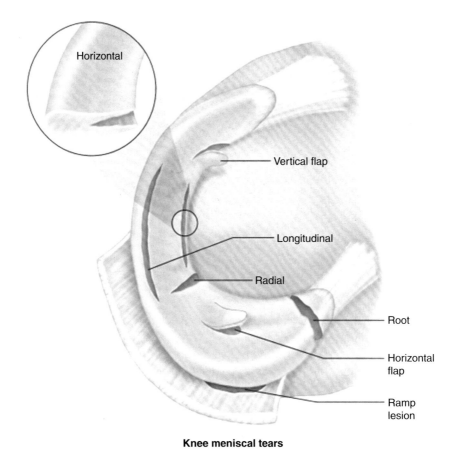

Knee meniscal tears

Figure 1G.15. Typical anatomic representation of different meniscus tears.

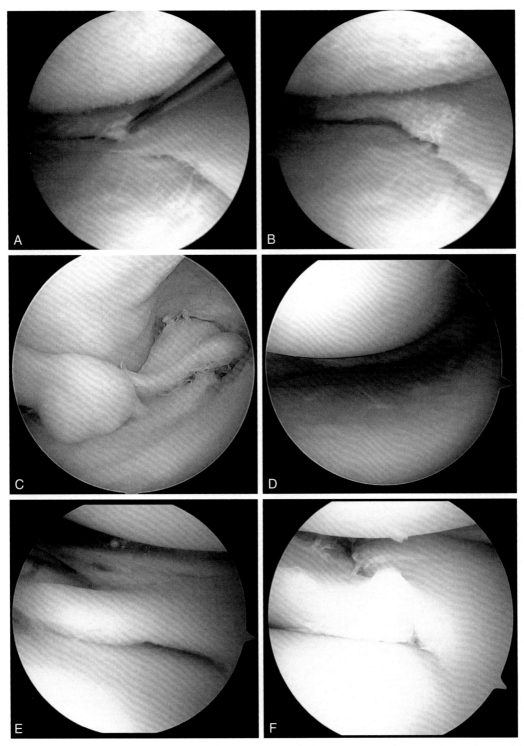

Figure 1G.16. Parrot beak tear of the medial meniscus (A) with arthroscopic probe within tear (B), displaced bucket handle medial meniscus tear around medial femoral condyle before (C) and after reduction with partial medial menisectomy (D), incomplete longitudinal tear of the lateral meniscus (E) and after repair, ramp lesion of the medial meniscus (G) and after repair (H), lateral meniscal root tear (I) and after repair (J), and previous subtotal medial meniscectomy (K) and after medial meniscus transplant (L).

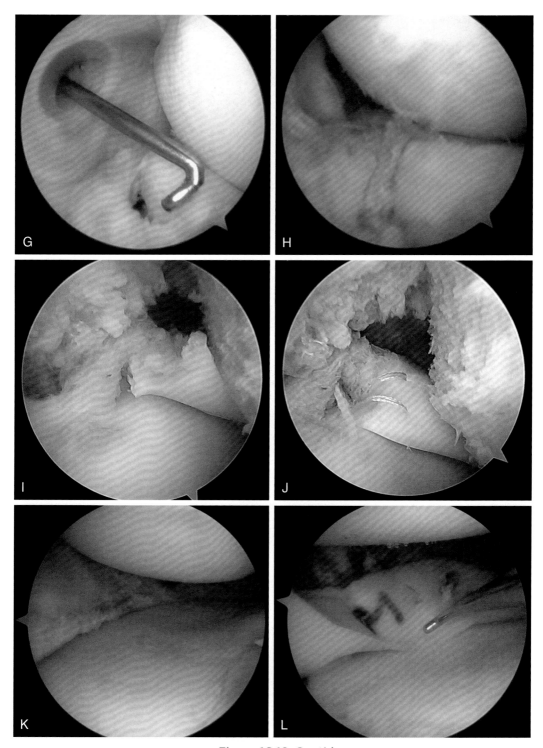

Figure 1G.16. Cont'd

REFERENCES

1. Apley AG. The diagnosis of meniscus injuries. *J bone joint Surg Am*. 1947;29(1):78-84.
2. Childress HM. Diagnosis of posterior lesions of the medial meniscus: description of a new test. *Am J Surg*. 1957;93(5):782-787.
3. Helfet AJ. *The Management of Internal Derangements of the Knee*. Lippincott; 1963.
4. Karachalios T, Hantes M, Zibis AH, et al. Diagnostic accuracy of a new clinical test (the Thessaly test) for early detection of meniscal tears. *J Bone Joint Surg*. 2005;87(5):955-962.
5. McMurray TP. The diagnosis of internal derangements of the knee. In: *The Robert Jones Birthday Volume*. London: Humphrey Milford; 1928:301-306.
6. Payr E. Einfaches und schonendes Verfahren zur beliebig breiten Eröffnung des Kniegelenkes. *Zentralbl Chir*. 1917;44:921.
7. Springorum PW. Die Diagnose der Meniskusläsion. *Dtsch Med Wochenschr*. 1964;89(3):111-114.
8. Bragard K. Die Nervendehnung als diagnostisches Prinzip ergibt eine Reihe neuer Nervenphänomene. *Münchener Medizinische Wochenschrift*. 1929;76:1999-2003.

SECTION H
Patellar Instability

Ian J. Dempsey and Mark D. Miller

HISTORY

- Most commonly occurs in ages 20s to 30s
- Lateral subluxation is by far the most common but medial subluxation, which has been described secondary to an overaggressive lateral retinacular release of the knee
- Acute instability is usually as a result of a trauma such as a noncontact twisting event with the knee extended or a direct blow from a cleat or helmet
- An initial instability event may lead to repeated instability events
- More common to occur in individuals with general ligamentous laxity like Ehlers-Danlos syndrome; this is typically chronic
- Another cause of chronic instability is "miserable malalignment syndrome" which is a result of increased femora anteversion, genu valgum, and external tibial torsion
- The combination of these 3 physical features leads to an increased Q-angle
- Habitual instability is usually painless and occurs during flexion of the knee and may be due to a tight iliotibial band, vastus lateralis, or perhaps trochlear dysplasia
  - Dejour et al in 1994[4] noted that anatomic differences in the trochlear may predispose certain patients to repeated dislocation events
  - They discussed a trochlear "bump" or "spur" as a major cause of these instability events
  - He later created a classification system to demonstrate the different trochlear morphology that may be seen (Figure 1H.1)

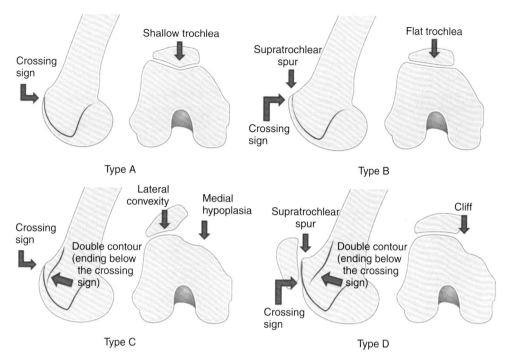

Figure 1H.1. Trochlear dysplasia classification according to D. Dejour. Type A, presence of crossing sign in the lateral true view. The trochlea is shallower than normal but still symmetric and concave. Type B, crossing sign and trochlear spur. The trochlea is flat or convex in axial images. Type C, presence of the crossing sign and the double-contour sign, representing the densification of the subchondral bone of the medial hypoplastic facet. In axial CT scan views, the lateral facet is convex. Type D, combines all the mentioned signs: crossing sign, supratrochlear spur, and double-contour sign going below the crossing sign. In axial CT scan views, there is a cliff pattern. (From Johnson DL. *Master Techniques in Orthopaedic Surgery: Reconstructive Knee Surgery*. Philadelphia: Wolters Kluwer Health; 2017.)

PHYSICAL EXAMINATION

- There are multiple soft tissue and bony features of a patient's lower extremity that may predispose the patient to patellar instability events

KEY EXAMINATION MANEUVERS

- **Fairbanks Apprehension and Modified Apprehension Test** (Sensitivity 0.39, Specificity not reported) (Figure 1H.2A-B)
  - First described by Fairbanks in 1937[11]
  - A more detailed description was later given by Hughston in 1968[12]
  - **Maneuver:**
    - The patient is supine with the knee relaxed in 30° of flexion
    - The examiner uses one hand to push the patella laterally
    - It is considered a positive test if it reproduces the patient's pain or apprehension occurs with involuntary muscle contraction for fear of dislocation
    - The modification has the knee in the same position except that the force on the patella is applied to the superior pole of the patella in a distal and lateral direction at approximately 45° toward the fibular head
    - This is thought to isolate possible ligamentous damage to the MPFL, as it prevents the lateral prominence of the trochlea from impeding translation of the patella

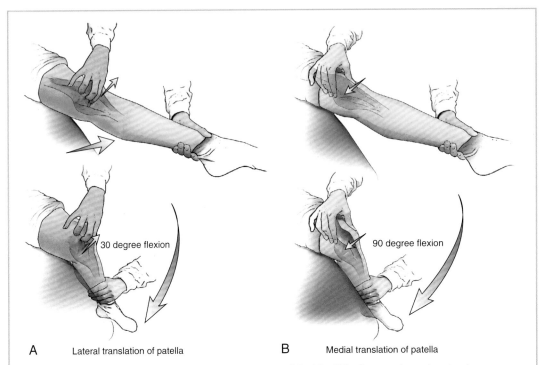

A   Lateral translation of patella   B   Medial translation of patella

Figure 1H.2. A and B, Apprehension test. C and D, Modified apprehension test.

- **Bassett Sign** (Figure 1H.3)
  - First described by Bassett at an instructional course lecture[1] in 1976
  - **Maneuver**:
    - The patient is supine with the knee relaxed
    - Palpation of the adductor tubercle and medial epicondyle elicits tenderness that may indicate rupture of the MPFL from its femoral insertion
    - Not to be confused with Bassett sign for patellar tendinitis where the patient elicits pain with palpation of the inferior pole of the patella in full extension but not in full flexion

- **Lateral and Medial Patellar Glide Test** (Figure 1H.4)
  - First described in conjunction with the Fairbanks apprehension test in the 1930s, as the examination maneuvers have similarities
  - Again discussed by Hughston in the 1968[12], but the actually grading was not mentioned until 1990 by Kolowich[8]
  - **Maneuver**:
    - The patient is supine with the knee relaxed in 30° of flexion
    - The examiner moves the patella medially and laterally with the patella divided into 4 quadrants
    - A glide greater than or equal to 3 quadrants may represent damage to the MPFL
    - Decreased mobility is manifested by less than 1 quadrant of displacement, which may represent a tight lateral retinaculum

- **Patellar Tilt Test** (Figure 1H.5)
  - First mentioned by Hughston in 1964[13] as he noted the lateral tilt of the patella and named this position the "grasshopper eye patella"
  - **Maneuver:**
    - The patient is supine with the knee relaxed in 20° of flexion
    - The examiner holds the patella between the thumb and forefinger and pushes the patella downward in an attempt to flip the lateral edge of the patella upward
    - Elevation of the patella to less than neutral suggests an excessively tight lateral retinaculum
    - The patella normally elevates from 0° to 20°

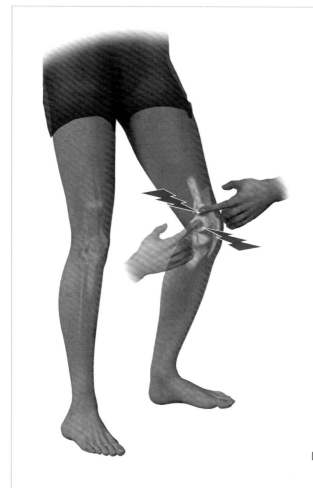

Figure 1H.3. Bassett sign.

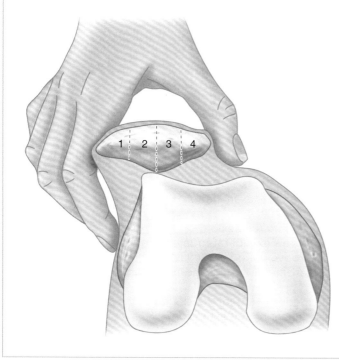

Figure 1H.4. Patellar glide. Passive lateral glide of the patella demonstrating subluxation to its second quadrant. Hypomobility is manifested by less than 1 quadrant of displacement; hypermobility is manifested by 3 or more quadrants (greater than half of patellar width). (From Anderson MK, Barnum M. *Foundations of Athletic Training: Prevention, Assessment, and Management*. Wolters Kluwer Health; 2017.)

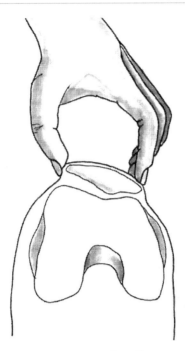

Figure 1H.5. Patellar tilt test.

- **Gravity Subluxation Test** (Figure 1H.6)
  - First discussed by Hughston JC[5] in 1988 as a complication of lateral retinacular release
  - First described as an examination maneuver by Nonweiler and DeLee[10] in 1994
  - Commonly used to diagnose medial subluxation of the patella
  - **Maneuver**:
    - The patient is in the lateral decubitus position
    - If the affected leg is the left one, this means the patient is left side up in the lateral position
    - The knee is in full extension with the patient relaxed
    - The examiner abducts the patient's leg
    - The test is positive if the patella visibly shifts medially
    - The examiner then asks the patient to contract the quadriceps; if the patella does not reduce, there is likely complete dissociation of the vastus lateralis from the patella
    - This may be a product of overaggressive release of the lateral retinaculum

- **J-Sign** (Figure 1H.7)
  - First mentioned in the literature as the J-sign in 1998 by Johnson et al[7] but has been discussed regarding patellar instability since the 1960s[3]
  - **Maneuver**:
    - The patient sits on the edge of the examination table with the knee in full extension
    - The patient then brings the knee into full flexion
    - The examiner then observes for an exaggerated lateral to medial translation of the patella into the trochlear groove during early flexion
    - Conversely, the patient can start in full flexion and then bring the knee into full extension
    - There will be an exaggerated medial to lateral translation of the patella out of the trochlear groove, as the knee is nearing full extension

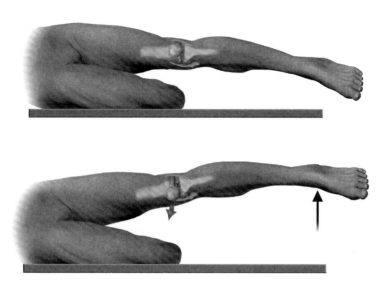

Figure 1H.6. Gravity subluxation test.

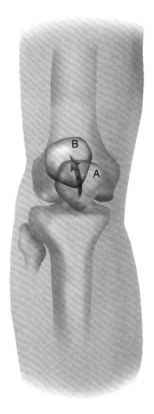

Figure 1H.7. J-sign. As the knee extends (A to B) the patella tracks laterally (red arrow).

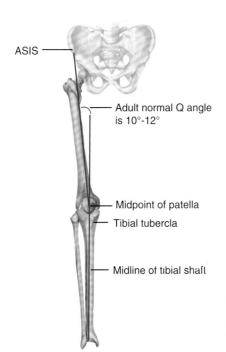

ASIS

Adult normal Q angle
is 10°-12°

Midpoint of patella

Tibial tubercla

Midline of tibial shaft

Figure 1H.8. Q-angle. ASIS, anterior superior ili-ac spine. (From Chila AG, American Osteopathic Association. *Foundations of Osteopathic Medicine.* Philadelphia: Wolters Kluwer Health/Lippincott Williams & Wilkins; 2011.)

- **Q-Angle** (Figure 1H.8)
  - First described by Brattström[2] in 1964
  - **Maneuver**:
    – The patient is supine
    – A vertical line drawn from the tibial tuberosity up through the middle of the patella and a second line that connects the anterior superior iliac spine with the midpoint of the patella
    – A normal Q-angle is typically 10° to 15° for men and 15° to 20° for women
    – An increased Q-angle may increase the laterally directed force on the patella, which may predispose to patellar instability

- **Patella Position** (Figure 1H.9)
  - First described by
  - **Maneuver**:
    – Tested both with the patient supine and sitting with the knee flexed to 90°
    – The examiner looks at the overall position of the patella
    – A patella that excessively distal or close to the tibial tubercle is considered patella baja
    – A patella that is excessively proximal or far from the tibial tubercle is considered patella alta
    – These can also be confirmed with specific measurements using a lateral radiograph

- **Vastus Medialis Obliquus (VMO) Strength** (Figure 1H.10)
  - **Maneuver:**
    – The patient sits on the edge of the examination table with the knee flex to 90°
    – The patient is asked to actively extend the knee
    – The examiner looks at the overall muscle bulk of the VMO during this activity
    – Atrophy of the VMO may lead to an overly lateral pull on the patella by the competing vastus lateralis, which may contribute to patellar instability

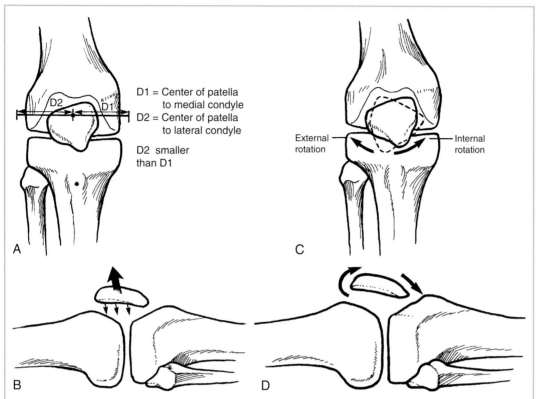

D1 = Center of patella
to medial condyle
D2 = Center of patella
to lateral condyle

D2 smaller
than D1

External
rotation

Internal
rotation

Figure 1H.9. Patella position. Patellar glide (A), patellar tilt (B), patellar rotation (C), and anteroposterior position (D). (From Hertling D, Kessler RM. *Management of Common Musculoskeletal Disorders: Physical Therapy Principles and Methods*. Philadelphia: Lippincott Williams & Wilkins; 2006.)

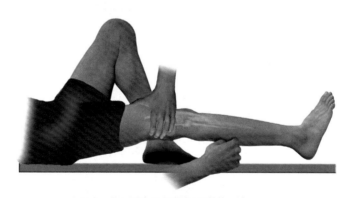

Figure 1H.10. Vastus medialis obliquus strength. (From Hertling D, Kessler RM. *Management of Common Musculoskeletal Disorders: Physical Therapy Principles and Methods*. Philadelphia: Lippincott Williams & Wilkins; 2006.)

IMAGING

Plain Radiographs

- AP and lateral radiographs are obtained to understand the basic morphology of the patella and femur
- Patella height can be assessed using the lateral radiograph of the knee
  - Multiple methods can be used to determine if the patella is high riding called patella alta or low riding called patella baja
    - Patella alta is associated with patellar instability
    - The Insall-Salvati[6] method and Caton-Deschamps method are commonly used (Figure 1H.11)
- A Merchant view can be used to assess the congruence angle (Figure 1H.12)
- A Laurin view can be used to determine lateral opening of the patella (Figure 1H.13)

Stress Radiographs

- Not typically used for isolated patellar instability

Computed Tomography

- Used in conjunction with radiography to determine the morphology of the trochlea and to appropriately assess for trochlear dysplasia (Figure 1H.14)
- Also used to calculate the tibial tubercle, trochlear groove distance (TT-TG)
  - A value of >20 mm is considered abnormal (Figure 1H.15)

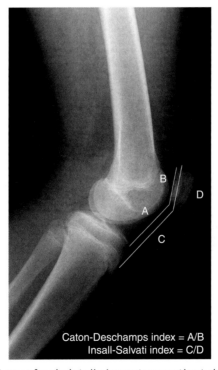

Caton-Deschamps index = A/B
Insall-Salvati index = C/D

Figure 1H.11. Lateral knee X-ray of a skeletally immature patient demonstrating measurement techniques for Caton-Deschamps (A and B) and Insall-Salvati (C and D) to determine patellar height. A ratio greater than 1.2 is considered patella alta. (From Cordasco FA, Green DW, Wolters Kluwer (Haga). *Pediatric and Adolescent Knee Surgery*. Philadelphia: Wolters Kluwer; 2015.)

Magnetic Resonance Imaging

- Used to determine status of the MPFL in addition to any possible chondral injury with the medial facet of the patella and lateral femoral condyle (Figure 1H.16)

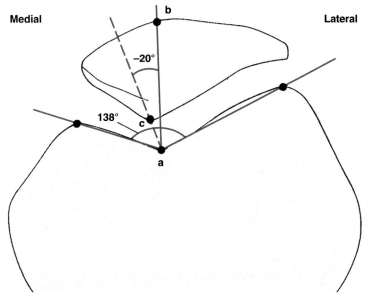

Figure 1H.12. Sulcus and congruence angles. Two specific measurements can be obtained from the Merchant axial view: the sulcus angle and the congruence angle. The sulcus angle, formed by lines extending from the deepest point of the intercondylar sulcus (a) medially and laterally to the tops of the femoral condyles, normally measures approximately 138°. To determine the congruence angle, the sulcus angle is bisected to establish a reference line (ba), which is drawn to connect the apex of the patella (b) with the deepest point of the sulcus (a). In normal subjects, this line is close to vertical. A second line (ca) is then drawn from the lowest point on the articular ridge of the patella (c) to the deepest point of the sulcus (a). The angle formed by this line and the reference line is the congruence angle. If the lowest point on the patellar articular ridge is lateral to the reference line, then the congruence angle has a positive value; if it is medial to the reference line, as in the present example, then the angle has a negative value. In the Merchant study, the average congruence angle in normal subjects was −6° (standard deviation [SD], ±11°). (Modified from Merchant AC, Mercer RL, Jacobsen RH, Cool CR. Roentgenographic analysis of patello-femoral congruence. *J Bone Joint Surg Am.* 1974;56A:1391-1396.)

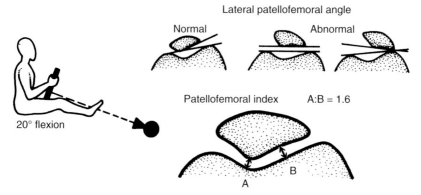

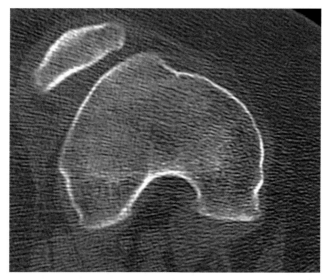

Figure 1H.13. Laurin view assessing lateral opening of the patella using the lateral patellofemoral angle and patellofemoral index. (From Bucholz RW, Heckman JD, eds. *Rockwood and Green's Fractures in Adults*. 5th ed. Baltimore: Lippincott Williams & Wilkins; 2002.)

Figure 1H.14. Selected CT cut demonstrating a type D trochlea in trochlear dysplasia with a "cliff" separating the medial and lateral facets.

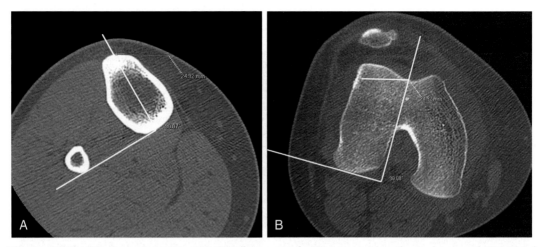

Figure 1H.15. CT demonstrating TT-TG distance of ~25 mm with selected cuts of the tibial tubercle (A) and trochlear groove (B).

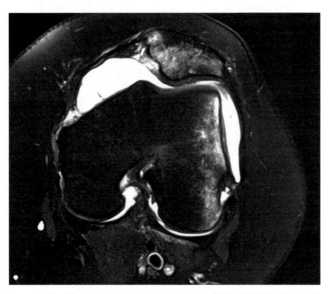

Figure 1H.16. MRI demonstrating high-grade tearing of the MPFL from the patellar insertion and complete avulsion from the femoral origin with associated bony edema and chondral injury of the medial facet of the patella and bony edema lateral femoral condyle.

Classic Arthroscopic Findings (Figure 1H.17)

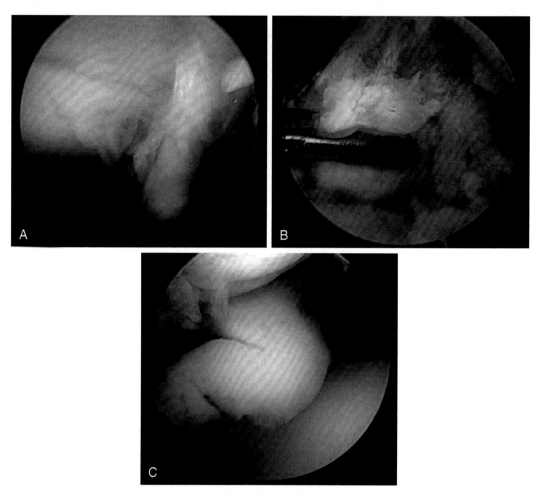

Figure 1H.17. High-grade tearing of patellar insertion of MPFL, patella on left (A); complete tearing of MPFL off femoral insertion pulled into the joint by an arthroscopic grabber (B); large free chondral fragment from medial patella (C).

REFERENCES

1. Bassett FH. Acute dislocation of the patella, osteochondral fractures, and injuries to the extensor mechanism of the knee. *Instr Course Lect*. 1976;25:40-49.
2. Brattström H. Shape of the intercondylar groove normally and in recurrent dislocation of patella: a clinical and x-ray anatomical investigation. *Acta Orthop Scand*. 1964;35(suppl 68):1-148.
3. Dandy DJ. Recurrent subluxation of the patella on extension of the knee. *Bone Joint J*. 1971;53(3):483-487.
4. Dejour H, Walch G, Nove-Josserand L, et al. Factors of patellar instability: an anatomic radiographic study. *Knee Surg Sports Traumatol Arthrosc*. 1994;2(1):19-26.
5. Hughston JC, Deese M. Medial subluxation of the patella as a complication of lateral retinacular release. *Am J Sports Med*. 1988;16(4):383-388.
6. Insall J, Goldberg V, Salvati E. Recurrent dislocation and the high-riding patella. *Clin Orthop Relat Res*. 1972;88:67-69.
7. Johnson LL, van Dyk GE, Green 3rd JR, et al. Clinical assessment of asymptomatic knees: comparison of men and women. *Arthroscopy*. 1998;14(4):347-359.
8. Kolowich PA, Paulos LE, Rosenberg TD, et al. Lateral release of the patella: indications and contraindications. *Am J Sports Med*. 1990;18(4):359-365.
9. Merchant AC, Mercer RL, Jacobsen RH, Cool CR. Radiographic analysis of patellofemoral congruence. *J Bone Joint Surg Am*. 1974;56:1391-1396.

10. Nonweiler DE, DeLee JC. The diagnosis and treatment of medial subluxation of the patella after lateral retinacular release. *Am J Sports Med*. 1994;22(5):680-686.
11. Fairbank HAT. Internal derangement of the knee in children and adolescents. *Proc R Soc Med*. 1937;30:427-432.
12. Hughston JC. Subluxation of the patella. *J Bone Joint*. 1968;50A:1003-1026.
13. Hughston JC, Stone MM. Recurring dislocations of the patella in athletes. *South Med J*. 1964;57:623-628.

SECTION I
Osteochondritis Dissecans and Osteochondral Injuries

Ian J. Dempsey and Mark D. Miller

HISTORY

- Osteochondritis dissecans (OCD) is an articular cartilage and subchondral bone lesion that affects both juvenile and adult populations
- Most commonly seen on the posterolateral aspect of the medial femoral condyle
- May be related to heredity and vascular status (proposed for adults)
- Osteochondral injuries are likely due to a combination of degeneration from aging and trauma sustained by the knee
- They can occur in the medial, lateral, and patellofemoral compartments, which include the femur, tibia, and patella

PHYSICAL EXAMINATION

- There are few clinical examination maneuvers helpful to diagnose OCD and osteochondral injuries
- Most commonly diagnosed using advanced imaging

KEY EXAMINATION MANEUVERS

- **Wilson Test** (Figure 1I.1)
  - First described by Wilson[4] in 1967, revisited in 2003 by Conrad et al[2] who demonstrated that the test may have minimal clinical significance
  - **Maneuver:**
    - The patient lies supine and the affected knee is flexed
    - The examiner grabs the flexed knee at the ankle and knee and slowly internally rotates the foot and extends the knee completely, which attempts to impinge the ACL against the posterolateral aspect of the medial femoral condyle where OCD lesions classically are found
    - The test is positive if the patient elicits pain with the knee internally rotated and knee extended
    - The pain should subside if the internal rotation is relaxed

- **Passive and Active Patellar Grind Test** (Figure 1I.2 A-B)
  - First described by Fründ[3] in 1926 with striking the patella with the knee flexed to elicit pain
  - Owre also described pressure over the patella eliciting pain with chondral injury in 1936[5]
  - Also can be used with instability evaluation

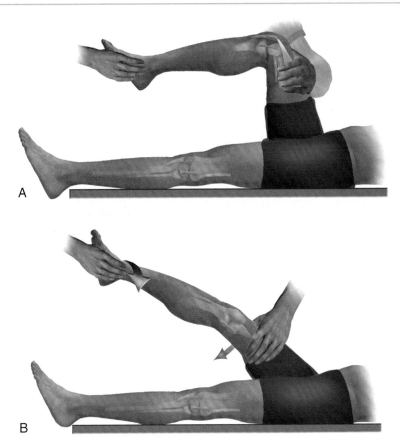

Figure 1I.1. Wilson test. A, Knee flexion and internal rotation. B, Knee extension and internal rotation.

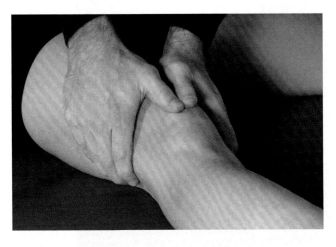

Figure 1I.2. Passive patellar grind test. (From Anderson MK, Barnum M. *Foundations of Athletic Training: Prevention, Assessment, and Management*. Wolters Kluwer Health; 2017.)

- **Maneuver:**
  - For the passive test, the patient lies supine with the knee relaxed
  - The examiner uses the palm of his/her hand to press the patella against the femur while passively flexing the knee with the other
  - For the active test, the patient is at the edge of the table with the knee flexed
  - The examiner uses his/her fingers to applied pressure to the patella while the patient actively extends and flexes the knee

- For both test, if there are chondral irregularities, crepitus will be felt in addition to eliciting pain
- Crepitus may be felt at different points of flexion and extension
- If crepitus is felt near full extension, it is likely due to chondral irregularities at the inferior pole of the patella
- If crepitus is felt near full flexion, it is likely due to chondral irregularities at the inferior trochlear groove or superior pole of the patella

IMAGING

Plain Radiographs

- Weight-bearing AP and lateral radiographs are typically obtained
- A tunnel (notch) view with the knee bent between 30° and 50° can be used to demonstrate evidence of an OCD (Figure 1I.3)

Stress Radiographs

- Not typically used for OCDs

Magnetic Resonance Imaging

- Used to determine location and characteristics of the OCD; may also demonstrate loose bodies
- OCDs are most commonly found on the posterolateral aspect of the medial femoral condyle (Figure 1I.4) but also be found in other places (Figure 1I.5)

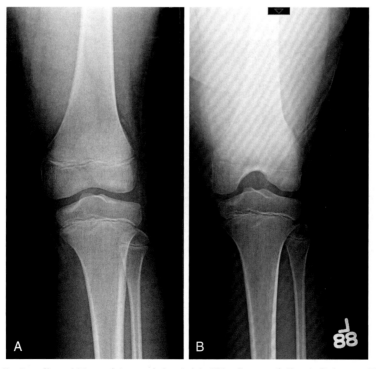

Figure 1I.3. AP standing (A) and tunnel (notch) (B) views of the left knee. There is some evidence of a possible OCD on the lateral femoral condyle of the femur.

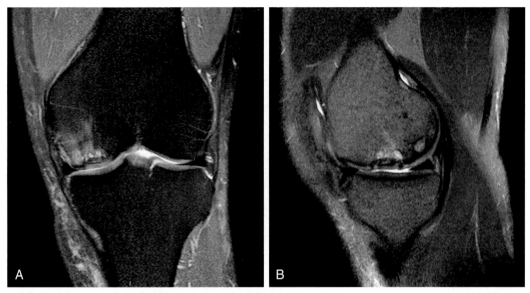

Figure 1I.4. Coronal (A) and sagittal (B) T2 imaging of an unstable OCD in the classic position of the posterolateral aspect of the medal femoral condyle.

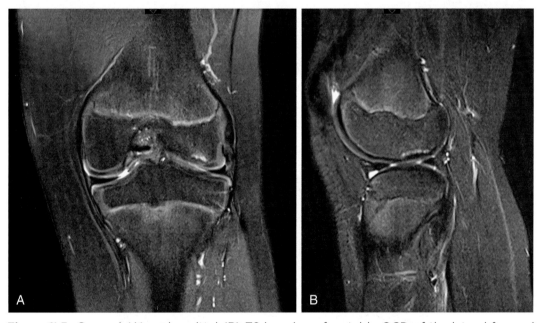

Figure 1I.5. Coronal (A) and sagittal (B) T2 imaging of a stable OCD of the lateral femoral condyle.

- Osteochondral injures in general can be found throughout the medial, lateral, and patellofemoral compartments
- Dipaola et al[1] developed an MRI based grading system to help guide treatment
  - Grade 1: thickening of cartilage without disruption
    - 1a: bone marrow edema present
    - 1b: fluid at lesion-bone interface
  - Grade 2: cartilage breached, fluid at interface, but not entire interface
  - Grade 3: cartilage completely disrupted with fluid interface surrounding lesion
  - Grade 4: displaced fragment

- In general, nondisrupted OCDs could attempt a trial of non–weight-bearing to allow the lesion to heal vs back drilling the OCD to promote healing
- Disrupted or breached cartilage would require an arthroscopic debridement with microfracture, microfracture and reimplantation of cartilage with bone graft, autologous transplant of articular cartilage, or transplant of cadaveric cartilage to fill the defect

Classic Arthroscopic Findings of OCDs (Figure 11.6-11.12)

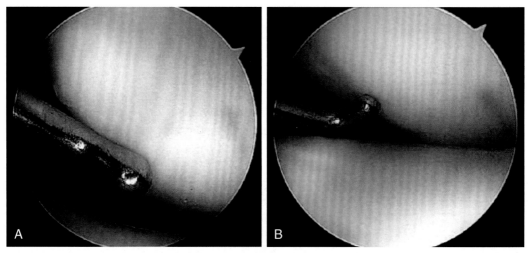

Figure 11.6. A subtle cleft is noted upon arthroscopic inspection of the lateral femoral condyle (A) and (B) seen on MRI. An arthroscopic probe is used, and there is a subtle softening of this area, but it is otherwise stable.

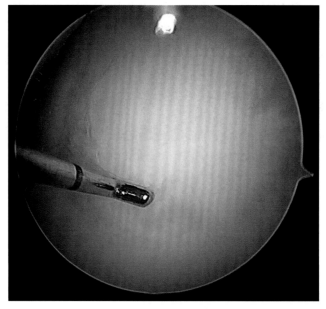

Figure 11.7. Arthroscopic evaluation of the medial femoral condyle reveals an unstable chondral flap on the posterolateral surface of the medial femoral condyle.

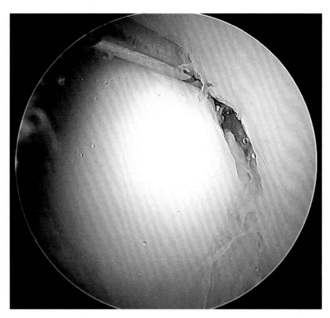

Figure 1I.8. An arthroscopic knife is used to remove the unstable cartilage, which was saved for later reimplantation.

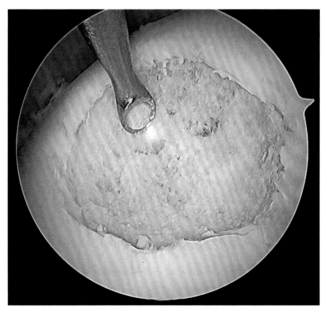

Figure 1I.9. A curette is used to remove any articular cartilage remnants and subchondral bone.

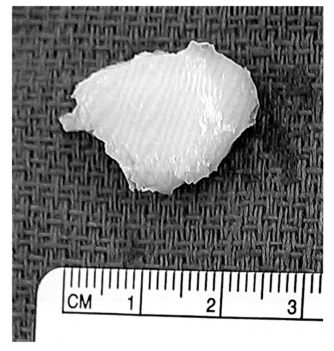

Figure 1I.10. The fragment was measured to be 18 mm × 16 mm.

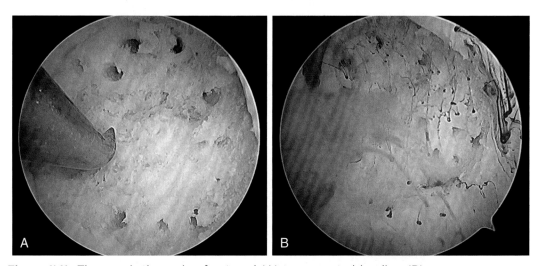

Figure 1I.11. The area is then microfractured (A) to promote bleeding (B).

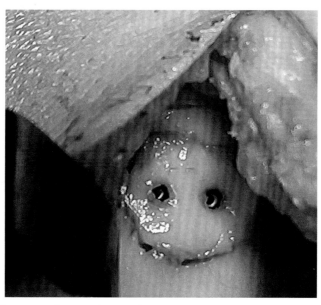

Figure 1I.12. Local bone graft was obtained (not shown) from the medial distal femur, packed into the defect, and then the articular cartilage was placed and affixed with 2 headless screws.

REFERENCES

1. Dipaola JD, David WN, Colville MR. Characterizing osteochondral lesions by magnetic resonance imaging. *Arthroscopy.* 1991;7(1):101-104.
2. Conrad JM, Stanitski CL. Osteochondritis dissecans: Wilson's sign revisited. *Am J Sports Med.* 2003;31(5):777-778.
3. Fründ H. *Zentralbl Chir.* 1926;53:707.
4. Wilson JN. A diagnostic sign in osteochondritis dissecans of the knee. *J Bone Joint Surg Am.* 1967;49(3):477-480.
5. Owre A. Chondromalacia Patellae. *Acta Chirurgica Scandinavica.* 1936;77(suppl 41).

2
SECTION

The Shoulder

Section Editor
Brian C. Werner

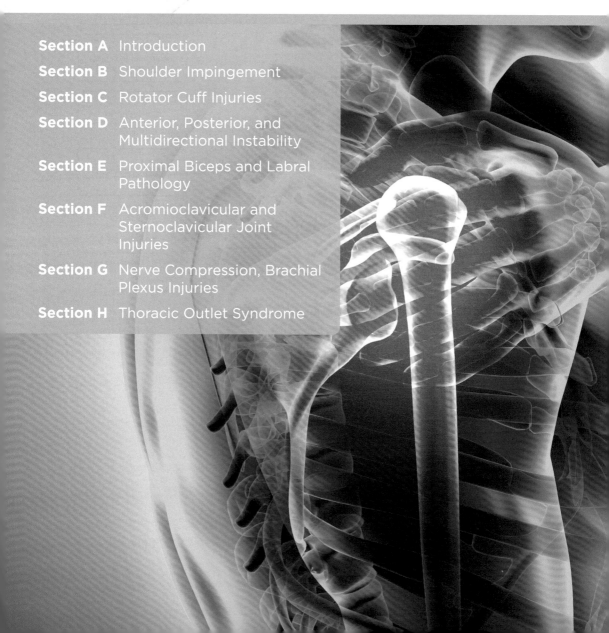

QUICK REFERENCE FLOW CHARTS

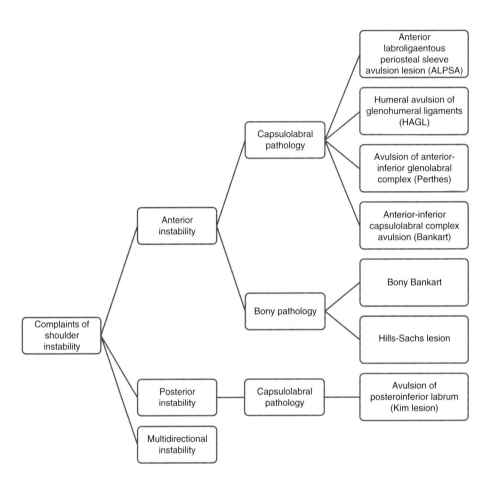

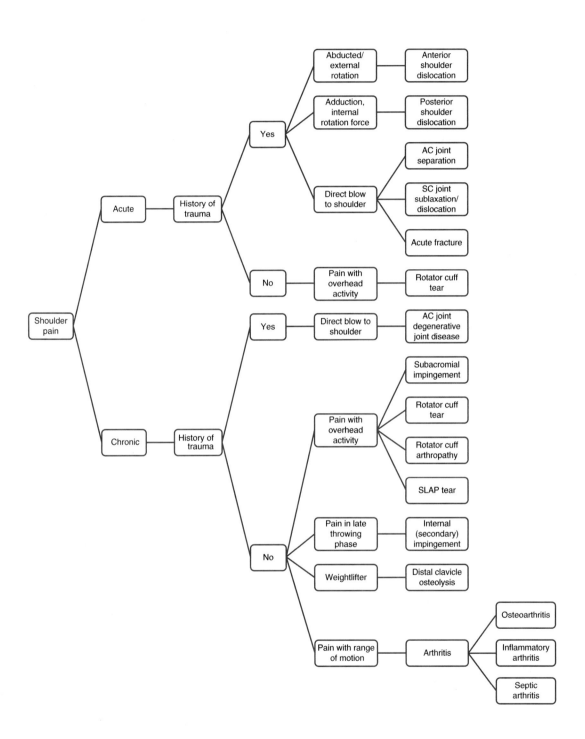

SECTION A
Introduction

Michelle E. Kew

HISTORY

It is important to consider the following parameters when a patient presents to the clinic with a shoulder complaint:

- Patient age
  - Younger patients (age <30 y) are more likely to have an acute labral tear, instability, acromioclavicular (AC) joint injury
  - Older patients (age >50 y) are more likely to have osteoarthritis and/or rotator cuff arthropathy, adhesive capsulitis
- Chronicity of symptoms
  - Acute injuries may represent AC joint separation, shoulder dislocation, labral pathology, and acute rotator cuff tear
  - Chronic pain may represent adhesive capsulitis (if stiffness is present), rotator cuff tear, and osteoarthritis
- Mechanism of injury (if any)
  - Shoulder dislocation
    - Determine arm position at the time of injury
    - Initial mechanism (posteriorly directed force with arm in forward flexion and adduction versus force with arm in abduction and external rotation)
  - Evaluate for repetitive overhead throwing motion (pitchers)
- Mechanical symptoms (crepitus)
  - May indicate subacromial bursitis, rotator cuff pathology, or osteoarthritis
- History of shoulder dislocation
- History of shoulder surgery
  - One must critically analyze the prior surgery to determine if there may have been any technical errors. Obtain prior operative reports, images; patient reports are often incomplete or inaccurate
- Prior treatment
- Current medications
- One-finger test: Ask patients to point, with 1 finger, to the area where it hurts (they often cannot do so, but it can be helpful)

PHYSICAL EXAMINATION

Observation

- Remove shirt
- Observe for symmetry, soft tissue deformity, atrophy, hypertrophy, scapular winging
- Evaluate posture

Palpation

- Bony prominences (Figure 2A.1)
  - Acromion
  - Clavicle
  - Sternoclavicular joint
  - AC joint
  - Coracoid process
  - Scapular borders
    - Supraspinatus and infraspinatus fossae
  - Proximal humerus
    - Lesser and greater tuberosities
    - Bicipital groove
    - Subacromial space
- Muscles and soft tissues
  - Deltoid
  - Rotator cuff muscles
  - Trapezius
  - Biceps tendon in groove

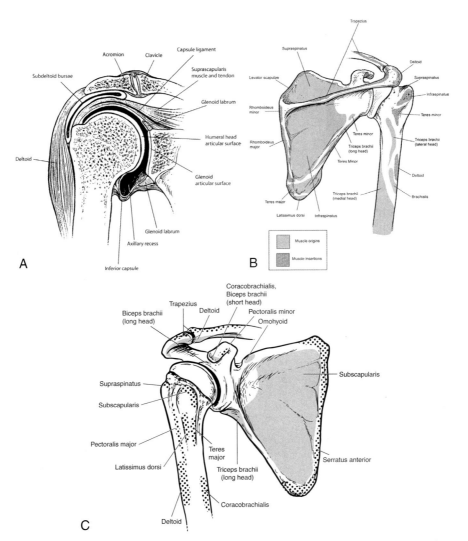

Figure 2A.1. A, Shoulder bony landmarks. B, Posterior shoulder muscle attachments. C, Anterior shoulder muscle attachments.

Range of Motion ▶

- Normal range of motion (degrees) (Figure 2A.2)
  - Forward elevation: 0 to 150 to 180
  - Abduction: 0 to 90
  - External rotation, arm adducted: 0 to 70

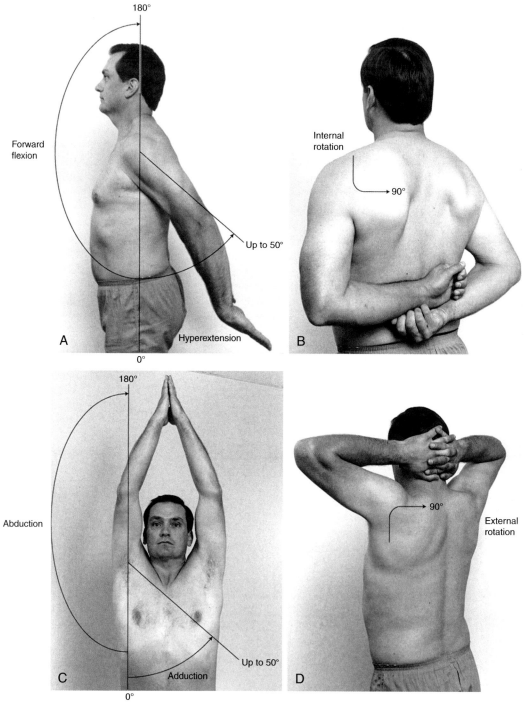

Figure 2A.2. A-D, Shoulder range of motion. A, Forward flexion, hyperextension. B, Internal rotation. C, Abduction, adduction. D, External rotation. (Borrowed from Jones RM, Jones RM. *Patient Assessment in Pharmacy Practice*. Wolters Kluwer Health; 2016.)

TABLE 2A.1 Medical Research Council Muscle Grading Scale; Used for Rotator Cuff Strength Evaluation

Medical Research Council Score
0 = No movement is observed
1 = Visible contraction, no segment movement
2 = Active movement upon resistance of gravity removed
3 = Active movement, against gravity
4 = Active movement against gravity and examiner's resistance
5 = Normal strength
Evaluate shoulder abduction, elbow flexion, wrist extension, hip flexion, knee extension, ankle dorsal flexion; addition of score from 0 (complete tetraparesis) to 60 (normal muscle strength)

- External rotation, arm abducted: 0 to 100
- Internal rotation in abduction: 0 to 70
- Internal rotation to vertebral height
  - T4-T8 is normal
- Horizontal adduction: 0 to 50
- Assess ROM with the patient in the upright position
- To isolate glenohumeral motion, evaluate horizontal adduction and IR/ER in 90° abduction in a supine position, as this stabilizes the scapulothoracic joint
- Evaluate for hypermobility (refer to section D)

Muscular Strength

- Rotator cuff strength is graded with Medical Research Council rating scale (Table 2A.1)
  - Supraspinatus
    - Evaluated in 70° to 90° of abduction in the plane of the scapula
    - Evaluated in internal rotation with the forearm maximally pronated (empty can test; Figure 2A.3)
      - Downward pressure is applied to the forearm, and the patient is asked to resist

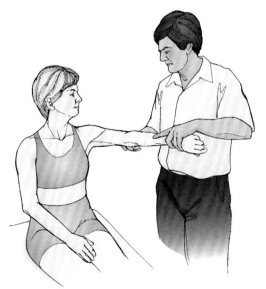

Figure 2A.3. Empty can test for supraspinatus pathology. (Borrowed from Hendrickson T, Hendrickson T. *Massage and Manual Therapy for Orthopedic Conditions.* Philadelphia: Wolters Kluwer Health/Lippincott Williams & Wilkins; 2009.)

- Infraspinatus
  - Tested in adduction with elbow at 90° flexion
  - The patient tries to externally rotate the arm from 45° IR against counterforce
  - Positive drop sign
    - The patient cannot maintain the arm in 45° external rotation and the arm falls spontaneously back to 0°
    - Indicates infraspinatus insufficiency
- Teres minor
  - Isolated when the arm is in 90° ER and 90° abduction
  - The examiner tries to rotate the arm internally
- Subscapularis
  - Tested with belly-press, lift-off, bear-hug test (outlined below)

Sensation

- Can be viewed as dermatomes C5-T1 (Figure 2A.4A) or as peripheral nerves (Figure 2A.4B) listed below:
- Axillary
- Musculocutaneous
- Medial brachial and antebrachial cutaneous
- Median
- Radial
- Ulnar

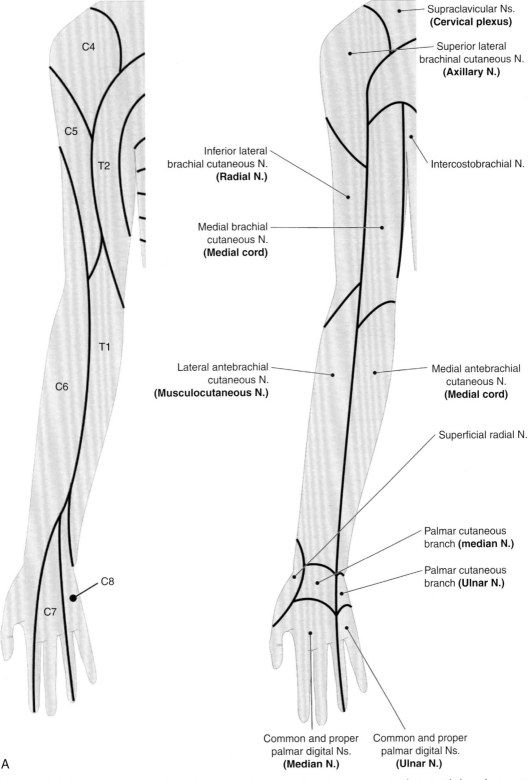

Figure 2A.4. A, Upper extremity dermatomes. B, Upper extremity peripheral nerve distributions. (Borrowed from Olinger AB. *Human Gross Anatomy*. Philadelphia: Wolters Kluwer; 2016 and Moore KL, Dalley AF, Agur AMR. *Clinically Oriented Anatomy*. 7th ed. Philadelphia: Wolters Kluwer/Lippincott Williams & Wilkins Health; 2014.)

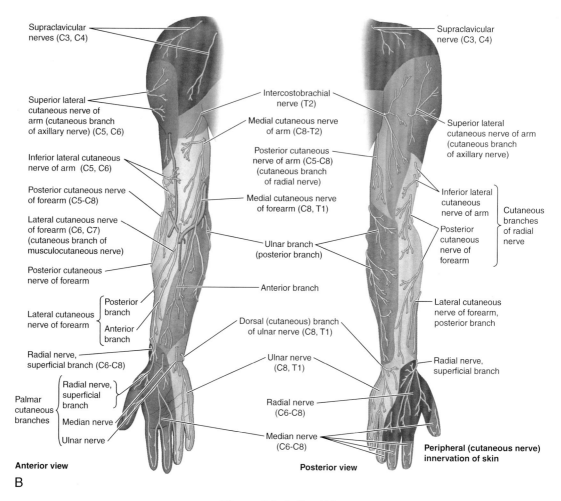

Figure 2A.4. Cont'd

- **Impingement**
  - Neer impingement sign
  - Impingement test
  - Hawkins test

- **Rotator Cuff**
  - Jobe test
  - Drop-arm test
  - External rotation lag sign or dropping sign
  - Drop-arm sign
  - Hornblower's sign
  - Lift-off test
  - Belly-press/push test or Napoleon test
  - Internal rotation lag sign or modified lift-off test or subscapularis lag sign
  - Bear-hug test

- **Anterior, Posterior, and Multidirectional Instability**
  - Beighton criteria
  - Gagey hyperabduction test
  - Apprehension test
  - Relocation test
  - Load and shift test
  - Modified load and shift test
  - Jerk test
  - Sulcus sign

- **Biceps/Labrum**
  - O'Brien test or active compression test
  - Resisted thrower's test
  - Anterior slide test
  - Biceps load test
  - Crank test
  - Speed's test
  - Yergason test

- **AC and Sternoclavicular Joint**
  - Cross-body adduction test
  - AC resisted extension test
  - Buchberger test
  - O'Brien test or active compression test
  - Paxinos test

- **Miscellaneous**
  - Spurling maneuver
  - Wright test
  - Medial scapular winging
  - Lateral scapular winging

IMAGING

Plain Radiographs

- AP view
  - Evaluate glenohumeral joint space
- Glenohumeral "true" AP view
  - Evaluate glenohumeral joint space (Figure 2A.5A)
  - Evaluate for proximal migration of humerus (Figure 2A.5B)
- Axillary lateral view
  - Evaluate glenohumeral dislocation (Figure 2A.6A and 2A.6B)
  - Best view to evaluate for glenohumeral arthritis
  - Use Velpeau view if unable to abduct the arm
- Scapular Y view
  - Use to classify acromion, evaluate for glenohumeral subluxation and dislocation
  - Can show scapular body abnormalities
- Acromioclavicular AP view
- Additional views
  - Rotational views
  - Supine/prone
  - Tilted

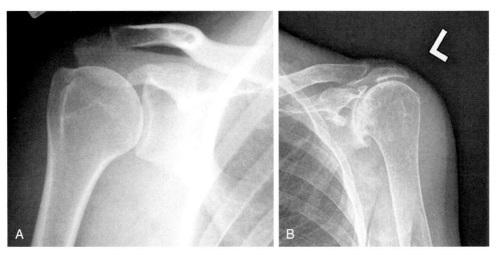

Figure 2A.5. A, Normal right shoulder radiograph. B, Proximal migration of the right humeral head with associated acetabularization of the glenohumeral joint.

Magnetic Resonance Imaging

MRI is useful for evaluating soft tissues, bony edema, and occult fractures.

- T1-weighted images
  - Often combined with MR arthrogram
  - Also useful to evaluate Hill-Sachs lesions
- T2-weighted images
  - Useful to visualize rotator cuff (Figure 2A.7)
- Short tau inversion recovery (STIR)
  - Helps to determine fatty infiltration versus edema in rotator cuff
  - Allows visualization of rotator cuff pathology
- Abduction external rotation (ABER) position
  - The patient places the hand behind the head
  - Tensions anteroinferior glenohumeral ligament (IGHL) and labrum

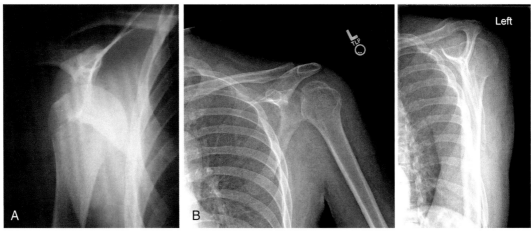

Figure 2A.6. A, Anterior dislocation. B, Posterior dislocation. (Borrowed from Staheli LT. *Fundamentals of Pediatric Orthopedics.* 5th ed. Philadelphia: Wolters Kluwer; 2016 and Dodson CC, Dines DM, Dines JS, Walch G, Williams GR. *Controversies in Shoulder Surgery.* 2014.)

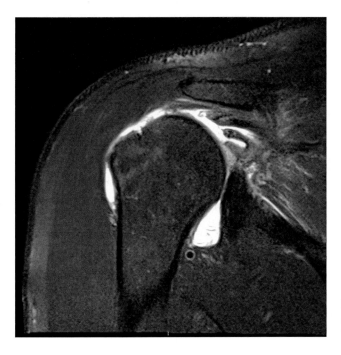

Figure 2A.7. T2-weighted MRI arthrogram showing supraspinatus tear.

- Relaxes the capsule
- Useful to visualize Bankart lesions, partial- and full-thickness tear of rotator cuff, internal impingement
- MR arthrogram
  - Used to augment MRI to diagnose soft tissue problems
  - Best modality for
    - Bankart lesion
    - Superior labrum anterior-posterior tear (SLAP)
    - Glenoid labral articular disruption (GLAD)
    - Anterior labral periosteal sleeve avulsion (ALPSA)
    - Humeral avulsion of glenohumeral ligament (HAGL)

CT

It allows improved evaluation of bony structures over MRI.

- Axial images
  - Evaluate Hill-Sachs lesions
- Coronal images
  - Evaluate fractures
- Sagittal images
  - Evaluate for anterior-inferior glenoid bone loss
- 3D reconstructions
  - Evaluate glenoid anatomy before total shoulder arthroplasty

Ultrasound

It can be used to evaluate rotator cuff and other soft tissue structures; however, its use limited by skill and experience of the technician.

- Anatomic structures that can be evaluated with ultrasound:
  - Long head biceps (LHB) tendon in groove
    - Biceps tendon subluxation or dislocation
  - Subscapularis, supraspinatus, infraspinatus, teres minor

- Rotator interval
- AC joint, subacromial-subdeltoid bursa
- Posterior labrum
- Can perform dynamic evaluation for subacromial impingement

Shoulder Arthroscopy

- Standard portals (Figure 2A.8)[1]
  - Posterior portal
    - 2 cm distal and medial to the posterolateral border of acromion, "soft spot"
    - Safest portal, provides adequate visualization of the entire joint
    - Used for viewing
    - Hazards: axillary nerve, suprascapular nerve, suprascapular artery

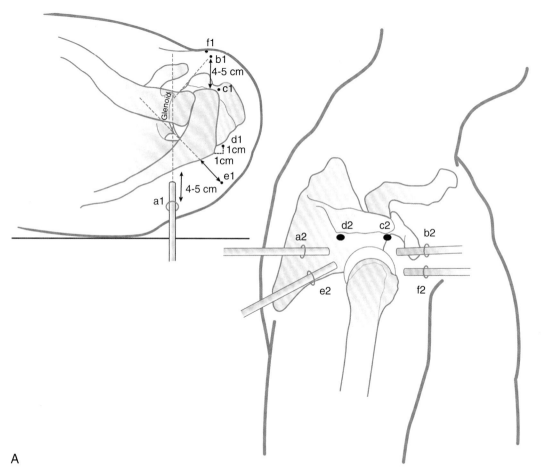

A

Figure 2A.8. A, Shoulder arthroscopy portals: a2-f2, diagram of portal placement, a1, posterior portal, b1, anterior portal, c1, anterosuperior portal, d1, Port of Wilmington portal, e1, low posterolateral portal, f1, 5-o'clock portal. B, Clinical photograph of portal placement (P, posterior portal; Pl, accessory posterolateral portal; PL, posterolateral portal; AS, anterosuperior portal; AL, accessory anterosuperior portal; A, anterior portal; LC, lateral portal; MA, low anterior portal). C, View from posterior portal, cannula is placed into the rotator interval. D, View from anterosuperior portal. E, View from Port of Wilmington (A, anterior capsule; BT, biceps tendon; G, glenoid; H, humerus). ((A, D, and E) Borrowed from Burkhart SS, Lo IKY, Brady PC, Denard PJ, Burkhart SS. *The Cowboy's Companion: A Trail Guide for the Arthroscopic Shoulder Surgeon.* Wolters Kluwer/Lippincott Williams & Wilkins; 2012. (B) Johnson D, Amendola NA, Barber F. *Operative Arthroscopy.* Philadelphia: Wolters Kluwer; 2015. (C) Koval KJ, Zuckerman JD. *Atlas of Orthopaedic Surgery: A Multimedia Reference.* Philadelphia: Lippincott Williams & Wilkins; 2004.)

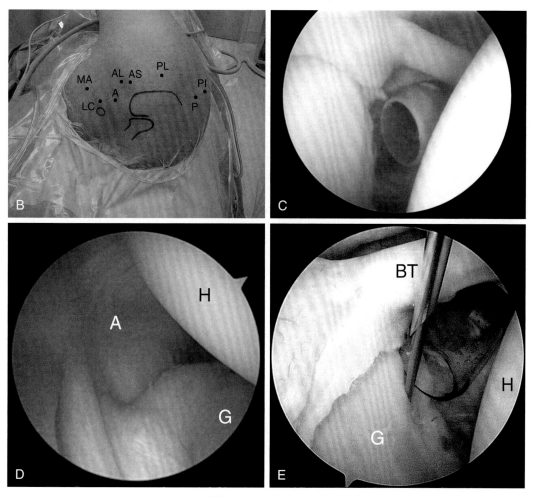

Figure 2A.8. Cont'd

- Anterior portal
  – Just anterior and lateral to AC joint, 1 to 2 cm inferomedial to anterolateral acromion, adjusting based on a planned procedure
  – Working portal for most arthroscopic procedures
  – Hazards: cephalic vein, axillary artery, musculocutaneous nerve
- Lateral portal
  – 1 to 2 cm distal to lateral acromion edge
  – Hazards: axillary nerve if too distal
- Accessory portals
  - Supraspinatus (Nevasier) portal
    – Used for SLAP repair suture passage
    – Placed between clavicle, acromion, and scapular spine
    – Hazards: suprascapular nerve, suprascapular artery
  - Anterolateral portal
    – Used for AC joint and subacromial pathology
    – Can be used for posterior glenoid visualization and SLAP repair
    – 2 to 3 cm distal to anterolateral acromion
    – Hazards: axillary nerve
  - Posterolateral portal
    – Used for rotator cuff repair, labral repair
    – Just anterior to the posterolateral corner of acromion
    – Hazards: axillary nerve

- 5-o'clock portal
  - Used for anterior stabilization procedures
  - Portal placed lateral to conjoint tendon through lower subscapularis
  - Hazards: axillary nerve, musculocutaneous nerve, cephalic vein, humeral cartilage
- Anteroinferior portal
  - Use for Bankart repair and stabilization procedures
  - Hazards: cephalic vein, axillary nerve
- Posteroinferior (7-o'clock) portal
  - Used for loose body removal, posteroinferior labral repair
  - Placed 2 to 3 cm inferior to posterior viewing portal
  - Hazards: suprascapular nerve, suprascapular artery, axillary nerve, posterior humeral circumflex artery
  - Axillary pouch portal
    - Safe alternative to 7-o'clock portal
    - Placed 2 to 3 cm inferior to posterolateral acromion
- Portal of Wilmington
  - Transrotator cuff portal used for SLAP repair
  - Placed 1 cm anterior and 1 cm lateral to the posterolateral part of acromion
  - Hazards: axillary nerve
- Suprascapular nerve portal
  - Used to treat suprascapular nerve compression by cutting superior transverse scapular ligament
  - Placed 2 cm medial to Nevasier portal
  - Hazards: suprascapular nerve, suprascapular artery

REFERENCE

1. Paxton SE, Backus J, Keener J, Brophy R. Shoulder arthroscopy: basic principles of positioning, anesthesia, and portal anatomy. *J Am Acad Orthop Surg.* 2013;21(6);332-342.

SECTION B
Shoulder Impingement

Ian J. Dempsey and Jourdan M. Cancienne

HISTORY

- Shoulder impingement presents as part of continuum of disease often closely associated with rotator cuff disease whether it be rotator cuff tendinitis or tear
- Impingement in isolation is most frequently seen in middle-aged adults who are consistently involved in overhead movements
- In older adults, impingement signs are typically indicative of rotator cuff pathology
- Pain is often elicited with shoulder elevation greater than 90° with pain in the anterolateral arm[5]
- Can have either subacromial impingement or subcoracoid impingement or both
  - Subacromial impingement is much more common and is associated with supraspinatus and infraspinatus pathology
  - Subcoracoid impingement is associated with subscapularis pathology
- Both are often exacerbated by overhead movement with subcoracoid impingement worst with the arm in abduction
- Subacromial impingement syndrome (SIS) can be caused by both extrinsic compression and intrinsic degeneration
  - **Extrinsic compression**
    - Extrinsic compression, as proposed by Neer, is due to impingement of the rotator cuff and humeral head against the undersurface of the anterior acromion, which progresses in 3 stages
      - Stage I: acute bursitis with subacromial edema
      - Stage II: rotator cuff tendinopathy
      - Stage III: progression to partial-thickness or full-thickness rotator cuff tears
    - Bigliani[1] felt acromial morphology also plays a role (Figure 2B.1)
      - Type I: flat
      - Type II: curved
      - Type III: hooked, with hook having the highest association with rotator cuff degeneration

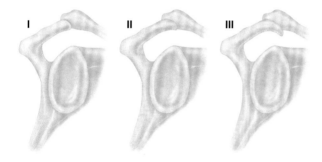

Figure 2B.1. Acromion morphology (I, flat; II, curved; III, hooked). (Borrowed from Williams A. *Massage Mastery: From Student to Professional.* Philadelphia, PA: Wolters Kluwer Health/Lippincott Williams & Wilkins; 2013.)

- Variations in the coracoacromial ligament anatomy may also play a role
  - Cadaveric studies have revealed an anterolateral and posteromedial band with osteophytes found in the anterolateral band more commonly
  - Variants with more than 1 band were associated with cuff degeneration
- **Intrinsic degeneration**: Multiple investigators have looked at aging, diminished vascular supply, and tensile forces on the rotator cuff as causes for SIS
  - A degenerated rotator cuff does not keep the humeral head depressed in the glenoid socket, and the resulting subtle superior migration can also result in SIS

PHYSICAL EXAMINATION

KEY EXAMINATION MANEUVERS

- **Neer Impingement Sign and Modified Impingement Sign** (Sensitivity: 0.75, Specificity: 0.47 for subacromial bursitis) (Figure 2B.2)
  - First described as diagnosing impingement by Neer in 1972[3]
  - **Maneuver:**
    - The examiner stands in front or to the side of either a standing or sitting patient and passively flexes the patient's shoulder to the position of maximal forward flexion while stabilizing the scapula with the other hand
    - Pain at maximal forward flexion is considered positive for impingement
    - The modified versus includes flexing the elbow to 90° while the shoulder is maximally forward flex with associated internal rotation of the arm again eliciting pain

- **Neer Impingement Test** 🔘
  - First described as diagnosing impingement by Neer in 1972[3] and used as a part of the Neer impingement sign
  - **Maneuver:**
    - If Neer impingement sign is positive, local anesthetic is injected into the subacromial space
    - The examiner then repeats the Neer impingement sign
    - If the pain is relieved, this is likely due to subacromial impingement and possibly rotator cuff pathology

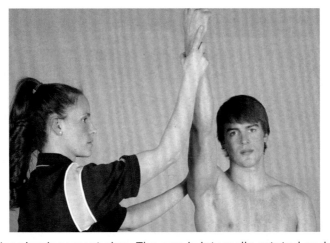

Figure 2B.2. Neer impingement sign. The arm is internally rotated and forcibly flexed forward to jam the greater tuberosity against the anteroinferior surface of the acromion. (Borrowed from Anderson MK, Parr GP. *Foundations of Athletic Training: Prevention, Assessment and Management*. Philadelphia: Lippincott Williams & Wilkins; 2013.)

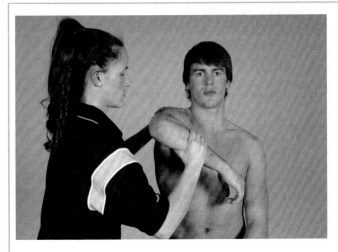

Figure 2B.3. Hawkins test. The arm is flexed to 90° and the arm is passively internally rotated with the elbow flexed at 90°. (Borrowed from Anderson MK, Parr GP. *Foundations of Athletic Training: Prevention, Assessment and Management.* Philadelphia: Lippincott Williams & Wilkins; 2013.)

- **Hawkins Test or Hawkins Impingement Reinforcement Test** 🔘 (Sensitivity: 0.92, Specificity: 0.44) (Figure 2B.3)
  - First described by Hawkins[6,7] in 1980
  - **Maneuver:**
    - The examiner stands in front of either a standing or sitting patient and passively flexes the patient's shoulder to 90°
    - The arm is then passively internally rotated
    - Pain from this motion is thought to be from driving the greater tuberosity into the acromion
    - The elbow may also be flexed to 90° to help internally rotate the shoulder

IMAGING

Plain Radiographs

- Obtain shoulder radiographs, including AP, axillary views, scapular Y view, or supraspinatus outlet view
  - Note: Supraspinatus outlet view is a variation of the scapular Y view with the same projection but the beam tilted 5° to 10° caudad
- Evaluate AP view for acromiohumeral interval (Figure 2B.4)
  - Normal: 7 to 14 mm
- Evaluate axillary view for evidence of dislocation, joint space pathology
- Evaluate scapular Y view or supraspinatus outlet view for acromial morphology (Figure 2B.5)
- May show changes within acromion or coracoacromial ligament

Magnetic Resonance Imaging

- Frequently obtained as impingement often has associated rotator cuff disease (Figures 2B.6 and 2B.7)
- Gold standard to evaluate rotator cuff disease

Arthroscopic Images

- Arthroscopic images of subacromial bursectomy with subsequent removal of subacromial spur (Figure 2B.8)

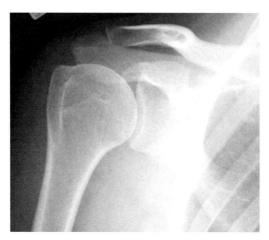

Figure 2B.4. AP radiograph of the right shoulder.

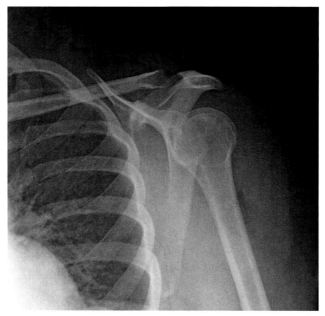

Figure 2B.5. Supraspinatus outlet view demonstrating a type III acromion. (Borrowed from Johnson D, Amendola NA, Barber F. *Operative Arthroscopy*. Philadelphia: Wolters Kluwer; 2015.)

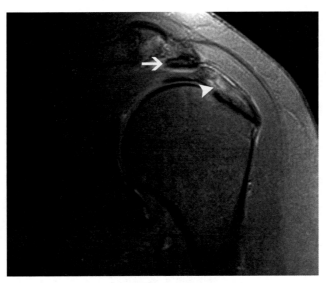

Figure 2B.6. MRI demonstrating subacromial impingement syndrome: Coronal PD-weighted MRI shows a large subacromial spur that has low signal (arrow). In addition, there is bursal side fraying and intermediate signal in the supraspinatus tendon, consistent with tendinosis (arrowhead), which is consistent with subacromial impingement syndrome. (Borrowed from Iannotti JP, Williams GR, Miniaci A, Zuckerman JD. *Disorders of the Shoulder: Diagnosis & Management.* 2014.)

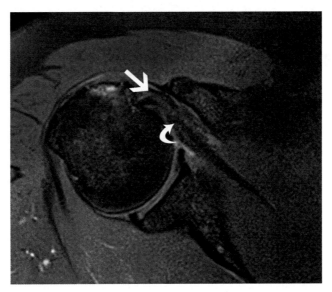

Figure 2B.7. MRI demonstrating subcoracoid impingement syndrome: axial T2-weighted MRI image in a patient with narrowed coracohumeral interval (straight arrow) and subscapularis tendinosis (curved arrow), suggestive of subcoracoid impingement. (Borrowed from Iannotti JP, Williams GR, Miniaci A, Zuckerman JD. *Disorders of the Shoulder: Diagnosis & Management.* 2014.)

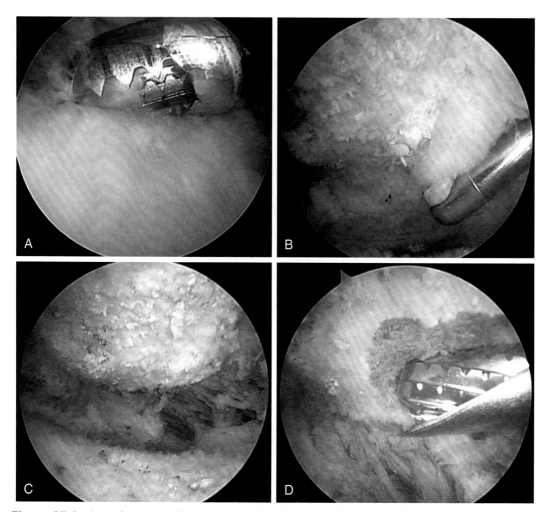

Figure 2B.8. A, Arthroscopic bursectomy. The bursa overlying the tendinous portion of the rotator cuff must be thoroughly resected to evaluate the tendons for bursal-side rotator cuff tear. B, Soft tissue on the undersurface of the acromion is denuded with a radiofrequency electrocautery. Removing the soft tissue will expose the bony undersurface of the acromion and facilitate acromioplasty by the burr's cutting flutes. C, The acromial spur is now completely visualized. The coracoacromial (CA) ligament must be completely resected from the anterolateral acromion. Failure to do so may result in residual impingement by the CA ligament. Visualization of the undersurface fibers of the deltoid indicates a complete CA ligament resection. D, The acromioplasty begins at the far anterolateral tip of the acromion. The burr's diameter, usually 5-6 mm, is used to assess the initial depth of the acromial resection. The acromioplasty proceeds in 5- to 6-mm strips from anterior to posterior and lateral to medial. E, Completed acromioplasty. The undersurface of the acromion is converted to a type I morphology. Any residual ridges or rough edges can be safely smoothed with the burr in the reverse cutting position. F, View of the acromioplasty from the lateral portal. At the procedure's completion, the arthroscope should be placed in the lateral portal to assess the acromion for any residual downslope or unresected bone. The AC joint is also well visualized from this portal and may be resected or coplaned via the anterior portal. G, Coplaning of the AC joint. The posterior or lateral portal is used for arthroscopic visualization. Coplaning is performed with the burr in the anterior or lateral portal. (Borrowed from Miller MD, Wiesel SW. *Operative Techniques in Sports Medicine Surgery*. Wolters Kluwer Health; 2016.)

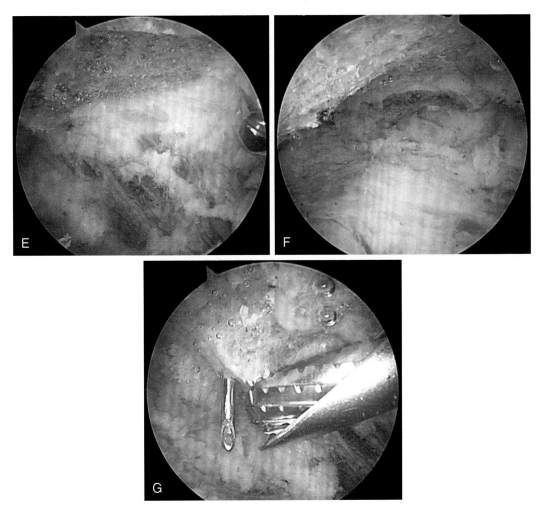

Figure 2B.8. Cont'd

REFERENCES

1. Bigliani LU, Levine WN. Subacromial impingement syndrome. *J Bone Joint Surg Am*. 1997; 79(12):1854-1868.
2. Neer II CS. Impingement lesions. *Clin Orthop Relat Res*. 1983;173:70-77.
3. Neer II CS. Anterior acromioplasty for the chronic impingement syndrome in the shoulder: a preliminary report. *J Bone Joint Surg Am*. 1972;54(1):41-50.
4. Bigliani BU, Morrison ES, April EW. The morphology of the acromion and its relationship to rotator cuff tears. *Orthop Trans*. 1986;10:216.
5. Gerber C, Galantay RV, Hersche O. The pattern of pain produced by irritation of the acromioclavicular joint and the subacromial space. *J Shoulder Elbow Surg*. 1998;7(4):352-355.
6. Hawkins RL, Hobeika P. Physical examination of the shoulder. *Orthopedics*. 1983;6(10):1270-1278.
7. Hawkins RJ, Kennedy JC. Impingement syndrome in athletes. *Am J Sports Med*. 1980;8(3):151-158.
8. MacDonald PB, Clark P, Sutherland K. An analysis of the diagnostic accuracy of the Hawkins and Neer subacromial impingement signs. *J Shoulder Elbow Surg*. 2000;9(4):299-301.

SECTION C
Rotator Cuff Injuries

Michelle E. Kew

HISTORY

- Patients present with insidious onset of pain worsened with overhead activity[1]
- Symptoms can include night pain, weakness, pain in deltoid region, changes in range of motion of affected extremity
- Etiology of the patient's symptoms can vary with age of presentation
  - Patients <40 years old may present with high-energy injury or dislocation
  - Patients 50 to 60 years old may present with history of trauma
  - Patients >60 years old usually present without history of trauma
- Should discuss current activity level and treatment expectations with each patient

PHYSICAL EXAMINATION[5]

- Important to assess for tenderness throughout the shoulder, including the following:
  - Greater tuberosity
  - AC joint
  - Bicipital groove
  - Coracoid process
- Assess passive and active range of motion on affected and unaffected extremity
- Perform thorough neurovascular examination
- May note muscle atrophy with chronic cuff dysfunction
- Massive rotator cuff tear may be detected as a defect in the supraspinatus tendon at the anterolateral shoulder
- Strength testing ▶
  - Supraspinatus[6] (Figure 2C.1)
    - The patient holds the arm in 90° elevation in the plane of the scapula in mild internal rotation
    - The examiner stands in front of the patient and provides resistant force to abduction and elevation in the scapular plane
  - Infraspinatus (Figure 2C.2)
    - The patient holds the arm at the side in neutral rotation with the elbow at 90°
    - The examiner stands in front of the patient and provides resistant force to external rotation
  - Teres minor (Figure 2C.3)
    - The patient holds the arm in 90° abduction with the elbow flexed to 90°
    - The examiner stands in front of the patient and provides resistant force to external rotation

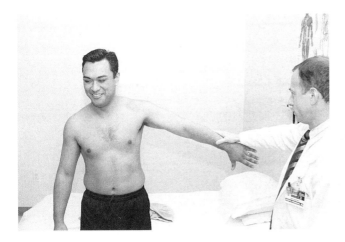

Figure 2C.1. Supraspinatus strength test. (Borrowed from DeLisa JA, Frontera WR, Ovid Technologies Inc. *DeLisa's Physical Medicine & Rehabilitation Principles and Practice*. Philadelphia: Wolters Kluwer Health/Lippincott Williams & Wilkins; 2010.)

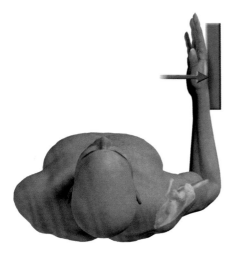

Figure 2C.2. Infraspinatus strength test.

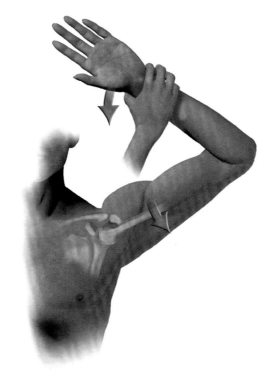

Figure 2C.3. Teres minor strength test.

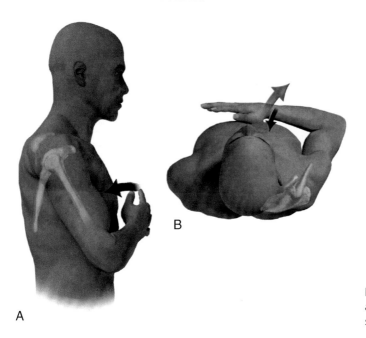

A

B

Figure 2C.4. "Belly-press" test assessing for subscapularis strength.

- Subscapularis (Figure 2C.4)
  - The patient places extremity in internal rotation with the elbow flexed to 90° and hand pressing into the abdomen
  - The examiner stands in front of the patient and provides posteriorly directed force on the patient's flexed elbow
- Important to evaluate for shoulder impingement using the Neer and Hawkins signs (See section B)

KEY EXAMINATION MANEUVERS

- **Jobe Test** ▶
  - Used to evaluate supraspinatus
  - First described by Jobe[11]
  - **Maneuver** (Figure 2C.5):
    - The patient's arm is placed in 90° abduction and neutral rotation
    - The shoulder is then internally rotated and the thumb is pointed to the floor
    - The examiner stands in front of the patient and provides a downward force on the affected extremity
    - Positive if the patient is unable to resist the force

- **Drop-Arm Test**
  - Tests the supraspinatus
  - Described by Codman[12]
  - **Maneuver** (Figure 2C.6):
    - The patient's arm is passively abducted to 180°
    - The patient is asked to slowly lower the arm to the side
    - The examiner stands in front of the patient and evaluates the patient's ability to lower the arm in a controlled fashion
    - Positive if the patient is able to lower the arm to 90° abduction, but unable to lower the arm further and the arm drops to the side
    - Also positive if the patient is unable to maintain the arm abducted to 180° and the arm falls to the side

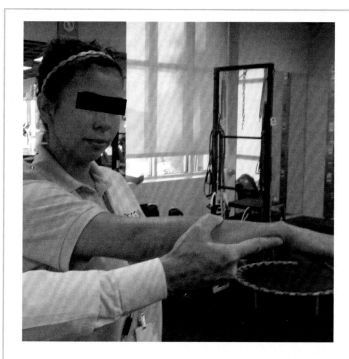

Figure 2C.5. Jobe test.

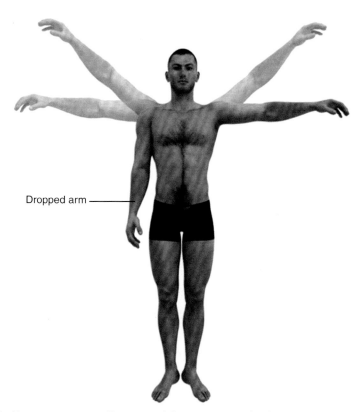

Dropped arm

Figure 2C.6. Drop-arm test. (Borrowed from Hoppenfeld JD. *Fundamentals of Pain Medicine How to Diagnose and Treat Your Patients*. Philadelphia: Wolters Kluwer Health; 2015.)

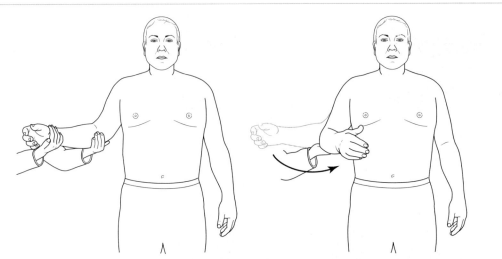

Figure 2C.7. External rotation lag sign. A, Starting point at full external rotation. B, Positive test: if the patient is unable to maintain external rotation. (Borrowed from Brunner UH, Scheibel M. Klinische Untersuchung der Schulter. In: Habermeyer P, Lichtenberg S, Magosch P, eds. *Schulterchirurgie.* Munich: Elsevier; 2010:63-98.)

- **External Rotation Lag Sign or Dropping Sign**
  - Used to evaluate the infraspinatus
  - First described in 1996 by Hertel et al[4]
  - **Maneuver** (Figure 2C.7):
    - The patient's elbow is passively flexed to 90° with the shoulder in 20° elevated and close to maximal external rotation
    - The examiner stands in front of the patient and supports the elbow of the affected extremity
    - Positive if the patient's extremity drops and cannot maintain external rotation
  - **Limitations of Maneuver:**
    - Patients must have full painless passive range of motion
    - False-negative results may occur if range of motion is reduced
    - May be negative in partial-thickness tear

- **Drop-Arm Sign[3]**
  - Used to evaluate the infraspinatus
  - First described in 1996 by Hertel et al[4]
  - **Maneuver** (Figure 2C.8):
    - The examiner stands in front of the patient and holds the affected extremity at 90° of elevation with the elbow flexed to 90° and almost full external rotation
    - The patient is asked to keep this position while the examiner releases the patient's wrist
    - Positive if the patient's arm cannot maintain external rotation and lags forward
  - **Limitations of Maneuver:**
    - Similar to external rotation lag sign
    - The patient must have full passive range of motion to prevent false-negative results

- **Hornblower's Sign[3]**
  - Evaluates teres minor
  - First described in 1972 by Arthuis[13] in obstetric brachial plexus palsy
  - Sensitivity 100%, specificity 93%
  - **Maneuver** (Figure 2C.9):
    - The patient's arm is abducted to 90°
    - The elbow is flexed to 90°

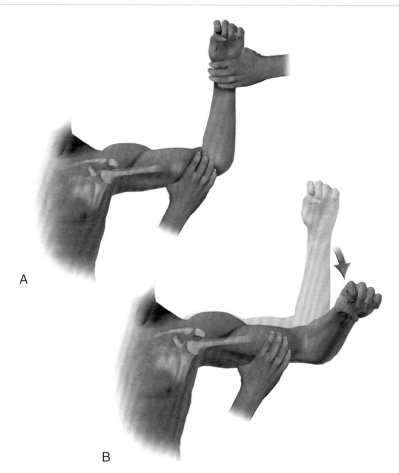

Figure 2C.8. Drop-arm sign. A, Initial maneuver, with extremity at 90° of elevation and maximal external rotation. B, Positive drop-arm sign—the patient cannot maintain external rotation.

- The examiner stands in front of the patient and provides a force against the patient's upper extremity as the shoulder is externally rotated
- The examiner asks places the arm in 90° of abduction and 90° of external rotation
- Positive if the patient cannot hold the arm in external rotation essentially falling into a "hornblower" position

- **Lift-Off Test**
  - Used to test subscapularis
  - Eliminates all internal rotators of the shoulder except for subscapularis
  - First described by Gerber and Krushell[2]
  - Tokish in 2003[9] found that this maneuver significantly activates the lower subscapularis
  - **Maneuver** (Figure 2C.10):
    - The patient placed the affected extremity fully extended and internally rotated behind the back
    - The patient is asked to lift the hand off the back
    - The examiner stands behind the patient and evaluates the position of the patient's hand
    - Positive if unable to maintain hand off the back

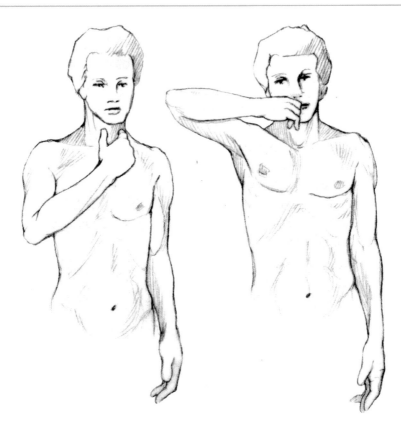

Figure 2C.9. Hornblower's sign. (From Brunner UH, Scheibel M. Klinische Untersuchung der Schulter. In: Habermeyer P, Lichtenberg S, Magosch P, eds. *Schulterchirurgie*. Munich: Elsevier; 2010:63-98.)

- **Belly-Press/Push Test** 🔊
  - Also called the Napoleon test
  - Used to test subscapularis (sensitivity: 0.40, specificity: 0.93)
  - Developed by Gerber and Krushell 1991[2] for use in shoulders that had decreased passive internal rotation
    - Allows its use where the lift-off test reports false-negative results
  - Tokish in 2003[9] found that this maneuver significantly activates the upper subscapularis
  - **Maneuver** (Figure 2C.11):
    - The patient is asked to press the abdomen with a flat hand
    - The extremity is maintained in maximum internal rotation
    - The examiner stands in front of the patient and evaluates the position of the patient's affected extremity
    - Positive if the patient is unable to maintain internal rotation and the elbow drops backward

- **Internal Rotation Lag Sign** Also Called the **Modified Lift-off Test** or **Subscapularis Lag Sign**
  - Used to evaluate the subscapularis
  - First described in 1996 by Hertel et al[4]
  - **Maneuver** (Figure 2C.12):
    - The examiner stands in front of the patient and holds the patient's affected extremity in close to full internal rotation with the elbow flexed to 90° and the shoulder in 20° elevation

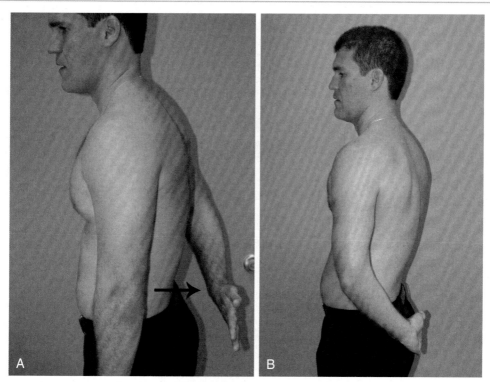

Figure 2C.10. Lift-off test. (Borrowed from Burkhart SS, Brady PC, Lo IKY. Ovid Technologies I. *Burkhart's View of the Shoulder: A Cowboy's Guide to Advanced Shoulder Arthroscopy*. 2006.)

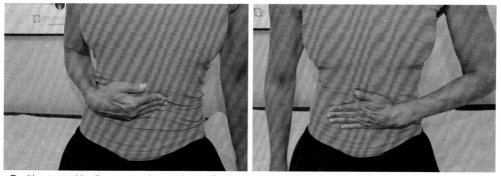

Positive test with elbow extension and wrist flexion   Normal comparison

Figure 2C.11. Right side, positive belly-press test; left side, negative belly-press test. (Borrowed from Snyder SJ, Bakh M, Burns J, eds. *SCOI Shoulder Arthroscopy*. 3rd ed. Wolters Kluwer Health; 2015.)

- The patient's hand is lifted off the back
- The patient is asked to maintain this position
- Positive if the patient is unable to maintain internal rotation

- **Bear-Hug Test** ▶
  - Used to evaluate the subscapularis, specifically the upper part
  - First described by Barth et al in 2006[10]

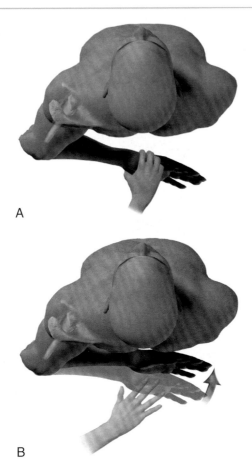

A

B

Figure 2C.12. Internal rotation lag sign. A, Initial maneuver with the arm in full internal rotation, the elbow flexed to 90°. B, Positive internal rotation lag sign—the patient is unable to maintain internal rotation.

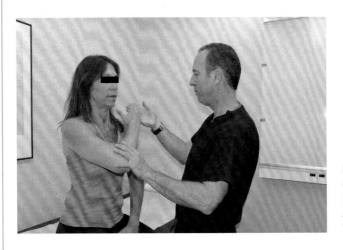

Figure 2C.13. Bear-hug test. (Borrowed from Snyder SJ, Bakh M, Burns J, eds. *SCOI Shoulder Arthroscopy*. 3rd ed. Wolters Kluwer Health; 2015.)

- **Maneuver** (Figure 2C.13):
  - The patient starts by placing the palm of the affected shoulder on the opposite shoulder with fingers extended and the elbow positioned anterior to the body
  - The examiner faces the patient and attempts to lift the affected arm off the shoulder with an external rotation force applied perpendicular to the forearm
  - Positive if the patient cannot hold the hand against the shoulder

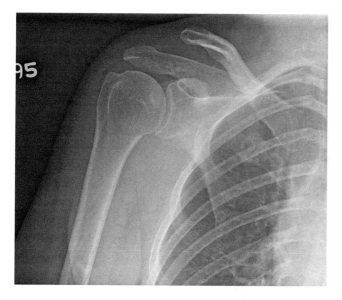

Figure 2C.14. AP radiograph of the right shoulder.

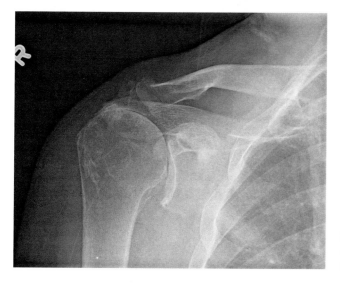

Figure 2C.15. Superior migration of the humeral head due to rotator cuff arthropathy.

IMAGING[7,8]

Plain Radiographs

- Obtain shoulder radiographs, including AP, axillary views, scapular Y view
- Evaluate AP view for acromiohumeral interval (Figure 2C.14)
  - Normal: 7 to 14 mm
- Evaluate axillary view for evidence of dislocation, joint space pathology
- Evaluate scapular Y view for acromial morphology
- May show changes within acromion or coracoacromial ligament
- Chronic, massive rotator cuff tear will manifest as superior migration of humeral head (Figure 2C.15)

Ultrasonography

- Used to evaluate for rotator cuff disease
- Provides dynamic assessment of rotator cuff

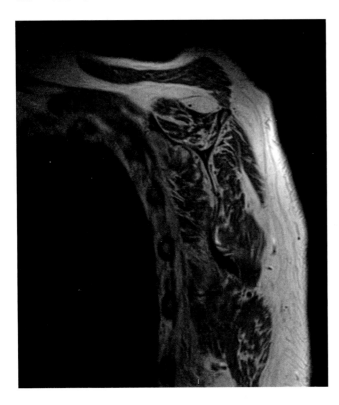

Figure 2C.16. Fatty atrophy of supraspinatus, infraspinatus, and subscapularis.

- Can be used as an adjunct for subacromial or intra-articular injections to confirm correct placement
- Dependent on the operator's skill and image interpretation

Magnetic Resonance Imaging

- Gold standard to evaluate rotator cuff disease, especially full-thickness tears
- Rotator cuff best viewed in T2-weighted images
- Used to define the tear, including degree of tear retraction and presence of muscular atrophy
- Important to evaluate for fatty atrophy of the affected muscle (Figure 2C.16)
  - Best seen on T1-weighted images
- Allows evaluation of other structures, including the labrum, capsule, and cartilage
- Magnetic resonance arthrography
  - Can be used as an adjunct to diagnose partial-thickness rotator cuff tears

Classic Arthroscopic Images

- Arthroscopic view demonstrating a full-thickness rotator cuff tear being prepared for repair (Figure 2C.17)
- Arthroscopic views demonstrating prepared rotator cuff and associated repair using a double-row repair (Figure 2C.18)

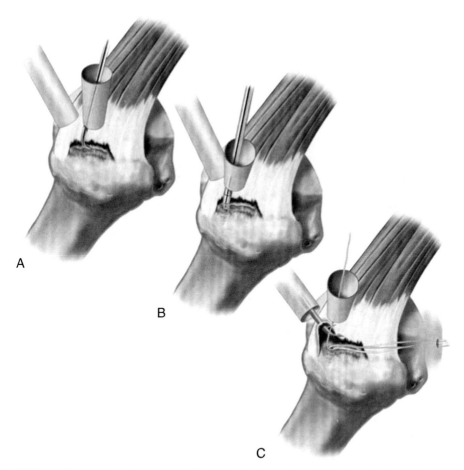

Figure 2C.17. Arthroscopic rotator cuff repair. A, Debridement of rotator cuff footprint. B, Screw-in anchors are placed at footprint. C-F, Bridging horizontal mattress sutures are shuttled through the rotator cuff tendon medially. G, Arthroscopic knots are used to bring rotator cuff tissue to footprint. H, Double-row repair is created using 2 lateral anchors. (Borrowed from Miller MD, ed. *Sports Medicine Conditions: Return to Play: Recognition, Treatment, Planning.* Philadelphia, PA: Lippincott Williams & Wilkins; 2014.)

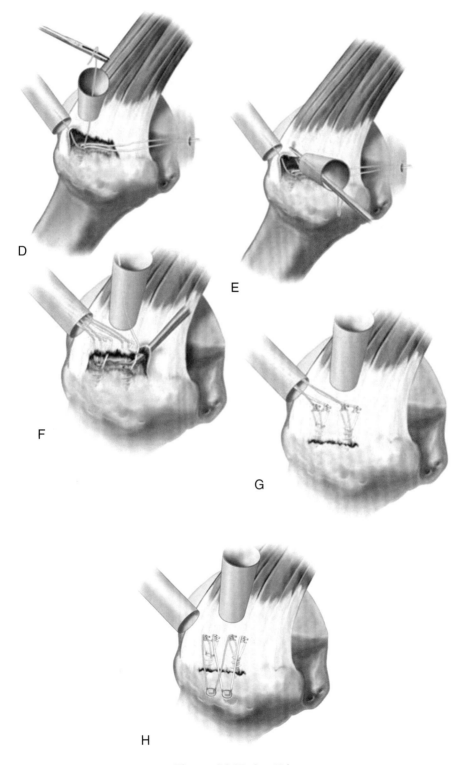

Figure 2C.17. Cont'd

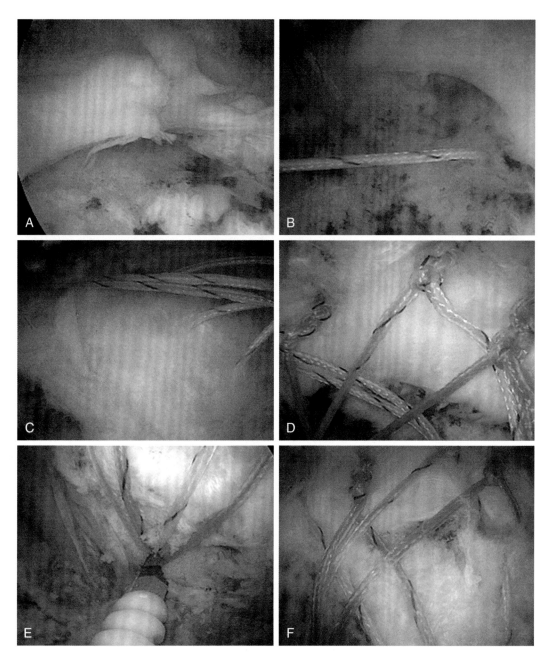

Figure 2C.18. Arthroscopic views. A, Rotator cuff tear viewed from lateral portal. B, Debrided greater tuberosity and 2 medial row anchors are inserted. C, Sutures passed through rotator cuff in horizontal mattress configuration. All sutures are exiting through the anterior cannula. D, Tied medial row sutures and planned suture configuration for lateral row anchor insertion. E, Lateral row anchor insertion with tensioning of the rotator cuff. F, Final double-row repair construct viewed from a lateral portal. (Borrowed from Miller MD, Wiesel SW. *Operative Techniques in Sports Medicine Surgery*. Wolters Kluwer Health; 2016.)

REFERENCES

1. Eiji I. Rotator cuff tear: physical examination and conservative treatment. *J Orthop Sci.* 2013;18(2):197-204.
2. Gerber C, Krushell RJ. Isolated rupture of the tendon of the subscapularis muscle. Clinical features in 16 cases. *J Bone Joint Surg.* 1991;73B(3):389-394.
3. Walch G, Boulahia A, Calderone S, Robinson A. The 'dropping' and 'hornblower's' signs in evaluation of rotator-cuff tears. *J Bone Joint Surg.* 1998;80B(4):624-628.

4. Hertel R, Ballmer FT, Lambert M, Gerber C. Lag signs in the diagnosis of rotator cuff rupture. *J Shoulder Elbow Surg.* 1996;5(4):307-313.

5. Jain NB, Wilcox R, Katz JN, Higgins LD. Clinical examination of the rotator cuff. *PM R.* 2013;5(1):45-56.

6. Lyons RP, Green A. Subscapularis tendon tears. *J Am Acad Orthop Surg.* 2005;13(5):353-363.

7. McConville OR, Iannotti JP. Partial-thickness tears of the rotator cuff: evaluation and management. *J Am Acad Orthop Surg.* 1999;7(1):32-43.

8. Green A. Chronic massive rotator cuff tears: evaluation and management. *J Am Acad Orthop Surg.* 2003;11(5):321-331.

9. Tokish JM, Decker MJ, Ellis HB, et al. The belly-press test for the physical examination of the subscapularis muscle: electromyographic validation and comparison to the lift-off test. *J Shoulder Elbow Surg.* 2003;12(5):427-430.

10. Barth JRH, Burkhart SS, De Beer JF. The bear-hug test: a new and sensitive test for diagnosing a subscapularis tear. *Arthroscopy.* 2006;22(10):1076-1084.

11. Jobe FW, Moynes DR. Delineation of diagnostic criteria and a rehabilitation program for rotator cuff injuries. *Am J Sports Med.* 1982;10:336-339.

12. Codman EA. *The Shoulder: rupture of the supraspinatus tendon and other lesions in or about the subacromial bursa.* Boston, T. Todd Company; 1934.

13. Arthuis M. Obstetrical paralysis of the brachial plexus. I. Diagnosis. Clinical study of the initial period. *Rev Chir Orthop Reparatrice Appar Mot.* 1972;58:124-136.

SECTION D
Anterior, Posterior, and Multidirectional Instability

Aaron J. Casp

HISTORY[1]

- Can either be posttraumatic, generally causing unidirectional instability, or atraumatic multidirectional instability (MDI)
- History of trauma or dislocation is important
- Which arm position aggravates the sense of instability?
  - This can differentiate anterior-posterior instability with MDI
- More common in athletic individuals, especially in sports more associated with dislocations
- Excessive glenohumeral translation can lead to pain or frank glenohumeral dislocation
- Generally a long-standing issue causing discomfort and limits activities
- Feeling of instability of the shoulder, especially with load-bearing or overhead activities
- Age at initial dislocation is an important prognostic indicator for recurrent instability
- Frequency of instability events
- Which sports does the patient play, and what is the patient's occupation?
- Question about any psychopathology for chronic voluntary dislocators

PHYSICAL EXAMINATION

- **Neer and Foster first described diagnosing MDI based on the following:**
  - Positive sulcus sign for inferior instability
  - For at least 1 direction (anterior and/or posterior), a positive result for at least 2 of the following:
    - Anterior and posterior draw tests (10°-30° abduction)
    - Anterior and posterior draw tests in (80°-120° abduction)
    - Anterior and posterior apprehension test

KEY EXAMINATION MANEUVERS

- **Assessment of General Laxity—Beighton Criteria** (Figure 2D.1)
  - First described in the literature in 1964 by Carter and Wilkinson[7], it was modified in 1973 by Beighton et al[8]
  - **Maneuver**:
    - Components of Beighton scale
      - Passive dorsiflexion of fifth MCP joint beyond 90°
      - Passive apposition thumb to flexor aspect of forearm
      - Passive hyperextension of elbow beyond 10°

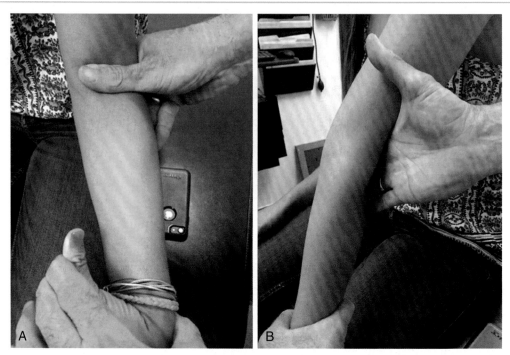

Figure 2D.1. Examples of hyperlaxity: thumb to forearm (A) and elbow hyperextension (B).

- Passive hyperextension of the knee beyond 10°
- Active forward flexion of the trunk with knees extended so that palms rest flat on the floor
- **Limitations of Maneuver:**
  - Many patients may have general ligamentous joint laxity without pathologic shoulder motion
  - May be difficult to assess if the patient is resisting you or has a painful shoulder or limb that limits assessment

- **Anterior and Posterior Draw**
  - First described by Gerber and Ganz[9]
  - **Maneuver:**
    - **Anterior Draw:**
      - The patient lies supine on the examination table
      - The examiner holds the patient's arm in varying amounts of abduction, 0° to 20° of forward flexion and 0° to 30° of external rotation
      - The examiner places the hand of the affected extremity in the examiner's axilla
      - One of the examiner's hand is on the humeral shaft to provide an anterior or posteriorly directed force, and the other is used to stabilize the scapula (the thumb along the coracoid anteriorly, fingers on the scapular spine)
      - **Limitations**: difficulty controlling rotation of the scapula
    - **Posterior Draw**:
      - The patient lies supine, with subtle differences to anterior draw test
      - The examiner holds the patient's proximal forearm and the elbow is flexed to 120° with the shoulder in 80° to 120° of abduction and 20° to 30° of forward flexion
      - Scapular spine held with the examiner's opposite index and long finger, with the thumb placed just lateral to the coracoid

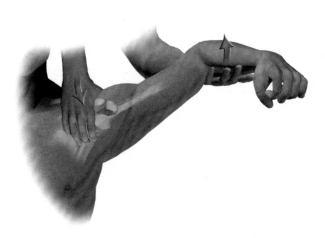

Figure 2D.2. Positive Gagey hyperabduction test.

- The shoulder is then flexed 60° to 80° with slight internal rotation, and the examiner's thumb exerts a posterior pressure to translate the humeral head posteriorly
- The fingers along the scapular spine can palpate the head, as it translates posteriorly

- **Gagey Hyperabduction Test** (Sensitivity 0.85) (Figure 2D.2)
  - First described by Gagey and Gagey
  - **Maneuver**:
    - The patient is generally seated
    - The examiner stands behind the patient on the affected side
    - The examiner places one hand or forearm on the superior shoulder of the patient to stabilize the scapula
    - The examiner uses the other hand to passively abduct the shoulder, while preventing scapular movement by applying a downward force to the arm on the superior shoulder
    - The examiner evaluates the maximum amount of glenohumeral abduction
    - More than 105° of abduction before initiation of scapulothoracic movement is associated with inferior laxity

- **Apprehension Test and Relocation Test (Jobe Relocation Test)** 🎥 (Sensitivity 0.44, Specificity 0.87) (Figure 2D.3)
  - First described by Jobe et al[11]
  - No significant modifications
  - **Maneuver**:
    - The patient lies supine at edge of the examination table with the affected shoulder close to the edge
    - The patient's shoulder is abducted at 90° and externally rotated to 90°
    - The examiner places a hand on the posterior aspect of the shoulder and applies an anteriorly directed force
    - The patient's subjective sensation of apprehension of dislocation indicates anterior instability
    - Relocation test (Jobe relocation test)—apprehension test is performed
    - The examiner places the hand on the anterior shoulder and applies a posteriorly directed force
    - Relief of apprehension with this posteriorly directed force again indicates anterior instability
  - **Limitations of Maneuver**
    - May be limited by patient guarding
    - Relies on the patient reporting subjective sensation of apprehension
    - Only moderate sensitivity

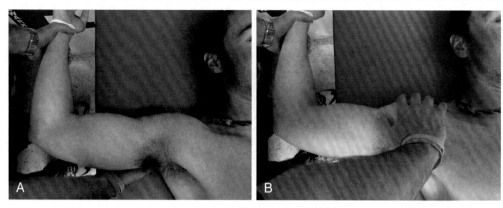

Figure 2D.3. Apprehension and Jobe relocation test. A, The arm is placed in the apprehension position and an anteriorly directed force is applied. B, The examiner's arm then applies a posteriorly directed force on the humeral head. If pain is elicited when this posteriorly directed force is released, the test is positive. (From Iannotti JP, Williams GR, Miniaci A, Zuckerman JD. *Disorders of the Shoulder: Diagnosis & Management.* Wolters Kluwer; 2014.)

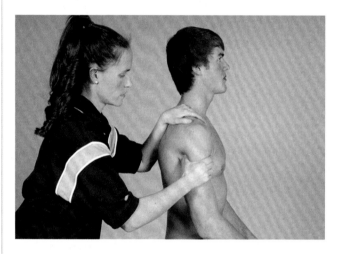

Figure 2D.4. Load and shift test. (From Anderson MK, Barnum M. *Foundations of Athletic Training: Prevention, Assessment, and Management.* Wolters Kluwer Health; 2017.)

- **Load and Shift Test and Modified Load and Shift Test** (Sensitivity 0.5 anterior, 0.14 posterior, Specificity 1.00, LR > 80) (Figure 2D.4)
  - First described by Hawkins, Schutte et al[12]
  - **Maneuver:**
    - The patient is seated with the arm adducted in a dependent position
    - The examiner stands behind the patient, with the corresponding hand on the humerus and the contralateral hand wrapping over the superior shoulder with the thumb on the posterior shoulder and fingers on the anterior shoulder
    - The examiner applies pressure with the hand that is on the humerus to "load" the glenohumeral joint
    - The examiner then stabilizes the shoulder with the opposite hand and shifts the humeral head anterior and posterior
    - Excessive translation of >25% anteriorly or >50% posteriorly suggests instability
  - **Alternative Maneuver** (Figure 2D.4):
    - The patient lies supine on the edge of the examination table with the center of the scapula on the edge of the table
    - The patient's shoulder is abducted to 90° and the elbow bent

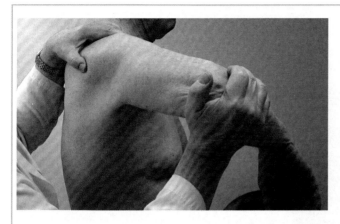

Figure 2D.5. Jerk test evaluating for torn posterior labrum. (From Williams GR, Ramsey ML, Wiesel BB, Wiesel SW. *Operative Techniques in Shoulder and Elbow Surgery*. Wolters Kluwer Health; 2016.)

- The examiner is seated next to the patient controlling the patient's humerus with both hands (the ipsilateral hand on the distal humerus or elbow and the other hand near the shoulder)
- The examiner applies a load to the glenohumeral joint through the elbow or distal hand and then shifts the humeral head anterior to posterior with the hand that is above the humeral head
- The shift is often graded with the modified Hawkins grading on a scale of 0 to 3:
  - Grade 0: Little or no movement of the humeral head
  - Grade 1: The humeral head can be shifted, so it begins to ride up anteriorly on the glenoid labrum
  - Grade 2: The humeral head can be shifted off the glenoid but spontaneously relocates
  - Grade 3: The humeral head can be shifted off the glenoid and remains dislocated once the manual pressure is released
- **Limitations of Maneuver**:
  - Depend on the examiner's subjective translation distance
  - Uncomfortable for the patient
  - May be limited by patient guarding

- **Jerk Test**—evaluation for torn posterior labrum (Sensitivity 0.73, Specificity 0.98) (Figure 2D.5)
  - Described by Jahnke[13]
  - **Maneuver**:
    - The patient is seated with the examiner standing behind the patient (may also be performed with the patient in a supine position)
    - One of the examiner's hands stabilizes the shoulder and scapula
    - The patient's arm is forward flexed 90° with the elbow bent, internally rotated, and an axial load along the humerus is applied by the examiner
    - As the arm is adducted while this axial load is applied, there may be palpable laxity of the humeral head or a click
    - Palpable laxity or click are considered positive results

- **Sulcus Sign (Figure 2D.6)**
  - First described by Neer and Foster[14]
  - **Maneuver**:
    - The patient is seated with the examiner standing on the affected side
    - The patient's arm rests in an adducted position along the side
    - The examiner applies an inferior force downward from above the elbow
    - Increased acromiohumeral distance demonstrates inferior laxity or instability, with a positive result being a visible sulcus in the acromiohumeral interval

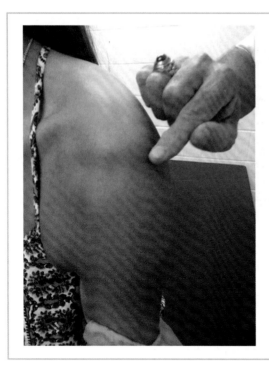

Figure 2D.6. Sulcus sign of inferior laxity.

IMAGING

Plain Radiographs

- AP, internal/external rotation, true AP (Grashey), and axillary view (**Figure 2D.7**)
  - Inspect for abnormal calcifications or Hill-Sachs lesions (external rotation and axillary views)
  - Glenoid bone loss visible on West Point view or Bernageau view
  - Hill-Sachs easily identified on Stryker notch view

Computed Tomography

- Determination of the bony anatomy and pathology
  - Indications include the following:
    - Multiple dislocations
    - Increasing ease of dislocations/relocation
    - Apprehension with the arm at less than 75° of abduction
    - Radiographic evidence of bone loss
  - 3D CT can quantitatively evaluate bone loss as the glenoid can be viewed *en face*
    - AP distance from the bare area method or perfect circle method (Figure 2D.8):
      - Estimate the bare area by first drawing a vertical line from supraglenoid tubercle and then a horizontal line at the widest AP distance
      - The intersection is the approximated bare area
      - Then draw the "best fit circle" centered at the bare area
        - Distance from the bare area to posterior glenoid rim and remaining anterior glenoid rim is measured
      - Percentage bone loss = [(posterior distance) − (anterior distance)]/(2× posterior distance)
        - In general, with more than 30% of percentage bone loss, one may have to treat with something more than standard arthroscopic stabilization[4]

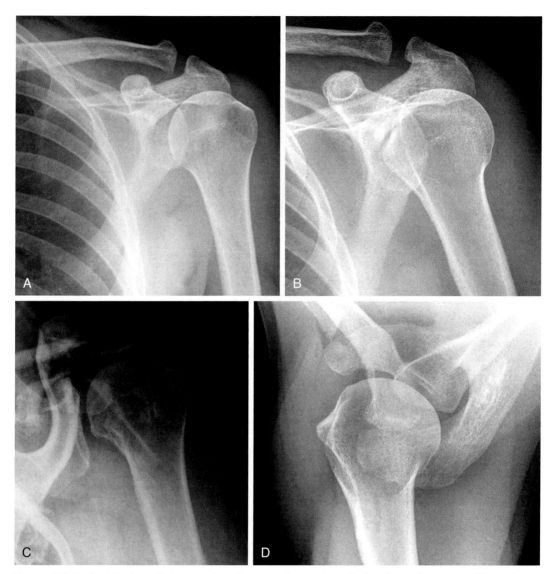

Figure 2D.7. A, AP view. B, Internal and external rotation. C, Grashey view. D, Axillary view.

Magnetic Resonance Imaging

- **MR arthrogram**: generally reserved for associated rotator cuff pathology, or if shoulder instability is in question
  - Intra-articular gadolinium increases the sensitivity to the mid 90% range for soft tissue pathologies
  - Having arm in abducted externally rotated position tensions IGHL, accentuating pathology
- **MRI** can detect HAGL
  - Important to identify preoperatively to determine if pathology can be treated open versus arthroscopically
- **CT arthrography**:
  - Recently found to be equivalent to MR arthrography at identifying HAGL lesions
  - Does not clearly identify soft tissue pathology and contributions to instability compared with MRI
- **Figure 2D.9** demonstrates an MRI cut of bony Bankart lesion
- **Figure 2D.10** demonstrates MRI examples of HAGL lesion

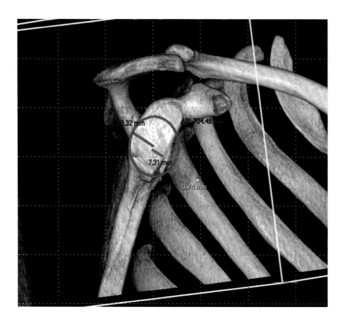

Figure 2D.8. Perfect circle method showing anterior glenoid bone loss.

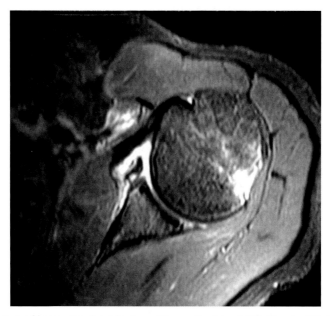

Figure 2D.9. MRI cut of bony Bankart lesion. (From Burkhart SS, Brady PC, Denard PJ, Adams CR, Hartzler RU. *The Cowboy's Conundrum: Complex and Advanced Cases in Shoulder Arthroscopy*. Wolters Kluwer Health; 2017.)

Classic Arthroscopic Findings

- **Figure 2D.11** demonstrates a diagram of anatomic variants that may be mistaken for labral tears. It is important to remember that a labral separation from 1 to 3 o'clock is not pathologic
- Glenoid labrum tears leading to shoulder instability are demonstrated in **Figure 2D.12A and 2D.12B**
- Bony Bankart: **Figure 2D.13** demonstrates an arthroscopic finding of a bony Bankart lesion on the anterior glenoid
- HAGL lesion: **Figure 2D.14** demonstrates arthroscopic views of an HAGL lesion

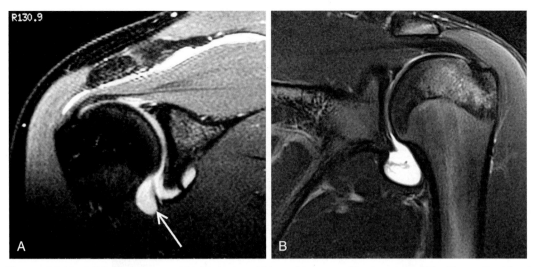

Figure 2D.10. MRI showing an HAGL lesion (A) and large axillary recess (B). (From Burkhart SS, Brady PC, Denard PJ, Adams CR, Hartzler RU. *The Cowboy's Conundrum: Complex and Advanced Cases in Shoulder Arthroscopy*. Wolters Kluwer Health; 2017.)

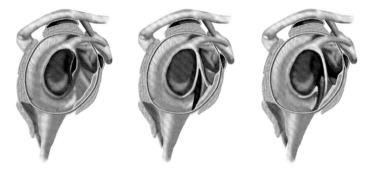

Figure 2D.11. Anatomic variants that may be encountered during arthroscopy. It is important to note that these are not pathologic and are not contributing to instability.

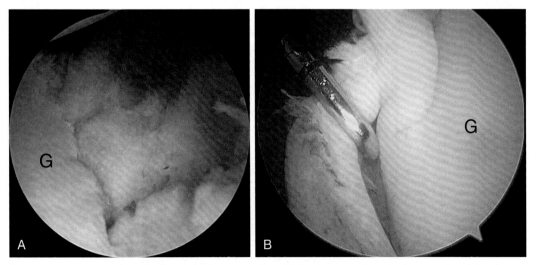

Figure 2D.12. A and B, Arthroscopic examples of large anterior and posterior labral tears leading to instability. G, glenoid. (From Burkhart SS, Brady PC, Denard PJ, Adams CR, Hartzler RU. *The Cowboy's Conundrum: Complex and Advanced Cases in Shoulder Arthroscopy*. Wolters Kluwer Health; 2017.)

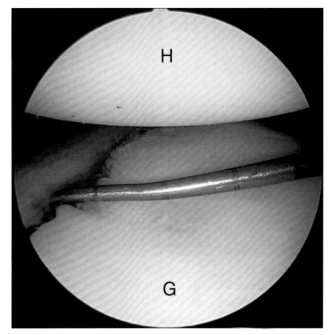

Figure 2D.13. Arthroscopic findings of bony Bankart lesion. G, glenoid; H, humerus. (From Burkhart SS, Brady PC, Denard PJ, Adams CR, Hartzler RU. *The Cowboy's Conundrum*: *Complex and Advanced Cases in Shoulder Arthroscopy*. Wolters Kluwer Health; 2017.)

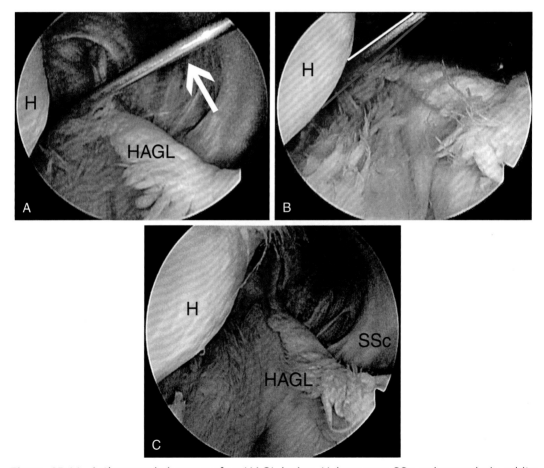

Figure 2D.14. Arthroscopic images of an HAGL lesion. H, humerus; SSc, subscapularis, white arrow showing expanded patulous capsule. (From Burkhart SS, Brady PC, Denard PJ, Adams CR, Hartzler RU. *The Cowboy's Conundrum*: *Complex and Advanced Cases in Shoulder Arthroscopy*. Wolters Kluwer Health; 2017.)

REFERENCES

1. Bahk M, Keyurapan E, Tasaki A, Sauers E, McFarland E. Laxity testing of the shoulder: a review. *Am J Sports Med*. 2007;35(1):131-144.
2. Spang J, Mazzocca A, Arciero R. The unstable shoulder. AAOS comprehensive orthopaedic review. In: Boyer M, ed. *American Academy of Orthopaedic Surgeons*. Vol 2, 2014.
3. Warren R, Craig E, Altchek D. *The Unstable Shoulder*. Philadelphia: Lipincott-Raven; 1998.
4. Provencher MT, Bhatia S, Ghodadra NS, et al. Recurrent shoulder instability: current concepts for evaluation and management of glenoid bone loss. *J Bone Joint Surg Am*. 2010;92(suppl 2):133.
5. Thompson SR, Al-Saatie M, Litchfield RB. Anterior shoulder instability. In: Miller MD, Thompson SR, eds. *DeLee and Drez's Orthopaedic Sports Medicine*: *Principles and Practice*. Philadelphia: Elsevier/ Saunders; 2015
6. Warby SA, Watson L, Ford J, Piari T. Multidirectional instability of the glenohumeral joint: etiology, classification, assessment, and management. *J Hand Therapy*. 2017;30(2):175-181.
7. Carter C, Wilkinson J. Persistent joint laxity and congenital dislocation of the hip. *J Bone Joint Surg Br*. 1964;46-B:40-45.
8. Beighton P, Solomon L, Soskolne CL. Articular mobility in an African population. *Ann Rheum Dis*. 1973;32:413-418.
9. Gerber C, Ganz R. Clinical assessment of instability of the shoulder. With special reference to anterior and posterior drawer tests. *J Bone Joint Surg Br*. 1984;66(4):551-556.
10. Gagey OJ, Gagey N. The hyperabduction test. *J Bone Joint Surg Br*. 2001;83(1):69-74.
11. Jobe FW, Kvitne RS, Giangarra CE. Shoulder pain in the overhand or throwing athlete. The relationship of anterior instability and rotator cuff impingement. *Orthop Rev*. 1989;18(9):963-975.
12. Hawkins RJ, McCormack RG. Posterior shoulder instability. *Orthopedics*. 1988;11(1):101-107.
13. Jahnke AH Jr, Greis PE, Hawkins RJ. *Orthop Clin North Am*. 1995;26(4):613-630.
14. Neer CS 2nd, Foster CR. Inferior capsular shift for involuntary inferior and multidirectional instability of the shoulder. A preliminary report. *J Bone Joint Surg Am*. 1980;62(6):897-908.
15. O'Brien SJ, Newman AM, Taylor SA. The accurate diagnosis of biceps-labral complex lesions with MRI and "3-pack" physical examination: A retrospective analysis with prospective validation. *Orthop J Sports Med*. 2013;1(4 suppl).
16. Liu SH, Henry MH, Nuccion SL. A prospective evaluation of a new physical examination in predicting glenoid labral tears. *Am J Sports Med*. 1996;24(6):721-725.
17. Gilecreest EL, Albi P. Unusual lesions of muscles and tendons of the shoulder girdle and upper arm. *Surg Gynecol Obstet*. 1939;68:903-917.
18. Yergason RM. Supination sign. *J Bone Joint Surg Br*. 1931;13:160.

SECTION E
Proximal Biceps and Labral Pathology

Aaron J. Casp

HISTORY

- Primarily anterior shoulder pain
- Pain with shoulder flexion or cross-body movements
- Common injuries in throwing athletes or repetitive overhead activity
  - When evaluating the throwing athlete or thrower's shoulder, there are several important pieces to keep in mind:
    - Where in the throwing motion do they have pain?
    - Is there associated weakness or tightness?
- Pain generators from several areas in the shoulder can present similarly
- LHB lesions in older patients often have concomitant pathology, such as rotator cuff tears
- Any acute tearing event for complete LHB ruptures

PHYSICAL EXAMINATION

Observation

- Evaluate range of motion
  - Especially in the throwing athlete, it is important to evaluate for a glenohumeral internal rotation deficit (GIRD)
    - Evaluate the internal and external rotation with the shoulder abducted to 90°, and compare with the contralateral side
  - Evaluate capsular tightness, especially posteriorly in the throwing or overhead athlete
- In LHB symmetry, evaluate for Popeye deformity

Palpation

- Tenderness along bicipital groove anteriorly and with palpation of LHB tendon
  - 10° of internal rotation with the arm adducted and elbow flexed
- Assess strength of all rotator cuff musculature, with special attention to subscapularis muscle, as subscapularis lesions are closely correlated with biceps tendon injuries and LHB tendon instability
- In the throwing shoulder, posterosuperior rotator cuff tears may be present due to internal impingement
  - The undersurface of the superior rotator cuff becomes impinged between the greater tuberosity and the glenoid rim, especially in maximal abduction/external rotation of the shoulder (late-cocking, early acceleration phase of throwing)
  - This can cause the "peel back" phenomenon of the posterosuperior labrum from a combination of overtightening of the posterior band of the IGHL and anterior microinstability
- Evaluate for GIRD in the throwing athlete by comparing internal and external rotation of the dominant and nondominant sides with the shoulder abducted to 90°
- Evaluate posterior capsular tightness by passive ROM testing

- **O'Brien Test or Active Compression Test**[10] 🎬 (Sensitivity 1.00, specificity 0.985 in the original paper; Sensitivity 0.63, specificity 0.73 in a subsequent study) (Figure 2E.1)
  - First described by O'Brien et al[9], initially called the active compression test
  - **Maneuver**:
    - The examiner stands on the opposite side of the affected shoulder
    - The patient is seated or standing with the shoulder forward flexed 90° with the elbow extended
    - The patient's shoulder is adducted 10° and maximally internally rotated (maximal forearm pronation)
    - The patient is then asked to resist a downward force applied to the arm by the examiner
    - Pain or clicking deep in the shoulder indicates a positive test
    - The patient is then asked to externally rotate (supinate) the arm in the same shoulder position and again resist the downward force applied by the examiner
    - If pain lessens with supination/external rotation, this is again suggestive of superior labral tear or pathology
    - If pain is present during the maneuver at the AC joint, this is likely due to AC pathology and not necessarily labral pathology
  - **Limitations of Maneuver**:
    - Diagnostic utility is not as accurate as possibly first described, as repeat studies have shown much lower sensitivity and specificity
    - May not fully isolate SLAP tears alone with other pain generators in the shoulder as in AC pathology
    - Somewhat dependent on subjective reports of pain with examination maneuver

- **Resisted Thrower's Test**[11] (Sensitivity 0.72-0.75, Specificity 0.67-0.78)
  - Most recently described by O'Brien[15]
  - **Maneuver:**
    - The patient's shoulder is abducted to 90°, elbow flexed to 90°, maximum external rotation
    - The patient steps forward with the contralateral leg, as if to perform a throwing motion, and moves into early acceleration of the arm
    - The examiner stops the throwing motion and provides an isometric resistance force with the hand on the patient's distal forearm

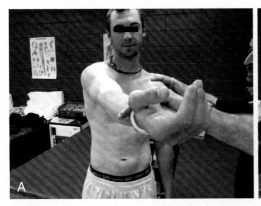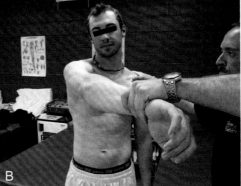

Figure 2E.1. O'Brien test or active compression test. Shoulder is (A) forward flexed to 90° and (B) then internally rotated and tested against resistance. Pain that is relieved when the same test is conducted with the shoulder in external rotation denotes a positive test. (Borrowed from Iannotti JP, Williams GR, Miniaci A, Zuckerman JD. *Disorders of the Shoulder: Diagnosis & Management*. Wolters Kluwer; 2014.)

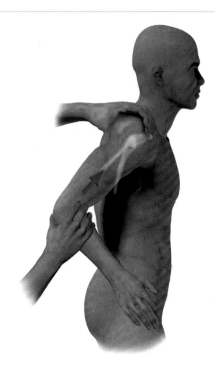

Figure 2E.2. Anterior slide test.

- **Anterior Slide Test** (Sensitivity 0.8-0.78, Specificity 0.85-0.91) (Figure 2E.2)
  - First described by Kibler[4]
  - **Maneuver**:
    - The patient is sitting or standing with the examiner standing behind the patient on the affected side
    - The patient places the hand on the ipsilateral hip/waist area, with the thumb pointing posterior (arm akimbo)
    - The examiner uses one hand to stabilize the scapula/clavicle with a hand on the superior shoulder, which enables him/her to palpate the humeral head
    - The examiner's other hand is placed on the patient's elbow, cupping the olecranon
    - The examiner exerts an anterosuperior force directed through the humerus into the glenohumeral joint
    - If the labrum is torn with a SLAP lesion, the humeral head will slide up over the labrum with a painful click or pop. Sometimes the examiner can palpate a click with the hand on the superior shoulder
  - **Limitations to Maneuver:**
    - Relies on the patient to relax and not guard
    - Wide-ranging sensitivity

- **Biceps Load Test and Biceps Load Test II** (Sensitivity 0.89-0.91, Specificity 0.97) (Figure 2E.3)
  - First described by Kim et al[6]
  - Modified by Kim et al[7] to include the biceps load test II
  - **Maneuver**:
    - The patient is positioned supine on the examination table
    - The examiner sits adjacent to the patient on the affected side and grasps the arm at the wrist and at the elbow
    - The patient's arm is abducted to 90°, externally rotated to the point of apprehension (or maximally externally rotated) with the forearm supinated
      - Note that, in biceps load test II, the patient places the arm at 120° of abduction, which is thought to more adequately isolate a SLAP tear

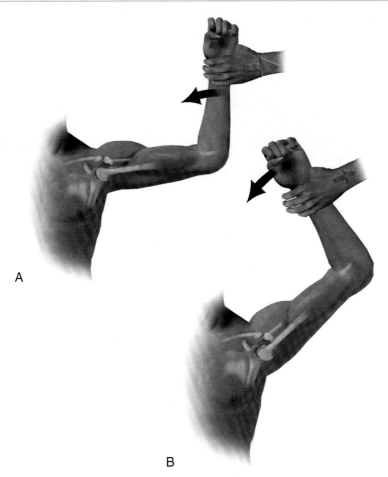

Figure 2E.3. Biceps load test (A) and biceps load test II (B).

- The patient is then asked to flex the elbow while the examiner resists
- The patient is then asked how the apprehension changed
- If the apprehension is relieved or the patient is more comfortable, the test is negative for a SLAP lesion
- The test is positive if the apprehension is unchanged or the shoulder becomes more painful

- **Crank Test** (Figure 2E.4)
  - First described by Liu et al[16]
  - **Maneuver:**
    - The examiner stands on the affected side
    - The patient is positioned supine on the examination table with the affected arm elevated to about 100° to 130° in the scapular plane and elbow to 90° with the humerus resting on the examination table (the patient may also be seated with the affected shoulder abducted to 100°-130° in the scapular plane)
    - The examiner applies an axial force along he humerus with one hand to load the glenohumeral joint while the examiner's other hand internally and externally rotates the humerus at the wrist
    - Reproduction of pain, catching, or clicking indicates a positive test
    - The patient may also be seated with the examiner on the affected side

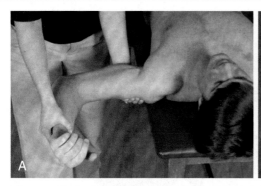
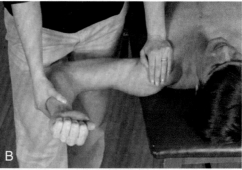

Figure 2E.4. Crank test. (Borrowed from Anderson MK, Barnum M. *Foundations of Athletic Training: Prevention, Assessment, and Management*. Wolters Kluwer Health; 2017.)

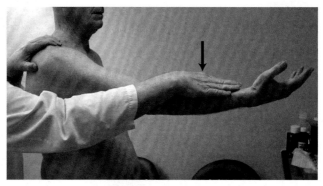

Figure 2E.5. Speed's test. (Borrowed from Miller MD, Wiesel SW. *Operative Techniques in Sports Medicine Surgery*. Wolters Kluwer Health; 2016.)

- **Speed's Test**[3] 🔊 (Sensitivity 0.31, PPV 75%, NPV 50%) (Figure 2E.5)
  - First described by Gilecreest and Albi[17]
  - **Maneuver**:
    - The patient's forearm is supinated, elbow extended, and shoulder forward flexed to 60° to 90° with the elbow straight
    - The examiner applies a downward force on the supinated arm while the patient resists
    - Positive if there is pain at the bicipital tendon area with this maneuver
    - The arm can then be pronated and the downward force is reapplied. This further localizes bicipital pathology if pain is less severe when the forearm is pronated compared with supinated

- **Yergason Test**[3] 🔊 (Sensitivity 0.43, Specificity 0.79) (Figure 2E.6)
  - First described by Yergason[18] in a *JBJS* article
  - **Maneuver**:
    - The examiner stands on the patient's affected side
    - The patient is seated with the elbow flexed to 90° and the forearm pronated, and the arm is adducted against the thorax
    - The examiner places a hand on the proximal portion of the humerus near the bicipital groove and the other hand on the distal forearm/wrist (the hand can also be grasped in a "handshake")
    - The patient is instructed to actively supinate the forearm and externally rotate at the humerus against resistance
    - Pain experienced in the anterior shoulder with this movement is considered a positive finding

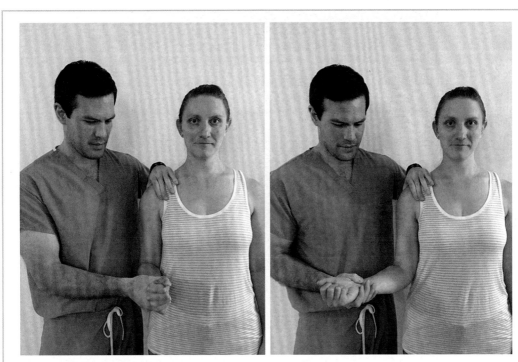

Figure 2E.6. Yergason test.

- **Limitations of Maneuver:**
  - There are multiple motions for the patient to perform simultaneously
  - There are many pain generators in the anterior shoulder and may not fully isolate one of them

IMAGING

Imaging is similar to anterior-posterior instability.

Plain Radiographs

- Not overly helpful for biceps and soft tissue labral lesions
- Complete biceps rupture can lead to subtle superior migration of the humeral head of the affected side with the loss of the downward pressure

Magnetic Resonance Imaging

- Remains the mainstay of diagnosing biceps and labral pathology
- MR arthrogram can highlight SLAP and labral tears, biceps tears near the anchor, and intra-substance biceps issues
- Figure 2E.7 demonstrates MRI findings of a sublabral recess, a normal anatomic variant
- Figure 2E.8 shows multiple MRI images of SLAP tears

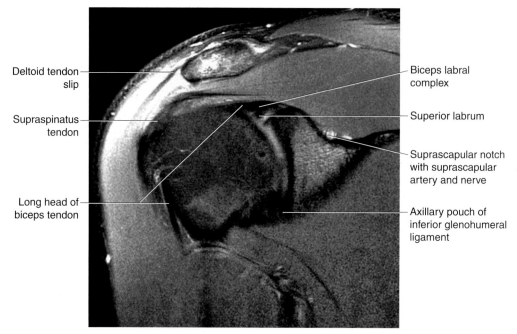

Figure 2E.7. Normal anatomic variant: sublabral recess.

- Lesions at the biceps-labral junction and bicipital groove are generally reserved for associated rotator cuff pathology or if shoulder instability is in question
- Intra-articular gadolinium increases the sensitivity to the mid 90% range for soft tissue pathologies
- Having arm in abducted externally rotated position tensions IGHL, accentuating pathology
- Important to identify preoperatively to determine if pathology can be treated open versus arthroscopically

Arthroscopic Findings

- Biceps tendon tearing (Figure 2E.9)
- SLAP tear (Figure 2E.10)
- Biceps anchor partial tears, fraying, or tendinosis (Figure 2E.11)
- Diagram of SLAP repair
- Arthroscopic biceps tenodesis as treatment of these injuries

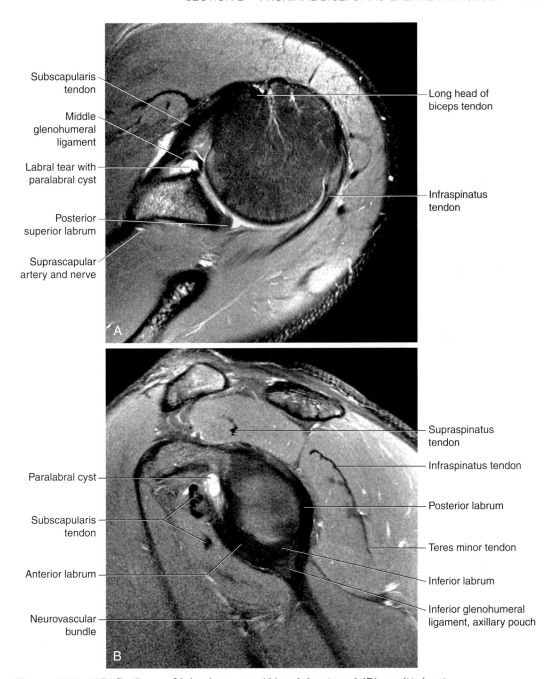

Figure 2E.8. MRI findings of labral tear on (A) axial cut and (B) sagittal cut.

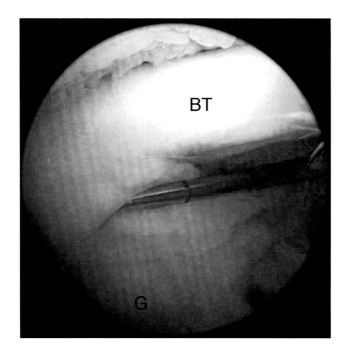

Figure 2E.9. Fraying at the biceps-labral junction and edema in biceps anchor. BT, biceps tendon; G, glenoid.

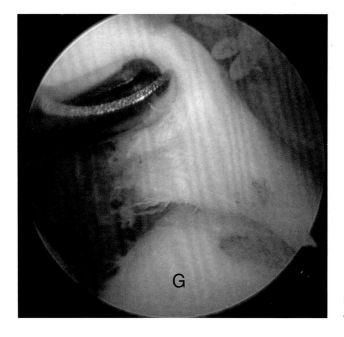

Figure 2E.10. Large labral tear and avulsion. G, glenoid.

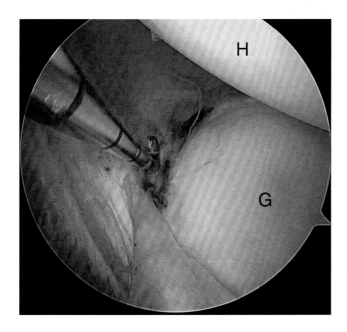

Figure 2E.11. Edematous and damaged to the superior labrum biceps anchor.

REFERENCES

1. Gill HS, El Rassi G, Bahk MS, Castillo RC, McFarland EG. Physical examination for partial tears of the biceps tendon. *Am J Sports Med.* 2007;35(8):1334-1340.
2. Guanche A, Jones DC. Clinical testing for tears of the glenoid labrum. *Arthroscopy.* 2003;19(5):517-523.
3. Holtby R, Razmjou H. Accuracy of the Speed's and Yergason's tests in detecting biceps pathology and SLAP lesions: comparison with arthroscopic findings, *Arthroscopy.* 2004;20(3):231-236.
4. Kibler WB. Specificity and sensitivity of the anterior slide test in throwing athletes with superior glenoid labral tears. *Arthroscopy.* 1995;11(3):296-300.
5. Kibler WB, Sciascia AD, Hester P, Dome D, Jacobs C. Clinical utility of traditional and new tests in the diagnosis of biceps tendon injuries and superior labrum anterior and posterior lesions in the shoulder. *Am J Sports Med.* 2009;37(9):1840-1847.
6. Kim SH, Ha KI, Han KY. Biceps load test: a clinical test for superior labrum anterior and posterior lesions in shoulders with recurrent anterior dislocations. *Am J Sports Med.* 1999;27(3):300-303.
7. Kim SH, Ha KI, Ahn JH, et al. Biceps load test II: a clinical test for SLAP lesions of the shoulder. *Arthroscopy.* 2001; 17(2): 160-164.
8. Matsen III FA, Kirby RM. Office evaluation and management of shoulder pain. *Orthop Clin North Am.* 1982;13(3):453-475.
9. O'Brien SJ, Pagnani MJ, Fealy S, McGlynn SR, Wilson JB. The active compression test: a new and effective test for diagnosing labral tears and acromioclavicular joint abnormality. *Am J Sports Med.* 1998;26(5):610-613.
10. Parentis MA, Glousman RE, Mohr KS, Yocum LA. An evaluation of the provocative tests for superior labral anterior posterior lesions. *Am J Sports Med.* 2006;34(2):265-268.
11. Taylor SA, Newman A, Dawson C, et al. The "3-pack" examination is critical for comprehensive evaluation of the biceps-labrum complex and the bicipital tunnel: a prospective study. *Arthroscopy.* 2017;33(1):28-38.
12. Thorsness R, Romeo AA. Diagnosis and management of the biceps-labral complex. *AAOS Instr Course Lect.* 2017;66:65-77.

SECTION F
Acromioclavicular and Sternoclavicular Joint Injuries

Michelle E. Kew

HISTORY

- Acute AC injuries are commonly caused by a direct blow to the shoulder
- AC osteoarthritis presents in patients with history of repetitive overhead activities or history of AC joint separation
  - Patients may report pain with lifting or while sleeping on the affected side
- Weightlifters or patients who have sustained a traumatic injury to the shoulder may present with distal clavicle osteolysis[8]
- Sternoclavicular (SC) joint injuries are typically caused by a high-energy force (motor vehicle collision, fall from height) and lead to subluxation and/or dislocation of the SC joint[7]
  - Less frequently caused by overhead elevation of the arm with spontaneous injury to the SC joint
  - Patients with posterior dislocation may present with mediastinal compromise, shortness of breath, dysphagia
    - If dislocation is present, the patient will present with the affected shoulder shortened and in a forward position/posterior position depending on the direction of dislocation
- Atraumatic SC joint pain can be attributed to a myriad of etiologies, including osteoarthritis, rheumatoid arthritis, septic arthritis, and Friedrich disease
- Patients may present with localized ecchymosis, tenderness, and swelling at the AC or SC joint

PHYSICAL EXAMINATION[6]

- Surface landmarks are useful to successfully identify the AC joint
  - AC joint is located at lateral apex of a triangle formed by the clavicle, base of the neck, and scapular spine (Figure 2F.1)
- Provocative tests outlined below may be performed before and after injection of local anesthetic to the AC joint to improve diagnostic accuracy

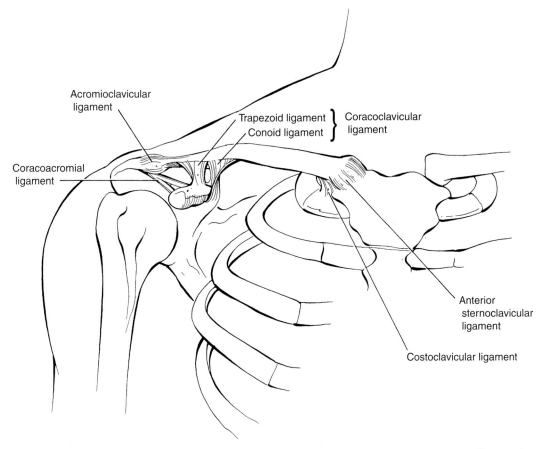

Figure 2F.1. Acromioclavicular joint anatomy. (Borrowed from Iannotti JP, Williams GR, Miniaci A, Zuckerman JD. *Disorders of the Shoulder: Diagnosis & Management*. Wolters Kluwer; 2014.)

KEY EXAMINATION MANEUVERS[1,5]

- **Cross-Body Adduction Test** (Figure 2F.2A)
  - **Maneuver:**
    - The patient's arm is passively elevated to 90° in a sagittal plane
    - The elbow is extended/flexed slightly
    - The examiner stands in front of the patient and pushes the patient's arm into horizontal adduction
  - Causes compression of medial acromial facet against distal clavicle
  - Positive if symptoms at the AC joint are reproduced
  - **Variation of Cross-Body Adduction Test (Bell-Van Riet Test)**[2]
    - Described in 2011 (Figure 2F.2B)
      - The patient's arm is passively elevated to 90° in maximal adduction and internal rotation
      - The elbow is in full extension and the arm is in full pronation
      - The examiner stands in front of the patient and resists upward translation of the arm
      - Positive if the patient reports pain and is unable to maintain the initial arm position

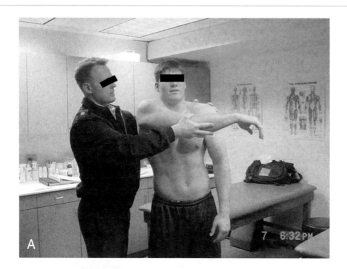

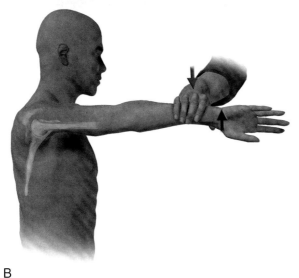

Figure 2F.2. A, Cross-body adduction test. B, Bell-Van Riet test.

- **AC Resisted Extension Test** (Figure 2F.3)
  - **Maneuver:**
    - The patient's arm is at 90° in a sagittal plane with 90° internal rotation, with the elbow flexed to 90°
    - The examiner stands behind the patient and provides resistance, as the patient horizontally abducts the arm
  - Positive if symptoms at the AC joint are reproduced

- **Buchberger Test** (Figure 2F.4)
  - First described in 1999[4]
  - Helps to identify the AC joint as the location of the patient's pain
  - **Maneuver:**
    - Neer impingement sign is performed first
    - The examiner then returns the patient's arm to neutral and places a hand on the lateral one-third clavicle
    - The patient's arm is externally rotated, adducted 10°, and passively forward flexed against the stabilizing force on the lateral clavicle

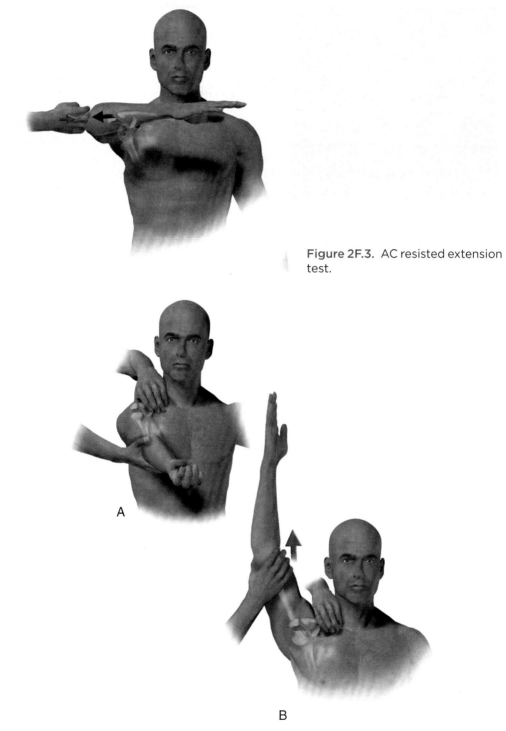

Figure 2F.3. AC resisted extension test.

A

B

Figure 2F.4. Buchberger test.

- External rotation of the patient's arm decreases subacromial impingement due to increased clearance for supraspinatus and biceps
- Forward flexion during this test creates shear on the AC joint
  - To further stress the AC joint, the patient's arm is forward flexed greater than 90°
  - Increased shear between acromion and distal clavicle

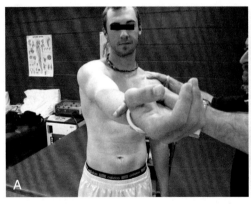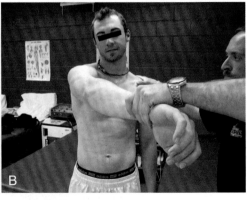

Figure 2F.5. O'Brien test or active compression test. Shoulder is (A) forward flexed to 90° and (B) then internally rotated and tested against resistance. Pain that is relieved when the same test is conducted with the shoulder in external rotation denotes a positive test. (Borrowed from Iannotti JP, Williams GR, Miniaci A, Zuckerman JD. *Disorders of the Shoulder: Diagnosis & Management*. Wolters Kluwer; 2014.)

- Positive Result:
  - If Neer sign is negative and Buchberger test causes AC joint pain
  - If Neer sign elicits AC joint pain with worsening pain and improved localization to the AC joint with Buchberger test

- **O'Brien Test or Active Compression Test** 🔵 (Sensitivity 1.00, Specificity 0.985 in the original paper; sensitivity 0.63, specificity 0.73 in a subsequent study) (Figure 2F.5)
  - First described by O'Brien and Pagnani in 1998[3] in *AJSM*, initially called the active compression test
  - **Maneuver**:
  - The examiner stands on the opposite side of the affected shoulder
  - The patient is seated or standing with the shoulder forward flexed 90° with the elbow extended
  - The patient's shoulder is adducted 10° and maximally internally rotated (maximal forearm pronation)
  - The patient is then asked to resist a downward force applied to the arm by the examiner
  - Pain or clicking deep in the shoulder indicates a positive test
  - The patient is then asked to externally rotate (supinate) the arm in the same shoulder position and again resist the downward force applied by the examiner
  - If pain lessens with supination/external rotation, this is again suggestive of superior labral tear or pathology
  - If pain is present during the maneuver at the AC joint, this is likely due to AC pathology and not necessarily labral pathology
  - **Limitations of Maneuver**:
    - Diagnostic utility is not as accurate as possibly first described, as repeat studies have shown much lower sensitivity and specificity
    - May not fully isolate SLAP tears alone with other pain generators in the shoulder as in AC pathology
    - Somewhat dependent on subjective reports of pain with examination maneuver

- **Paxinos Test** (Figure 2F.6)
  - **Maneuver:**
    - The examiner stands behind the patient
    - The thumb is placed over posterolateral acromion and the index finger is placed over midclavicle
    - Anterior pressure is applied by the thumb with inferior pressure applied by the index finger
  - Positive if symptoms at the AC joint are reproduced

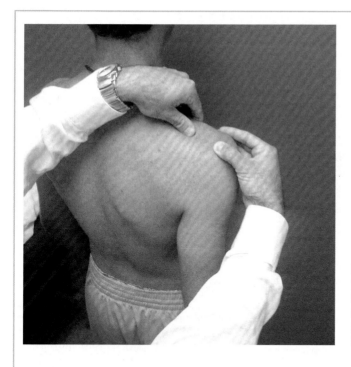

Figure 2F.6. Paxinos test. (Borrowed from Iannotti JP, Williams GR, Miniaci A, Zuckerman JD. *Disorders of the Shoulder*: *Diagnosis & Management*. Wolters Kluwer; 2014.)

- Hegeus et al performed a meta-analysis of commonly used physical examination tests for shoulder pathology
  - No AC joint–specific tests were found to be valuable as diagnostic tools
  - Active compression test, if positive, was found to rule in the AC joint as the etiology of the patient's pain

IMAGING

Plain Radiographs

- Images of the chest, clavicle, and shoulder should be taken
  - Useful to evaluate for AC separation and AC degenerative joint disease
  - Chest radiograph is important to rule out pneumothorax and hemothorax after high-energy trauma when evaluating for SC injury
- Axillary view
  - Used to evaluate for posterior translation of the distal clavicle
- Zanca view (Figure 2F.7A and 2F.7B)
  - Used to visualize the AC joint
  - Beam is directed 10° cephalad at 50% of normal penetrance
- Hobbs view (Figure 2F.8A and 2F.8B)
  - The patient is seated and leans forward over the imaging table
  - Beam is directed above the nape of the neck at 90°
  - Useful to evaluate for SC joint injury
- Heinig view (Figure 2F.9A and 2F.9B)
  - Beam is directed perpendicular to the joint
  - Useful for SC joint injury
- Serendipity view (Figure 2F.10A-2F.10D)
  - Beam is tilted 40° cephalad and centered on the sternum
  - Useful for SC joint injury

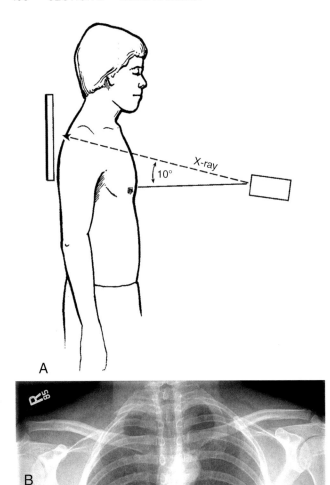

A

B

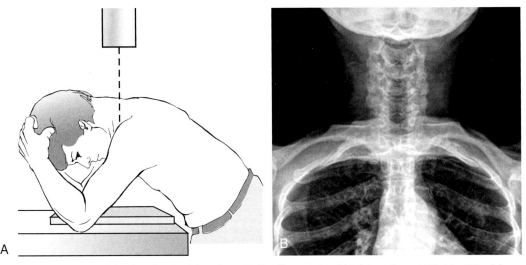

Figure 2F.7. A, Positioning for Zanca view. B, Radiograph of Zanca view. ((A) Borrowed from Acromioclavicular joint injuries. In: Bucholz RW, Heckman JD, Court-Brown C, eds. *Rockwood and Green's Fractures in Adults*. 6th ed. Philadelphia, PA: Lippincott Williams & Wilkins; 2006:1335 and (B) Iannotti JP, Williams GR, Miniaci A, Zuckerman JD. *Disorders of the Shoulder: Diagnosis & Management*. Wolters Kluwer; 2014).

A

B

Figure 2F.8. A, Positioning for Hobbs view. B, Radiograph of Hobbs view. ((A) Modified from Hobbs DW. Sternoclavicular joint: a new axial radiographic view. *Radiology*. 1968;90:801-802 and Bucholz RW, Heckman JD, Court-Brown C, et al, eds. *Rockwood and Green's Fractures in Adults*. 6th ed. Philadelphia: Lippincott Williams & Wilkins; 2006.)

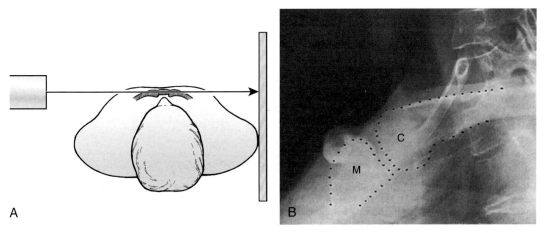

A

B

Figure 2F.9. A, Positioning for Heinig view. B, Radiograph of Heinig view. M, manubrium; C, clavicle. (Borrowed from Court-Brown CM, Heckman JD, McQueen MM, et al. *Rockwood and Green's Fractures in Adults*. Philadelphia: Wolters Kluwer Health; 2015.)

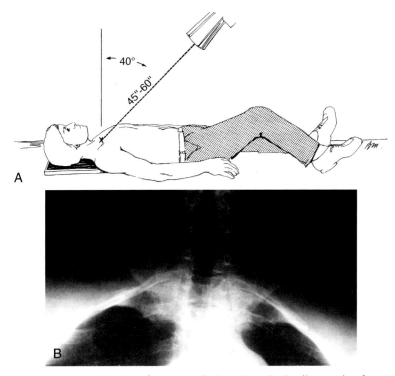

Figure 2F.10. A, Patient positioning for serendipity view. B, Radiograph of serendipity view. ((A) Courtesy of Columbia University Center for Shoulder, Elbow and Sports Medicine. and (B) Iannotti JP, Williams GR, Miniaci A, Zuckerman JD. *Disorders of the Shoulder: Diagnosis & Management*. Wolters Kluwer; 2014.)

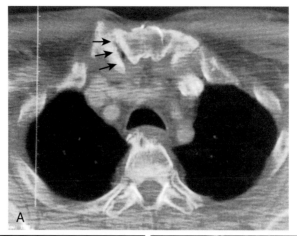

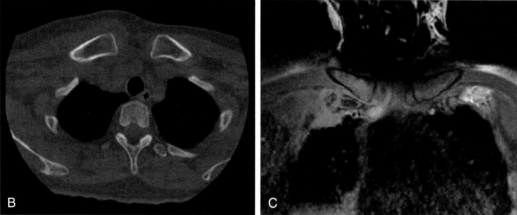

Figure 2F.11. A, Osteoarthritis of sternoclavicular joint. B and C, Septic arthritis of sternoclavicular joint. ((A) From Iannotti JP, Williams GR. *Disorders of the Shoulder Diagnosis and Management*. Philadelphia: Lippincott Williams & Wilkins; 2007 and (B) Waldman SD, *Waldman's Comprehensive Atlas of Diagnostic Ultrasound of Painful Conditions*. Lippincott Williams & Wilkins; 2016.)

Computed Tomography

- Useful to evaluate for SC joint injury, as radiographs may be difficult to interpret (Figure 2F.12)
- May show joint destruction in inflammatory conditions of the SC joint or evidence of osteo-arthritic changes (Figure 2F.11A and 2F.11B)
- CT angiograms or venograms may be required to evaluate vasculature after SC joint injury

Magnetic Resonance Imaging

- Routine use of MRI for AC joint pathology is not recommended, as radiographs are able to accurately confirm a diagnosis
- Pediatric patients may require MRI to distinguish physeal separations from SC joint dislocations
- Useful to evaluate for inflammatory conditions of the SC joint

Ultrasound

- Guided joint aspirations can be diagnostic in AC and SC joint septic arthritis and crystalline arthropathy

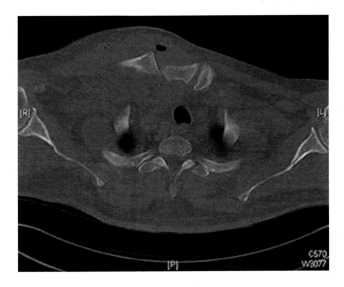

Figure 2F.12. Anterior dislocation of the sternoclavicular joint. (Courtesy of Columbia University Center for Shoulder, Elbow and Sports Medicine.)

REFERENCES

1. Walton J, Mahajan S, Paxinos A, et al. Diagnostic values of tests for acromioclavicular joint pain. *J Bone Joint Surg.* 2004;86A(4):807-812.
2. Van Riet RP, Bell SN. Clinical evaluation of acromioclavicular joint pathology: sensitivity of a new test. *J Shoulder Elbow Surg.* 2011;20(1):73-76.
3. O'Brien SJ, Pagnani MJ, Fealy S, McGlynn SR, Wilson JB. The active compression test: a new and effective test for diagnosing labral tears and acromioclavicular joint abnormality. *Am J Sports Med.* 1998;26:610-613.
4. Buchberger DJ. Introduction of a new physical examination procedure for the differentiation of acromioclavicular joint lesions and subacromial impingement. *J Manip Physiol Ther.* 1999;22(5):316-321.
5. Hegedus EJ, Goode A, Campbell S, et al. Physical examination tests of the shoulder: a systematic review with meta-analysis of individual tests. *Br J Sports Med.* 2008;42(2):80-92.
6. Simovitch R, Sanders B, Ozbaydar M, Lavery K, Warner J. Acromioclavicular joint injuries: diagnosis and management. *J Am Acad Orthop Surg.* 2009;17(4):207-219.
7. Higginbotham TO, Kuhn JE. Atraumatic disorders of the sternoclavicular joint. *J Am Acad Orthop Surg.* 2005;13(2):138-145.
8. Wirth MA, Rockwood CA. Acute and chronic traumatic injuries of the sternoclavicular joint. *J Am Acad Orthop Surg.* 1996;4(5):268-278.

SECTION G
Nerve Compression, Brachial Plexus Injuries

Michelle E. Kew

NERVE COMPRESSION SYNDROMES

HISTORY

- Patients may report a traction injury, compression injury, or direct blow to the shoulder
- Athletes who participate in overhead activities may present with weakness of deltoid, pain/paresthesias that worsen with overhead activity
- Pain may be present to superior, posterior, lateral shoulder with radiation to neck or arm
  - Adduction and internal rotation will worsen pain in suprascapular nerve compression

Note: Forearm, wrist, and hand nerve compression syndromes will be addressed in the Elbow or Hand and Wrist Sections.

PHYSICAL EXAMINATION

Long Thoracic Nerve Palsy[1]

It presents with medial scapular winging due to serratus anterior dysfunction (Figure 2G.1A).

- Scapula will be translated medially with inferior angle rotated toward midline
- Winging increased if the patient pushes against a wall
- If complete serratus anterior paralysis is present, the patient will be unable to raise the arm above the horizontal plane

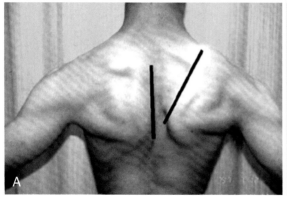 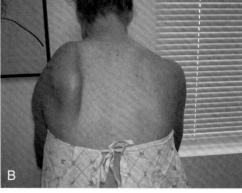

Figure 2G.1. Lateral (A) and medial (B) scapular winging. (From Iannotti JP, Williams GR, Miniaci A, Zuckerman JD. *Disorders of the Shoulder: Diagnosis & Management*. 2014.)

Spinal Accessory Nerve Palsy[2,3]

It presents with lateral scapular winging due to trapezius dysfunction (Figure 2G.1B).

- The scapula will be translated laterally with inferior angle rotation away from the midline
- Winging increased if the arm is abducted
- Weakness of arm abduction will be present

KEY EXAMINATION MANEUVERS:

- **Resisted Active External Rotation Test** (Figure 2G.2)
  - The shoulder is adducted and in a neutral rotation
  - The elbow flexed to 90°
  - The patient externally rotates the shoulder against a force
  - Positive if medial winging of scapula is present

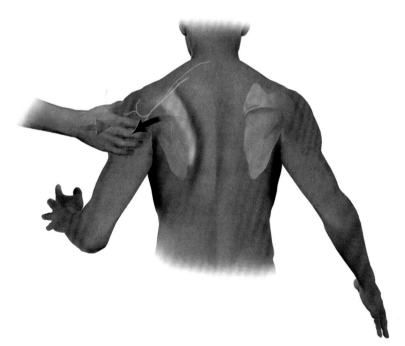

Figure 2G.2. Spinal accessory nerve palsy; resisted active external rotation test.

Suprascapular Nerve Palsy[4,5]

Compression occurs at either spinoglenoid notch or suprascapular notch (Figure 2G.3). In spinoglenoid notch, paralabral cyst or ganglion causes compression of nerve and leads to weakness and atrophy of infraspinatus. In suprascapular notch, ganglion or fracture callus in the area of transverse scapular ligament causes nerve compression and weakness and atrophy of supraspinatus and infraspinatus.

- Patients will exhibit loss of abduction and external rotation strength
- Atrophy of supraspinatus and/or infraspinatus may be present (Figure 2G.4)
- Patients may have associated rotator cuff or labral injury; therefore, a thorough shoulder examination is critical (refer to sections C and G, respectively)

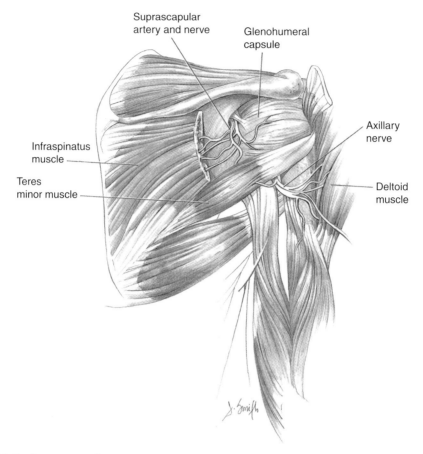

Figure 2G.3. Suprascapular nerve anatomy. (From Iannotti JP, Williams GR, Miniaci A, Zuckerman JD. *Disorders of the Shoulder: Diagnosis & Management.* 2014.)

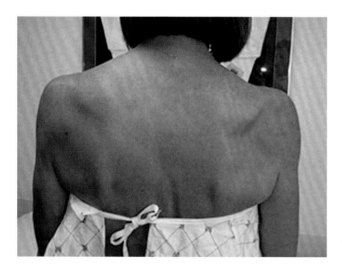

Figure 2G.4. Supraspinatus and infraspinatus muscle wasting. (From Iannotti JP, Williams GR, Miniaci A, Zuckerman JD. *Disorders of the Shoulder: Diagnosis & Management.* 2014.)

Quadrilateral Space Syndrome

It is the compression of the axillary nerve or posterior humeral circumflex artery.

- Reproduction of symptoms with arm abduction
- Weakness of teres minor
- Weakness of deltoid

IMAGING

Plain Radiographs

- Radiographs of the cervical spine, chest, and shoulder should be taken

Magnetic Resonance Imaging

- Useful in visualization of paralabral cyst, ganglion, or other space-occupying lesion in spino-glenoid and suprascapular notches for evaluation of suprascapular nerve compression and quadrilateral space syndrome (Figures 2G.5 and 2G.7)
- Used to evaluate degree of atrophy of supraspinatus and intraspinatus

Electromyography/Nerve Conduction Studies

- Confirm specific nerve injury
  - Example: long thoracic nerve palsy

Arteriography

- Used to confirm compression of posterior humeral circumflex artery in quadrilateral space syndrome (Figure 2G.6)

BRACHIAL PLEXUS[6]

HISTORY

- Injuries are usually due to high-energy mechanisms, resulting in nerve root avulsions or rupture of entire segments of the plexus
  - MVC
  - High-energy sport activity
  - Gunshot wounds
    - Severity depends on the caliber, velocity, and angle of entry

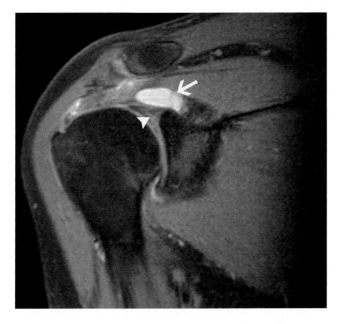

Figure 2G.5. Magnetic resonance imaging showing paralabral cyst, denoted by arrows. (From Iannotti JP, Williams GR, Miniaci A, Zuckerman JD. *Disorders of the Shoulder: Diagnosis & Management.* 2014.)

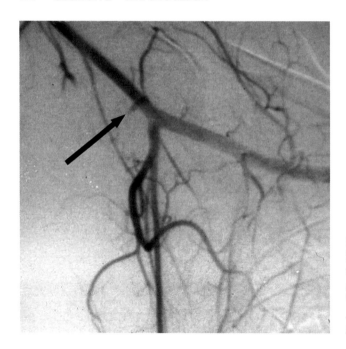

Figure 2G.6. Occlusion of posterior humeral circumflex artery (arrow) with abduction in quadrilateral space syndrome. (From Iannotti JP, Williams GR, Miniaci A, Zuckerman JD. *Disorders of the Shoulder: Diagnosis & Management*. 2014.)

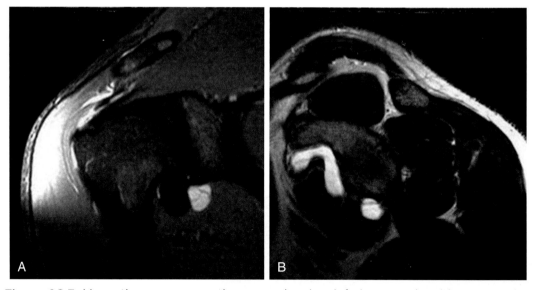

Figure 2G.7. Magnetic resonance arthrogram showing inferior paraglenoid cyst causing quadrilateral space syndrome. (From Kosy JD, White A, Redfern AC, et al. Arthroscopic removal of paraglenoid cyst causing quadrilateral space syndrome. *Shoulder Elbow*. 2010; 2(1):23-26.)

- Direction of force dictates injury
  - Force pushes shoulder caudally (fall on the shoulder)
    - Upper parts of plexus
    - High energy can disrupt all roots
  - Force pushes the shoulder into abduction (restraining a fall)
    - Lower parts of the plexus
    - Can have variable degree of injury to the upper plexus

- Signs of severe injury
  - Complete sensory loss
  - Global motor dysfunction
  - Neuropathic pain
  - Horner sign: ptosis, miosis, anhidrosis

PHYSICAL EXAMINATION

Strength Examination

- Determine the location of lesion with careful strength assessment (Figure 2G.8)
  - Median, ulnar, radial nerves: hand and wrist motion
  - Musculocutaneous, high radial nerves: elbow flexion, extension
  - Axillary nerve: shoulder abduction
  - Thoracodorsal nerve: latissimus dorsi; the patient was asked to cough
  - Medial and lateral pectoral nerves: abduct the arm against resistance
  - Suprascapular nerve: assess the shoulder external rotation
  - Long thoracic nerve: scapular winging, suggesting preganglionic injury
- Important to evaluate function of potential muscles and nerves for transfer

Sensory Examination

- Evaluate all sensory dermatomes of the neck and upper extremity (Figure 2G.9)
- Horner syndrome may indicate preganglionic injury with root avulsion at the C8-T1 level

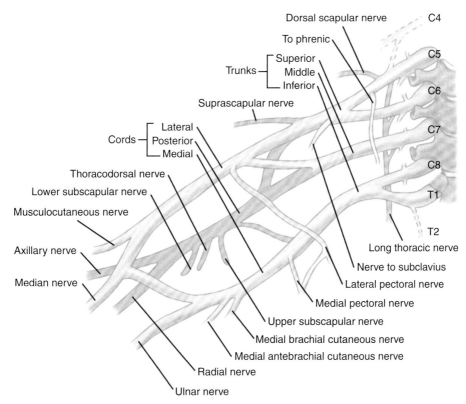

Figure 2G.8. Brachial plexus anatomy. (From Wiesel SW. *Operative Techniques in Orthopaedic Surgery. Sports Medicine; Pelvis and Lower Extremity Trauma; Adult Reconstruction.* Philadelphia: Wolters Kluwer; 2016.)

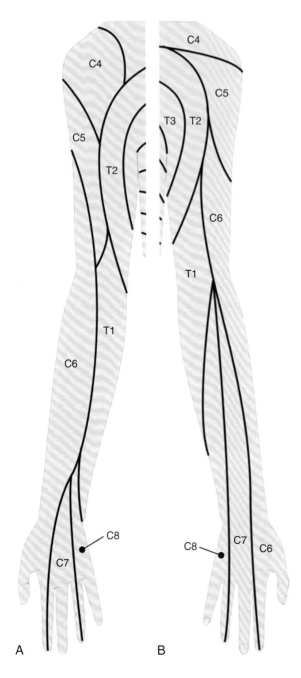

Figure 2G.9. Upper extremity derma-tomes. (From Olinger AB. *Human Gross Anatomy*. Philadelphia: Wolters Kluwer; 2016.)

Vascular Examination

- Full pulse examination to evaluate for associated axillary artery injury

IMAGING

Plain Radiographs

- Cervical spine
  - Evaluate for any cervical fractures associated with trauma
  - Transverse spinal process fractures may indicate root avulsions

- Chest
  - May demonstrate paralyzed hemidiaphragm, which indicates severe upper nerve root injury
  - Clavicle or rib fracture may indicate adjacent plexus injury
- Shoulder
  - Scapulothoracic dissociation is linked to multiple root avulsions and major vascular injury

Computed Tomography Myelography (Figure 2G.10A)

- Used to define the level of nerve root injury
- Immediately after injury, hematoma at the site can displace dye from myelogram
  - Perform CT myelogram 3 to 4 weeks after injury
- Cervical root avulsion causes the dural sheath to heal with a pseudomeningocele

Magnetic Resonance Imaging (Figure 2G.10B)

- Advantages over CT myelography
  - Noninvasive
  - Able to visualize whole plexus
  - CT myelography only shows nerve root-type brachial plexus injuries
- MRI can be used to evaluate for neuromas after trauma

Arteriography

- Used if vascular injury is suspected to axillary artery, subclavian artery, and subclavian vein

Electromyography/Nerve Conduction Studies

- Used to confirm diagnosis, localize lesions, and monitor recovery
- Best performed 3 to 4 weeks after injury
- Presence of few fibrillations at rest associated with good prognosis

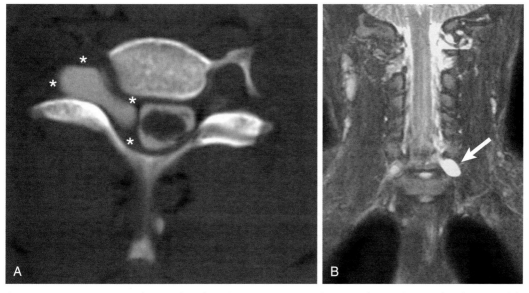

Figure 2G.10. A, CT myelography showing posttraumatic pseudomeningocele, the asterisks delineate the pseudomeningocele. B, Magnetic resonance imaging showing posttraumatic pseudomeningocele. ((A) From Schwartz ED, Flanders AE. *Spinal Trauma: Imaging, Diagnosis, and Management*. Philadelphia: Lippincott Williams & Wilkins; 2007 and (B) From Castillo M. *Neuroradiology Companion: Methods, Guidelines, and Imaging Fundamentals*. 4th ed. Philadelphia: Wolters Kluwer Health, Lippincott Williams & Wilkins; 2012.)

Somatosensory Evoked Potentials (SSEPs)/Nerve Action Potentials (NAPs)

- Used intraoperatively to evaluate nerves directly
- SSEPs
  - Presence associated with intact dorsal root, creating a connection between peripheral and central nervous system
  - Absent in postganglionic lesions
- NAPs
  - Presence associated with preserved axons or significant regeneration
  - Suggest that recovery will likely occur without need for grafting
  - Faster conduction velocity with large amplitude and short latency suggests preganglionic injury

REFERENCES

1. Wiater JM, Flatow EL. Long thoracic nerve injury. *Clin Orthop Relat Res*. 1999;368:17-27.
2. Martin RM, Fish DE. Scapular winging: anatomical review, diagnosis, and treatments. *Curr Rev Musculoskeletal Med*. 2008;1(1):1-11.
3. Chan PK, Hems TE. Clinical signs of accessory nerve palsy. *J Trauma Inj Infect Crit Care*. 2006; 60(5):1142-1144.
4. Moen TC, Babatunde OM, Hsu SH, Ahmad CS, Levine WN. Suprascapular neuropathy: what does the literature show? *J Shoulder Elbow Surg*. 2012;21(6):835-846.
5. Boykin RE, Friedman DJ, Higgins LD, Warner JJ. Suprascapular neuropathy. *J Bone Joint Surg*. 2010;92(13):2348-2364.
6. Shin AY, Spinner RJ, Steinmann SP, Bishop AT. Adult traumatic brachial plexus injuries. *J Am Acad Orthop Surg*. 2005;13(6):382-396.

SECTION H
Thoracic Outlet Syndrome

Michelle E. Kew

HISTORY[1]

- Symptoms can be attributed to the neurovascular structure that is compressed (Figure 2H.1)
  - vTOS: subclavian vein
  - aTOS: subclavian artery
  - nTOS: nerve root
- Vague symptoms
  - Arterial TOS: hand fatigue, mild edema, temperature sensitivity
  - Venous TOS: painful, swollen extremity with color changes (cyanosis, rubor), may also have arm fatigue, heaviness
  - Nerve TOS: back/arm/shoulder pain, headaches, arm paresthesias
- May present with vascular or neurologic symptoms
  - Vascular: venous congestion, Raynaud phenomenon, arterial ischemia
    - May see venous collaterals on skin in the ipsilateral shoulder, neck, and chest wall
  - Neurologic: sensory/motor dysfunction
    - Upper plexus: involve C5-C7, localized to lateral arm, occiput, scapula
    - Lower plexus: involve C8-T1, localize to scapula, axilla, medial arm, and forearm

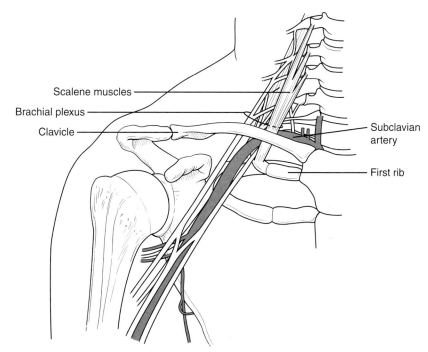

Figure 2H.1. Thoracic outlet anatomy. (From Iannotti JP, Williams GR, Miniaci A, Zuckerman JD. *Disorders of the Shoulder: Diagnosis & Management*. 2014.)

- May see muscle atrophy or winged scapula
  - Muscle atrophy seen in intrinsic muscles, thenar muscles
- May elicit tenderness over anterior scalene with palpation
- Arterial TOS may manifest as lower systolic blood pressure in the affected extremity with decreased distal pulses
- Patients will have a history of repetitive upper extremity motions, especially overhead activities
  - Example: swimmers, pitchers, laborers

PHYSICAL EXAMINATION

KEY EXAMINATION MANEUVERS

- Specificity has been shown to be ~80%

- Examination findings suggest a diagnosis but are not diagnostic

- **Adson Test**
  - Described in 1927 by Alfred Adson[2] and has been critically evaluated over the years by many studies
    - Wright et al noted that distal pulses could be diminished with turning the head to both sides
    - Woods et al noted that the Adson test was positive when the head was turned to the contralateral side more often (Figure 2H.2A)
  - Helpful to evaluate for arterial compression
  - **Maneuver** (Figure 2H.2B):
    - The patient keeps the arm at the side, hyperextends the neck, and rotates the head to the affected side
    - The examiner stands in front of the patient and palpates radial pulse
    - Positive if there is diminished radial artery pulse and if symptoms are reproduced with inhalation
  - **Limitations of Maneuver**:
    - As multiple disease processes can produce positive test, this maneuver is not diagnostic

- **Wright Maneuver**
  - Described by Wright as a modification of the Adson test in 1945[3]
  - **Maneuver** (Figure 2H.3):
    - The examiner stands in front of the patient and places the affected extremity in abduction and external rotation
    - Positive if patient's symptoms are reproduced, change in radial pulse

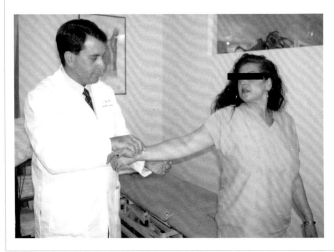

Figure 2H.2. Adson test. (From Iannotti JP, Williams GR, Miniaci A, Zuckerman JD. *Disorders of the Shoulder: Diagnosis & Management*. 2014.)

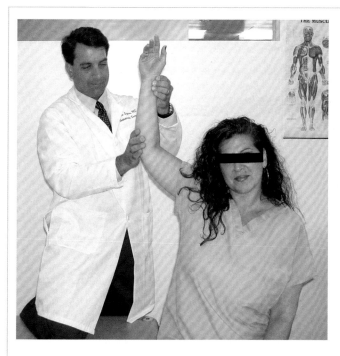

Figure 2H.3. Wright maneuver. (From Iannotti JP, Williams GR, Miniaci A, Zuckerman JD. *Disorders of the Shoulder: Diagnosis & Management*. 2014.)

- **Upper limb tension test of Elvey (modified)**
- Test both limbs simultaneously
  - Asymptomatic side is the control
- Useful to assist with diagnosis of nTOS
- **Original Test**
  - First described by Elvey[5]
  - First step: abduct the arm to 90° with the forearm flexed to 90°
  - Have found that this position is not needed for diagnosis; therefore, start with position 1 as listed below
- **Maneuver** (Figure 2H.4):
  - The examiner stands in front of the patient and abducts both arms to 90° with elbows straight
  - The patient then dorsiflexes wrists bilaterally and tilts the head to one side, then to other side
  - Positive if there is pain down the arm and paresthesias in hand
    - Strongest positive test: if symptoms occur with position 1 and symptoms worsen with positions 2 and 3
    - Indicate compression of nerve roots or brachial plexus branches
- **Limitations of Maneuver**:
  - Positive test is not diagnostic of TOS and suggests nerve root irritation only
  - Test may be negative in aTOS

- **Roos Test**
  - First described by Gilroy and Meyer in 1963[6] as modification of the Adson test; 90° abduction in external rotation test
  - Popularized by Roos in 1966[7], referred to as Roos test or elevated arm stress test (EAST)
  - **Maneuver (Figure 2H.5)**:
    - The examiner asks the patient to abduct both arms to 90° and externally rotate to 90°. The patient holds hands above the head for 1 minute
    - Positive if symptoms are reproduced in 60 seconds
  - **Modified Roos Test**
    - Same maneuver as above with opening and closing of fist
    - Symptoms are reproduced with continued flexion/extension of fingers

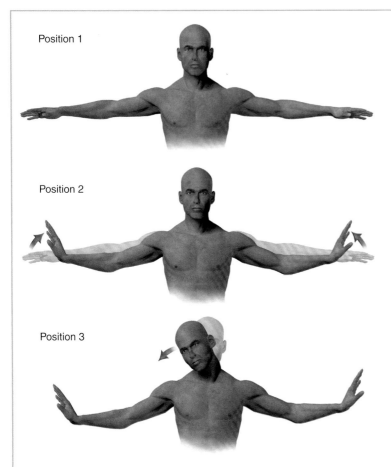

Position 1

Position 2

Position 3

Figure 2H.4. Upper limb tension test of Elvey.

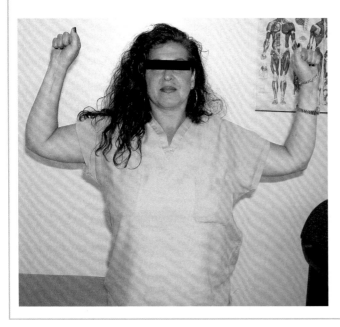

Figure 2H.5. Roos test. (From Iannotti JP, Williams GR, Miniaci A, Zuckerman JD. *Disorders of the Shoulder: Diagnosis & Management*. 2014.)

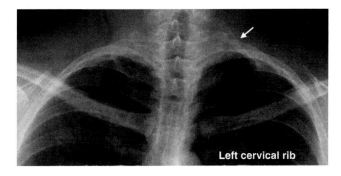

Figure 2H.6. Chest radiograph showing left cervical ribs (arrow). (From Dalman R, *Operative Techniques in Vascular Surgery*. Wolters Kluwer Health; 2016.)

IMAGING[4]

Plain Radiographs

- Standard chest radiographs: Evaluate for presence of cervical ribs (Figure 2H.6), bony abnormalities, and apical masses
- Cervical spine radiographs: Evaluate for evidence of diskogenic disease and spinal causes of symptoms

Dynamic Ultrasound

- Initial imaging study
- Can visualize flow changes in subclavian vessels with abduction and adduction of the arm
- Evaluate for presence of aneurysm
- Evaluate for venous compression
  - Decreased venous velocity by 50% with abduction
  - Presence of venous thickening consistent with deep vein thrombosis
  - Presence of acute vs chronic thrombus

Computed Tomography

- CT of the chest: evaluate arterial anatomy
  - Only used if concerned for aneurysm formation
- Use 3D reconstruction to evaluate the point of vascular compression

Magnetic Resonance Imaging

- Performed in provocative arm position to evaluate vasculature
- Can use MR neurogram to detect brachial plexus compression

Arteriography

- Used if diagnosis is unclear
- Can obtain dynamic imaging with adduction and abduction of the affected extremity
- Rarely needed to evaluate true arterial compression

REFERENCES

1. Sanders RJ, Hammond SL, Rao NM. Diagnosis of thoracic outlet syndrome. *J Vasc Surg.* 2007;46(3):601-604.
2. Adson AW, Coffey JR. Cervical rib: a method of anterior approach for relief of symptoms by division of the scalenus anticus. *Ann Surg.* 1927;85(6):839-857.
3. Wright IS. The neurovascular syndrome produced by hyperabduction of the arms: the immediate changes produced in 150 normal controls, and the effects on some persons of prolonged hyperabduction of the arms, as in sleeping, and in certain occupations. *Am Heart J.* 1945;21(9):1-19.

4. Leffert RD. Thoracic outlet syndrome. *J Am Acad Orthop Surg*. 1994;2(6):317-325.
5. Elvey RL, Quintner JL, Thomas AN. A clinical study of RSI. *Aust Fam Physician*. 1986;15:1314-1322.
6. Gilroy J, Meyer JS. Compression of the subclavian artery as a cause of ischemic brachial neuropathy. *Brain*. 1963;86:733-745.
7. Roos DM, Owens JC. Thoracic outlet syndrome. *Arch Surg*. 1966;93:71-74.

3
SECTION

The Hip

Section Editor
F. Winston Gwathmey

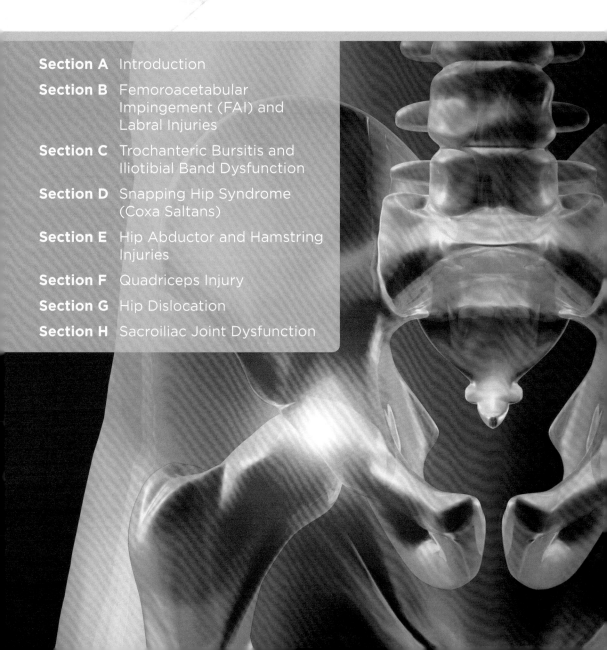

QUICK REFERENCE FLOW CHART

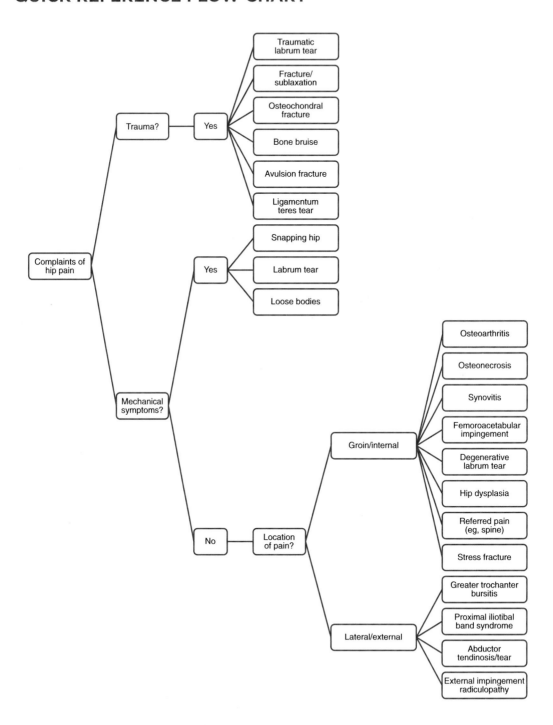

SECTION A
Introduction

James B. Carr, II

HISTORY

The hip joint is unique among lower extremity joints because it joins the axial skeleton to the appendicular skeleton. Smooth function of the hip is achieved through an appropriate balance of the surrounding bones, ligaments, and tendons. Injuries to these structures may cause pain, mechanical symptoms, or loss of function. It is important to consider the following parameters when a patient presents to the clinic with a hip complaint:

- Patient age
  - Younger patients are more likely to have complaints related to abnormal development of the hip joint, such as dysplasia or impingement. They are also more likely to have acute injuries from trauma or sports participation
  - Older patients are more likely to have chronic pain from overuse or osteoarthritis
- Chronicity of symptoms
  - Acute injuries may involve labrum tears, fractures, hip dislocation/subluxation, or synovitis
  - Chronic injuries may represent femoroacetabular impingement (FAI), osteoarthritis, posttraumatic arthritis, untreated labrum tears, stress fracture, or avascular necrosis of the femoral head
- Mechanism of injury (if any)
  - Rotation sports, such as golf, tennis, baseball, ballet, or martial arts, often lead to intra-articular injury
  - Contact sports, such as football and rugby, can lead to both extra-articular and intra-articular injuries depending on the exact mechanism of injury
  - Blow to lateral hip may result in chondral or labrum injury
  - Trauma can lead to high-energy injuries, including hip dislocation, hip subluxation, femoral head fracture, or chondral injury
  - Insidious onset of hip pain is very common and can indicate FAI, osteoarthritis, or bursitis
  - Worsening pain with activities of daily living that involve a deep squat, such as sitting down or getting out of a car, may suggest intra-articular pathology
- Associated swelling (effusion)
  - A clinically observable hip joint effusion is rarely evident. If present, one should think of bursitis, infection, or oncologic process
- Mechanical symptoms (locking, catching)
  - Commonly associated with intra-articular pathology, including labrum tears, chondral injuries, or instability
  - Must be delineated from "clunking," which is more commonly associated with extra-articular snapping hip syndromes
- History of hip injury
  - One must be concerned about reinjury
- History of hip surgery
  - Surgical treatment, including open and arthroscopic procedures, should be well documented and understood via previous operative reports and images when possible

- Prior treatment
  - Many patients with hip pain often have seen multiple doctors before presentation. It is important to understand the types of physicians previously seen along with any previous diagnoses
  - Treatment to date must be clearly defined, including both conservative and surgical measures
  - Conservative treatments often include rest, activity modification, ice, heat, oral or topical non-steroidal anti-inflammatory drugs (NSAIDs), physical therapy, injections, or shoe orthotics
  - Treatment and diagnostic workup for back pain, abdominal pain, or neurologic abnormality must be carefully noted to help rule out thoracolumbar etiology of pain, which is a common confounder when a patient presents with hip pain
- Current medications
- One-finger test: Ask patients to point, with 1 finger, to the area where it hurts (they often cannot do so, but it can be helpful)
  - Pain in the groin region often denotes intra-articular pathology, whereas pain in the lateral or posterior region may denote extra-articular pathology

PHYSICAL EXAMINATION

Observation

- Any soft tissue or bony contour abnormalities should be noted
  - Any asymmetry, including shoulder height, spinal alignment, or iliac crest height, may be indicative of scoliosis or a leg length discrepancy
- Overall lower extremity alignment and rotation should be carefully assessed
  - Excessive external rotation at the ankle may be indicative of excessive femoral retroversion
  - Excessive internal rotation at the ankle ("intoeing") may be indicative of excessive femoral anteversion
- The patient should be observed in both the standing and sitting positions
  - A stance of slight hip and knee flexion is often used by patients with intra-articular pathology to help offload the affected extremity
  - Similarly, patients may sit with less weight distributed to the affected extremity
- The patient should also be examined while ambulating
  - Hip hiking, circumduction, or excessive trunk extension or rotation may indicate muscle weakness, pain, or leg length discrepancy
  - A shortened stance phase or avoidance of hip extension may indicate pain from an intra-articular process
  - Abductor lurch occurs with shifting of the torso over the involved hip and may indicate abductor weakness

Palpation

- Effusion
- Palpation is a key part of the hip examination. Tenderness to palpation should be carefully noted to help isolate the location of pathology. Palpation of the following sites should be included with every hip examination:
  - Ischium: biceps femoris tendinitis, avulsion fracture, ischial bursitis
  - Anterior superior iliac spine: bone bruise, avulsion fracture
  - Anterior inferior iliac spine: bone bruise, avulsion fracture
  - Pubic symphysis: osteitis pubis, calcification, fracture
  - Adductor tubercle: adductor tendinitis, adductor strain/tear
  - Greater trochanter: greater trochanter bursitis, iliotibial (IT) band contracture
  - Gluteus maximus origin: gluteus maximus origin tendinitis
  - Gluteus maximus insertion: gluteus maximus tendinitis
  - Sacroiliac (SI) joint: sacroiliitis, distinguish between hip pain and back pain
  - Abdomen: fascial hernia, associated gastrointestinal or genitourinary pathology
  - Spine: mechanical pathology, rule out other spine pathology

Range of Motion ▶ (Figure 3A.1)

- Range of motion should be tested in both the seated and supine positions. The following values are commonly accepted as normal hip joint range of motion (degrees):
  - Seated internal rotation: 20 to 35
  - Seated external rotation: 30 to 45
  - Extended internal rotation: 20 to 35
  - Extended external rotation: 30 to 45
  - Supine hip flexion: 100 to 110
  - Supine adduction: 20 to 30
  - Supine abduction: 45

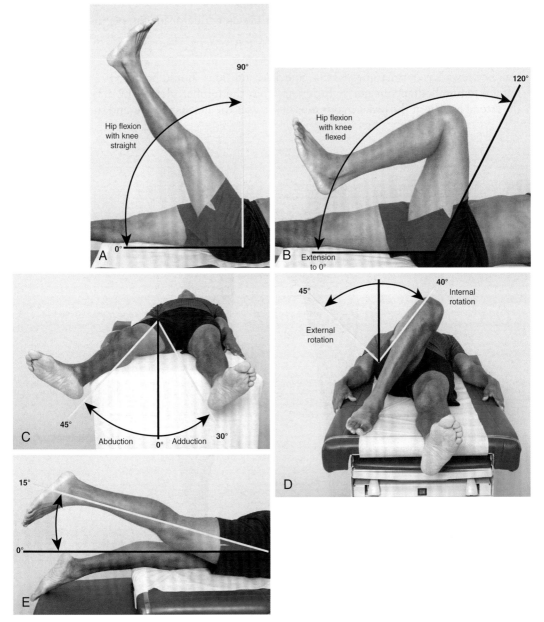

Figure 3A.1. Normal range of motion of the hips: A, hip flexion with extended knee straight; B, hip flexion with knee bent; C, abduction/adduction; D, internal and external rotation; and E, hyperextension.

- Any asymmetry in range of motion between the right and left sides should alert the examiner to the possible presence of pathology or anatomic differences between the 2 sides
- Loss of internal rotation of the hip joint is an early sign of intra-articular pathology

Muscular Strength

- Grading of the hip musculature follows the standard grade 1 to 5 scale
- Strength of the hip should be evaluated in every major plane of movement. Associated weakness in a plane may imply an injury to the following muscles:
  - Hip flexion: iliopsoas, rectus femoris, sartorius
  - Hip extension: gluteus maximus, biceps femoris, semitendinosus, semimembranosus, tensor fascia lata (TFL)
  - Hip abduction: gluteus medius, gluteus minimus
  - Hip adduction: adductor magnus, adductor brevis, adductor longus, pectineus, gracilis

Sensation (Figure 3A.2)

- Can be viewed as dermatomes L1-S4. Special conditions should be noted
- Lateral femoral cutaneous nerve: It derives from the lumbar plexus (L2-L3), emerges from the lateral border of the psoas major muscle, crosses the iliacus muscle, and then passes under

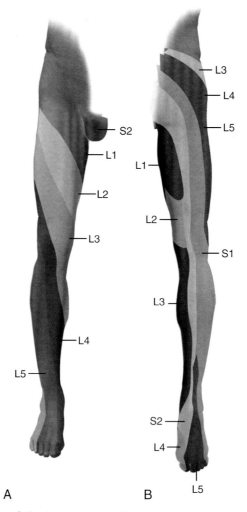

Figure 3A.2. Dermatomes of the lower extremity. A, Anterior view. B, Posterior view.

the inguinal ligament near the anterior superior iliac spine to supply sensation to the lateral thigh

- Meralgia paresthetica: tingling, numbness, and sometimes burning pain located in the outer thigh due to compression of the lateral femoral cutaneous nerve, which may be caused by trauma or tight clothing

KEY EXAMINATION MANEUVERS

- **FAI/Labral Injuries**
  - Asymmetric range of motion
  - Lateral rim impingement test
  - Posterior rim impingement test
  - Dynamic external rotatory impingement test (DEXRIT)
  - Dynamic internal rotatory impingement (DIRI) test
  - Stinchfield test
  - Passive supine rotation (log roll) test
  - Squat test
  - Flexion-abduction-external rotation (FABER) test
  - Flexion-adduction-internal rotation (FADDIR) test
  - Fitzgerald test

- **Trochanteric Bursitis/IT Band Dysfunction**
  - Greater trochanter palpation
  - Ober test
  - Resisted internal rotation of the thigh test

- **Snapping Hip Syndrome**
  - Ober test
  - Thomas test

- **Piriformis/Abductor/Hamstring Injury**
  - Active piriformis test
  - Piriformis stretch test
  - Lasègue sign (straight leg raise)
  - Trendelenburg test or sign
  - Resisted hip abduction
  - Puranen-Orava test
  - Bent knee stretch test

- **Quadriceps Injury**
  - Active extension test
  - Knee extension test

- **Hip Dislocation**
  - Supine external rotation test
  - Axial distraction test
  - Anterior apprehension test
  - Posterior apprehension test

- **SI Dysfunction**
  - Gaenslen test
  - Distraction (gapping) test
  - Compression test
  - FABER test
  - Thigh thrust test
  - Pressure over the sacral sulcus

IMAGING

Plain Radiographs (Figure 3A.3)

- Anteroposterior (AP) view (standing and sitting)
  - Neck shaft angle
    - Coxa varus vs coxa valgus
  - Lateral center edge angle
  - Tonnis angle
  - Crossover sign
- Frog-leg lateral view
  - Head-neck offset
  - Alpha angle
- Cross-table lateral view
- False profile view
  - Anterior center edge angle
- 45°- and 90° Dunn views
  - Head-neck offset
  - Alpha angle

Magnetic Resonance Imaging (Figure 3A.4)

- Labral tear
- Synovitis
- Effusion
- McKibbin instability index
- Alpha angle

Computed Tomography

- Femoral anteversion
- Helpful in assessing bony morphology in cam- and pincer-type impingement

Ultrasonography

- Dynamic assessment of snapping hip syndrome
- Evaluate hip joint effusion
- Evaluate iliopsoas tendon and bursa
- Evaluate hip abductor tendons and greater trochanter bursa

Hip Arthroscopy (Figure 3A.5)

- Portals
- Accessory portals
- Visualization

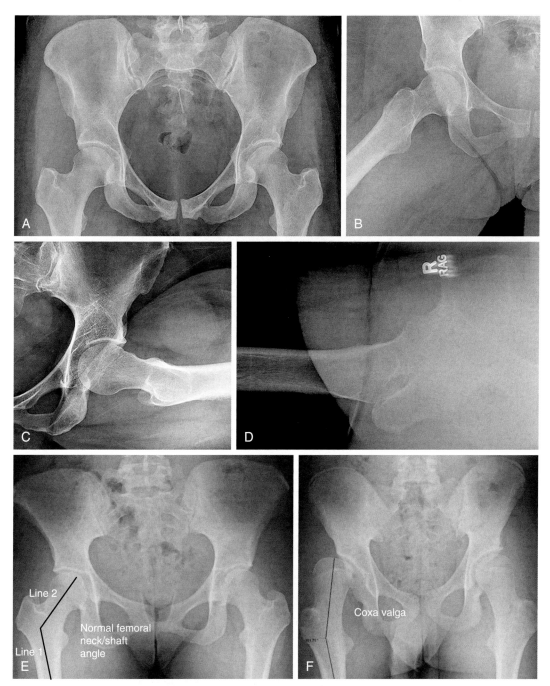

Figure 3A.3. Standard radiographs of the pelvis/hip. A, Anteroposterior (AP) view. B, Frog-leg lateral view of the hip. C, Dunn 90° lateral view, which optimizes visualization of the femoral neck and head-neck junction. D, Cross-table lateral view. E, A normal neck shaft angle. F, Coxa valga with an increased neck shaft angle. G, Coxa vara with a decreased neck shaft angle. H, AP pelvis radiograph displaying common radiographic measurements, including the lateral center edge angle (red), Tonnis angle (yellow), and lateral edge of the anterior (green) and posterior (blue) walls. I, Acetabular retroversion is seen when the acetabular rim (black dashed line) creates a crossover sign (black arrow), while the center of the femoral head (X) is lateral to the posterior wall and there is a prominent ischial spine sign (white dashed line and white arrow). J: False profile view. ((A–D) Borrowed from Callaghan JJ. *The Adult Hip: Hip Arthroplasty Surgery*. Wolters Kluwer Health; 2016; (E–G and J) Borrowed from Clohisy JC. *The Adult Hip: Hip Preservation Surgery*. Wolters Kluwer Health; 2015; (H) From SW, ed. *Operative Techniques in Orthopaedic Surgery*. 4 Vols. Wolters Kluwer Health; 2016; (I) From Barrack RL, Rosenberg AG. *The Hip*. Wolters Kluwer Health; 2016.)

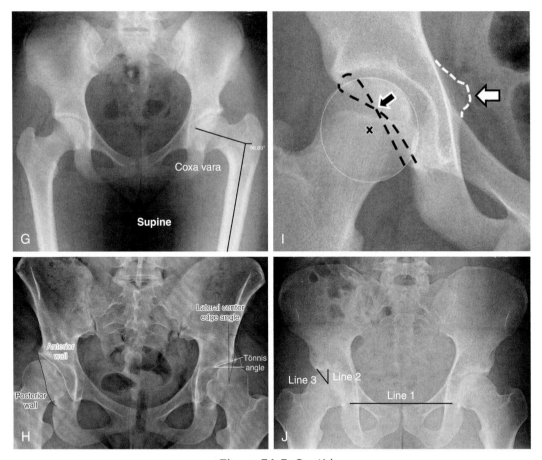

Figure 3A.3. Cont'd

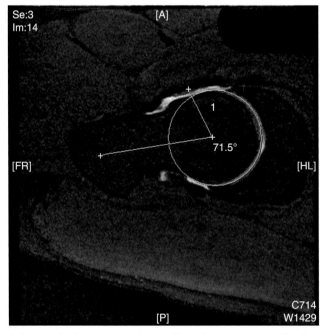

Figure 3A.4. The alpha angle is measured as a line drawn perpendicular to the narrow part of the femoral neck. A circle is drawn that most closely approximates the head size. A line is drawn from the center of the head to the point where the anterolateral femoral head exceeds the radius of the circle. The angle made by these 2 lines is the alpha angle. In this example, the alpha angle is 71°. An angle <50° or 55° is considered normal. (Figure used by permission of Marc R. Safran, MD.)

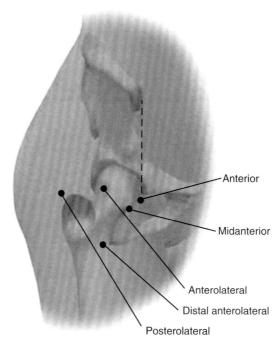

Figure 3A.5. Portals and landmarks for hip arthroscopy. The anterior superior iliac spine (ASIS) and greater trochanter are the landmarks for establishing arthroscopy portals. The dashed line represents a vertical line extending distally from the ASIS. This is a useful reference for portal placement. The anterolateral portal is usually established first with a spinal needle under fluoroscopic guidance, approximately 1 cm superior to the anterior edge of the greater trochanter. The anterior or midanterior portal is then established under direct visualization. The classic anterior portal was placed at the intersection of a line drawn distally from the greater trochanter and a line drawn perpendicularly from the greater trochanter at a 45° angle. The midanterior portal is located 6 to 8 cm distal and anteromedial to the anterolateral portal and has the advantage of being further away from the lateral femoral cutaneous nerve and rectus femoris tendon than the anterior portal. A posterolateral portal can be established if necessary, 1 cm posterior to the posterosuperior border of the greater trochanter and on a line parallel to the anterolateral portal. Care should be taken when establishing the posterior portal, as it lies close to the medial femoral circumflex artery and sciatic nerve. A distal anterolateral portal can be placed approximately 4 to 5 cm distal and in line with the lateral portal. The distal anterolateral portal allows more parallel positioning of the labral repair anchor along the acetabular rim and can also be used as the working portal for femoral osteochondroplasty. (Borrowed from Clohisy JC. *The Adult Hip: Hip Preservation Surgery*. Wolters Kluwer Health; 2015.)

SECTION B
Femoroacetabular Impingement (FAI) and Labral Injuries

Samuel Evan Carstensen

HISTORY

- FAI was first described by Mayers[9] in 1999, although Stulberg[10] described degenerative arthritis of the hip due to abnormal hip morphology in 1975
- Many patients have clicking +/– pain in their affected hip
- Labral tears classically are insidious in onset but may be related to trauma
  - FAI symptomatic in active patients, especially those who require extremes of hip range of motion
- Patients often present in the second or third decade of life

PHYSICAL EXAMINATION

KEY EXAMINATION MANEUVERS

- Asymmetric Range of Motion (Figure 3B.1)
  - Basic physical examination maneuver when examining the hip
  - Please refer to normal passive hip range of motion in the introduction (section 3A)
  - **Maneuver:**
    - The patient lies supine with both hips in a neutral position
    - The examiner then takes the unaffected hip through a full range of motion, including flexion, abduction, adduction, internal rotation, and external rotation
    - The contralateral (affected) leg is then tested in an identical manner
  - **Limitations of Maneuver:**
    - Patients may guard on the affected side due to anticipated or current pain

- Lateral Rim Impingement Test (Figure 3B.2)
  - The origin of the lateral rim impingement test is unknown
  - There have been no major modifications
  - **Maneuver:**
    - The patient lies supine with both hips in a neutral position
    - The examiner stands on the side of the affected limb and holds the leg with 1 arm while monitoring the hip joint with the other hand
    - The examiner passively abducts the involved hip, going through a full arc range of motion, while keeping the hip externally rotated
    - Positive test: reproduction of pain or symptoms

- Posterior Rim Impingement Test (Sensitivity 0.755, Specificity 0.85) (Figure 3B.3)
  - The origin of the lateral rim impingement test is unknown
  - There have been no major modifications

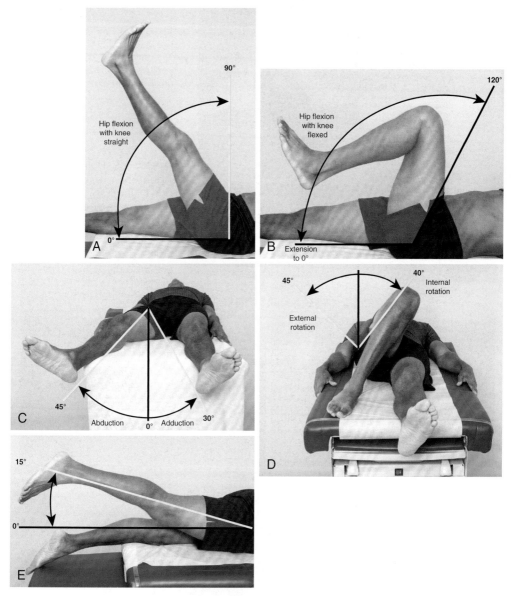

Figure 3B.1. Normal range of motion of the hip. (Borrowed from Weber J, Kelley J. *Health Assessment in Nursing*. Wolters Kluwer Health; 2014.)

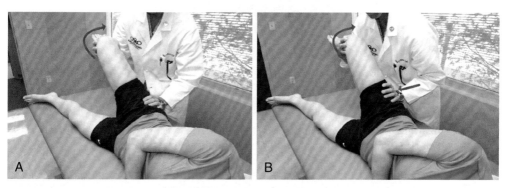

Figure 3B.2. Lateral rim impingement test. (Borrowed from Callaghan JJ. *The Adult Hip: Hip Arthroplasty Surgery*. Wolters Kluwer Health; 2016.)

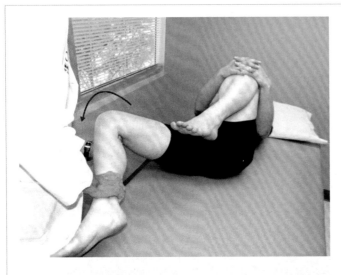

Figure 3B.3. Posterior rim impingement test. (Borrowed from Callaghan JJ. *The Adult Hip: Hip Arthroplasty Surgery.* Wolters Kluwer Health; 2016.)

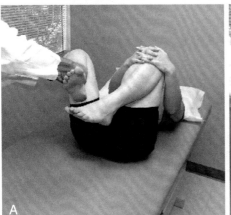

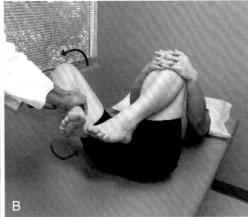

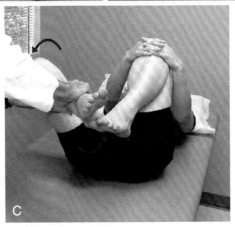

Figure 3B.4. Dynamic external rotatory impingement test (DEXRIT). (Borrowed from Callaghan JJ. *The Adult Hip: Hip Arthroplasty Surgery.* Wolters Kluwer Health; 2016.)

- **Maneuver:**
  - The examiner stands on the affected side of the patient with the patient on the edge of the examination table to permit full hip extension
  - The examiner has the patient start with both hips in full flexion
  - The examiner then extends the affected leg in full extension hanging off of the table then taken into abduction and external rotation
  - Positive test: reproduction of pain or symptoms

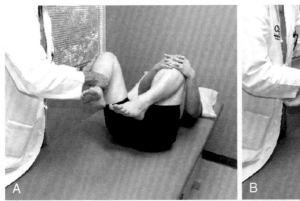
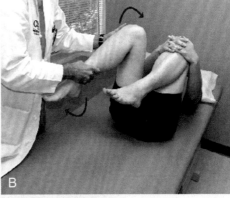
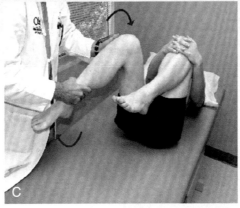

Figure 3B.5. Dynamic internal rotatory impingement (DIRI) test. (Borrowed from Callaghan JJ. *The Adult Hip: Hip Arthroplasty Surgery*. Wolters Kluwer Health; 2016.)

- DEXRIT (Sensitivity 0.50, Specificity 0.29) (Figure 3B.4)
  - First described by McCarthy in 2003[6]
  - There have been no major modifications
  - **Maneuver:**
    - The examiner stands on the affected side of the patient
    - The examiner then dynamically takes the hip from 90° flexion or beyond through an arc of abduction and external rotation through to extension
    - Positive test: production of pain or instability
- DIRI Test (Sensitivity 0.50, Specificity 0.29) (Figure 3B.5)
  - First described by McCarthy in 2003[6]
  - When combined with the DEXRIT, the combination is referred to as the McCarthy test
  - This test has been modified to the Scour test (as below)
  - **Maneuver:**
    - The examiner stands on the affected side of the patient
    - The hip is dynamically taken in a wide arc from abduction/external rotation to flexion, adduction, and internal rotation
    - Positive test: reproduction of symptoms
  - Modification of DIRI
    - Scour test (Sensitivity 0.50, Specificity 0.29) (Figure 3B.6)
      - **Maneuver:**
        - The examiner stands on the affected side of the patient
        - The examiner passively flexes and adducts the hip with knee in full flexion
        - A downward force is applied along the femoral shaft while adducting and externally/internally rotating the hip
        - Positive test: pain or apprehension in any range of motion
- Stinchfield Test (Sensitivity 0.59, Specificity 0.32) (Figure 3B.7)
  - Described by Frank Stinchfield although it was not labeled as such until the early 1990s[7]
  - There have been no major modifications

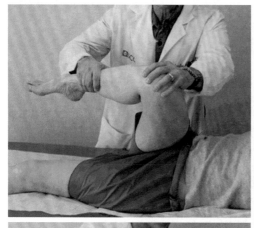
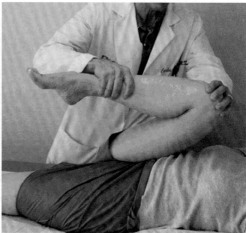
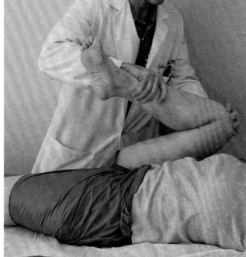

Figure 3B.6. Scour test (dynamic internal rotatory impingement [DIRI] modification). (Borrowed from Guanche CA. *Hip and Pelvis Injuries in Sports Medicine*. Philadelphia: Wolters Kluwer/Lippincott Williams & Wilkin; 2010.)

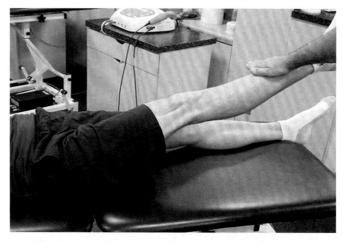

Figure 3B.7. Stinchfield test. (Borrowed from Johnson D, Amendola NA, Barber F. *Operative Arthroscopy*. Philadelphia: Wolters Kluwer; 2015.)

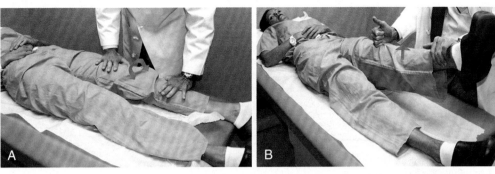

Figure 3B.8. Passive supine rotation (log roll) test. (Borrowed from Clohisy JC. *The Adult Hip: Hip Preservation Surgery*. Philadelphia: Wolters Kluwer; 2015.)

- **Maneuver:**
  - The examiner stands on the affected side
  - The patient lies supine and then actively flexes the hip to 20° to 30° with the knee in full extension
  - The examiner then applies resistance to the flexed thigh and leg simulating a joint force many times that of the patient's body weight
  - Positive test: pain in the anterior groin

- Passive Supine Rotation (Log Roll) Test 🔵 (Sensitivity 0.28, Specificity 0.91) (Figure 3B.8)
  - As this is a basic physical examination maneuver, there have been no major modifications
  - **Maneuver:**
    - The examiner stands on the affected side of the patient who lies supine on the examination table
    - With the hip in full extension, the lower extremity is internally and externally rotated
    - Positive pain: pain about hip or radiation of pain to the groin

- Squat Test (Sensitivity 0.75, Specificity 0.41) (Figure 3B.9)
  - This was described and clinically evaluated by Lamontagne et al in 2009[3]
  - There have been no major modifications
  - **Maneuver:**
    - The patient stands erect with feet shoulder width apart, back and shoulders neutral, arms forward flexed at the shoulder to 90° with elbows in full extension
    - The examiner stands facing the patient
    - The patient squats as deeply as possible with feet hip width apart
    - Positive test: pain in anterior thigh or groin on the affected side

- FABER Test 🔵 (Sensitivity 0.42-0.60, Specificity 0.18-0.75) (Figure 3B.10)
  - Also known as the Patrick test, it was first described by Hugh Talbot Patrick in 1917[8]
  - There have been no major modifications
  - **Maneuver:**
    - The patient lies supine with the examiner standing on the affected side
    - The patient's hip is fully flexed, abduct, and externally rotated
    - Positive test: recreation of symptoms of pain or impingement on the ipsilateral side, as the test is being performed upon

- FADDIR or Anterior Impingement Test 🔵 (Sensitivity 0.94-0.99, Specificity 0.05) (Figure 3B.11)
  - First described by Klaue and coworkers in 1991[2]
  - There have been no major modifications except that the test may also be performed in the lateral position
  - The most sensitive test for FAI

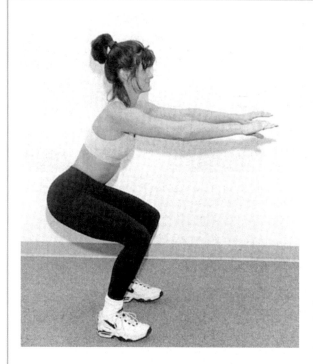

Figure 3B.9. Squat test. (Cox JM. *Low Back Pain: Mechanism, Diagnosis, and Treatment.* Philadelphia: Wolters Kluwer/Lippincott Williams & Wilkins; 2011.)

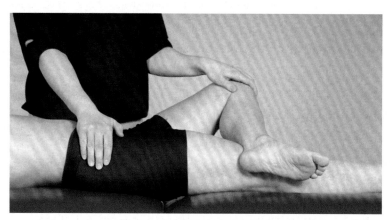

Figure 3B.10. Flexion-abduction-external rotation (FABER) test. (Borrowed from Anderson MK, Barnum M. *Foundations of Athletic Training: Prevention, Assessment, and Management.* Wolters Kluwer Health; 2017.)

- **Maneuver:**
  - The patient lies supine with the examiner standing on the affected side
  - The examiner fully flexes, adducts, and internally rotates the hip and takes it through an arc of motion
  - The contralateral hip should also be tested at this time
  - Positive test: recreation of symptoms of pain or impingement
- Fitzgerald Test (Sensitivity 0.98, Specificity unknown)
  - First described by Fitzgerald[1] in 1995

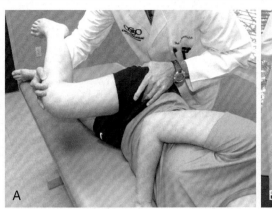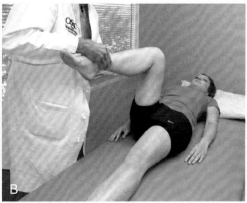

Figure 3B.11. Flexion-adduction-internal rotation (FADDIR) or anterior impingement test. (Borrowed from Callaghan JJ. *The Adult Hip: Hip Arthroplasty Surgery*. Wolters Kluwer Health; 2016.)

- **Maneuver:**
  - The examiner stands on the affect side with the patient in the supine position
  - The affected hip is brought into acute flexion, external rotation, and full abduction
  - The hip is then extended with internal rotation and adduction
  - Positive test: precipitated pain +/− clicking

IMAGING

Imaging is a mainstay in the workup for hip pathology.

Plain Radiographs (Figure 3B.12)

- Plain radiographs are the first step in radiographic evaluation of a painful hip. Specific views, as listed below, may reveal findings that may otherwise not be
- AP
  - Assess for an acceptable AP radiograph where the coccyx overlaps the pubic symphysis
    - Crossover sign: possible retroversion of the hip
    - Posterior wall sign: possible lack of posterior wall coverage
  - Obturators should be the same and ovoid in shape
- Lateral
  - Lateral radiographs of the affected hip are essential to evaluate the medial to lateral planes
- Dunn view
  - Pelvis neutral, hips flexed to 90° and abducted 20°
- Measurements (performed on AP and Dunn view):
  - Alpha angle: normal <55°
  - Lateral center-edge angle: normal 25° to 39°

Magnetic Resonance Imaging (MRI) (Figure 3B.13)

- MRI is essential for preoperative planning
- May reveal other pathology about the hip as well as provide significant insight as to the status of the labrum and chondral surfaces
- The sensitivity of 3.0T MRI is comparable with 3.0T magnetic resonance arthrography (MRA) in diagnosing labral tears, but not for articular surface handrail defects[4]

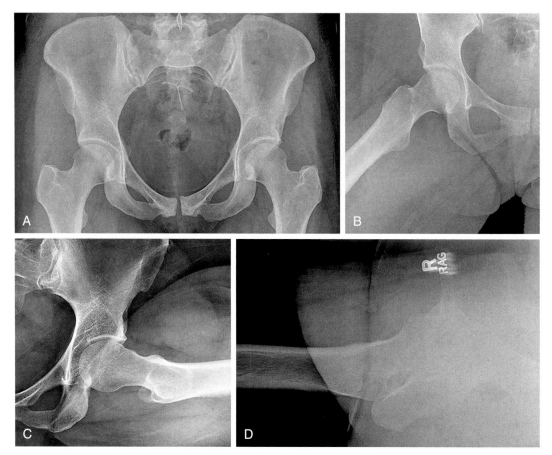

Figure 3B.12. Plain radiographs of the pelvis and hip in a patient with mixed-type FAI. A, Anteroposterior view of pelvis. B, Frog-leg lateral view of hip. C, Dunn 90° lateral view. The Dunn view optimizes visualization of the femoral neck and head-neck junction. As shown in this image, it can demonstrate abnormal bony proliferation and asphericity of the femoral head. D, Cross-table lateral view. (Borrowed from Callaghan JJ. *The Adult Hip: Hip Arthroplasty Surgery*. Wolters Kluwer Health; 2016.)

Computed Tomography (CT) (Figure 3B.14)

- CT is a modality not typically indicated for the assessment or treatment of FAI and labral tears but may provide more osseous detail regarding pincer and cam deformities

Ultrasonography (Figure 3B.15)

- Ultrasonography may be utilized in the setting of hip injections to provide immediate and dynamic feedback when accessing the hip joint
- Continued studies focus on the utility of ultrasonography to help diagnose hip and labral pathology

Hip Arthroscopy (Figure 3B.16)

Hip arthroscopy is often utilized in the treatment of FAI.

- Gold standard for intra-articular hip pathology
- Affords a minimally invasive approach by which to view and address pathology of the hip
- 30° and 70° scopes, much of the joint capsule can be viewed and examined

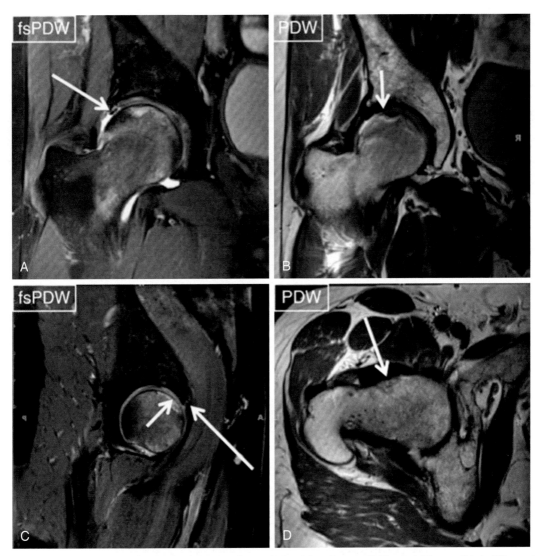

Figure 3B.13. Magnetic resonance imaging of the hip. Coronal (A and B), sagittal (C), and axial (D) images from the same individual show superolateral and anterosuperior labral tears (long arrows in A and C), a subchondral insufficiency fracture of the superior femoral head (short arrows in B and C), along with inadequate femoral head-neck offset with fibrocystic change (arrow in D), related to cam-type femoroacetabular impingement. (Borrowed from Chhabra A, Soldatos T. *Musculoskeletal MRI Structured Evaluation: How to Practically Fill the Reporting Checklist.* Wolters Kluwer Health; 2015.)

- Soft tissue and bony abnormalities may be addressed arthroscopically
  - Both cam and pincer lesions may be addressed by hip arthroscopy
    - Cam lesions require the femoral head-neck junction to be "normalized" by removing the excess bone in the anterosuperior aspect of the femoral neck
    - Pincer lesions require the acetabulum to be addressed
- Main portals (Figure 3B.17)
  - Anterior
  - Anterolateral
  - Posterolateral

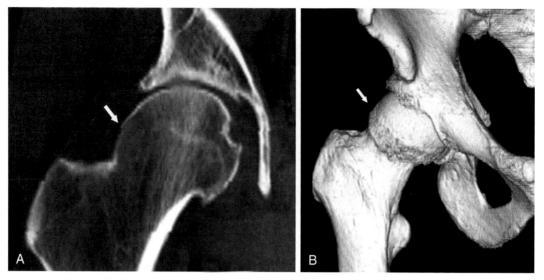

Figure 3B.14. Selected coronal CT of right hip (A) with 3D reconstruction (B). Arrow in both figures denotes the CAM deformity of the femoral head. (Borrowed from Greenspan A, Beltran J. *Orthopedic Imaging: A Practical Approach*. Wolters Kluwer Health; 2015.)

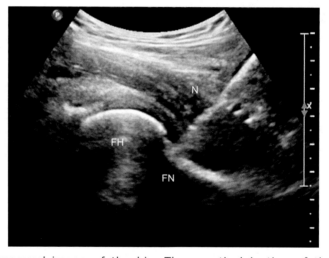

Figure 3B.15. Ultrasound image of the hip. Therapeutic injection of the hip is typically performed using a long-axis technique. The needle (N) is advanced to the femoral head-neck junction. A small injection of anesthetic may be used to confirm the position. FH, femoral head; FN, femoral neck. (Borrowed from Greenspan A, Beltran J. *Orthopedic Imaging: A Practical Approach*. Wolters Kluwer Health; 2015.)

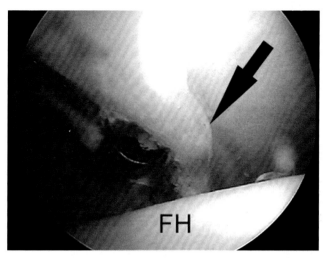

Figure 3B.16. Intra-articular view during hip arthroscopy. Initial view of unstable labral flap (arrow) laterally. FH, femoral head. (Borrowed from Johnson D, Amendola NA, Barber F. *Operative Arthroscopy*. Philadelphia: Wolters Kluwer; 2015.)

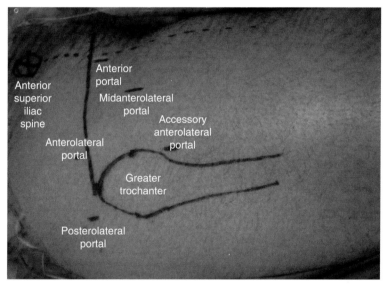

Figure 3B.17. Hip arthroscopy portals. Portals and landmarks for hip arthroscopy. The anterior superior iliac spine (ASIS) and greater trochanter are the landmarks for establishing arthroscopy portals. The dashed line represents a vertical line extending distally from the ASIS. This is a useful reference for portal placement. The anterolateral portal is usually established first with a spinal needle under fluoroscopic guidance, approximately 1 cm superior to the anterior edge of the greater trochanter. The anterior or midanterior portal is then established under direct visualization. The classic anterior portal was placed at the intersection of a line drawn distally from the greater trochanter and a line drawn perpendicularly from the greater trochanter at a 45° angle. The midanterior portal is located 6 to 8 cm distal and anteromedial to the anterolateral portal and has the advantage of being further away from the lateral femoral cutaneous nerve and rectus femoris tendon than the anterior portal. A posterolateral portal can be established if necessary, 1 cm posterior to the posterosuperior border of the greater trochanter and on a line parallel to the anterolateral portal. Care should be taken when establishing the posterior portal, as it lies close to the medial femoral circumflex artery and sciatic nerve 85. A distal anterolateral portal can be placed approximately 4 to 5 cm distal and in line with the lateral portal. The distal anterolateral portal allows more parallel positioning of the labral repair anchor along the acetabular rim and can also be used as the working portal for femoral osteochondroplasty. (Borrowed from Guanche CA. *Hip and Pelvis Injuries in Sports Medicine*. Philadelphia: Wolters Kluwer/Lippincott Williams & Wilkin; 2010.)

REFERENCES

1. Fitzgerald RH. Acetabular labrum tears: diagnosis and treatment. *Clin Orthop*. 1995;311:60-68.
2. Klaue K, Durnin CW, Ganz R. The acetabular rim syndrome: a clinical presentation of dysplasia of the hip. *J Bone Joint Surg Br*. 1991;73B:423-429.
3. Lamontagne M, Kennedy MJ, Beaulé PE. The effect of cam FAI on hip and pelvic motion during maximum squat. *Clin Orthop Relat Res*. 2009;467(3):645-650.
4. Magee T. Comparison of 3.0-T MR vs 3.0-T MR arthrography of the hip for detection of acetabular labral tears and chondral defects in the same patient population. *Br J Radiol*. 2015;88(1053):20140817.
5. Maslowski E, Sullivan W, Forster Harwood J, et al. The diagnostic validity of hip provocation maneuvers to detect intra-articular hip pathology. *Pharm Manag PM R*. 2010;2(3):174-181.
6. McCarthy JC, Busconi BD, Owens BD. Assessment of the painful hip. In: McCarthy JC, ed. *Early Hip Disorders*. New York, NY: Springer; 2003:3-6.
7. McGrory BJ. Stinchfield resisted hip flexion test. *Hosp Phys*. 1999;35:41-42.
8. Patrick HT. Brachial neuritis and sciatica. *J Am Med Assoc*. 1917;LXIX:2176-2179.
9. Mayers SR, Eijer H, Ganz R. Anterior femoroacetabular impingement after periacetabular osteotomy. *Clin Ortop*. 1999;363:93-99.
10. Stulberg SD, Cordell LD, Harris WH, et al. Unrecognised childhood disease: a major cause of idiopathic osteoarthritis of the hip. *The Proceedings of the Third Open Scientific Meeting of the Hip Society*. St Louis, MO: CV Mosby;1975;212-228.

SECTION C
Trochanteric Bursitis and Iliotibial Band Dysfunction

James B. Carr, II

HISTORY

- Patients with trochanteric bursitis or IT band dysfunction often present with a chief complaint of lateral hip pain
  - Caused by repetitive overuse plus acute inflammation in young patients and degenerative changes in older patients
- Greater trochanteric bursitis (GTB) refers to inflammation of the peritrochanteric bursa
  - Most commonly affected bursa is the subgluteus maximus bursa, which is the largest one along the lateral hip and located between the gluteus maximus muscle and the gluteus medius tendon (Figure 3C.1)
  - GTB is frequently diagnosed in patients with lateral hip pain, although imaging studies have revealed that these patients more commonly have abductor tears, tendinosis, and thickened IT bands with only a minority of patients actually having bursitis[1-3]
  - Proposed etiology is repetitive friction between the greater trochanter and IT band
    - Repetitive friction may be from overuse, leg length discrepancy, altered gait pattern, or trauma
  - Patients often report an insidious onset of lateral hip pain without known trauma
    - Pain may radiate along the IT band and even below the knee
  - Aggravating factors include sleeping on the affected side, side-bending, sitting with crossed legs, climbing stairs, running or other high-impact activities, and prolonged sitting or standing

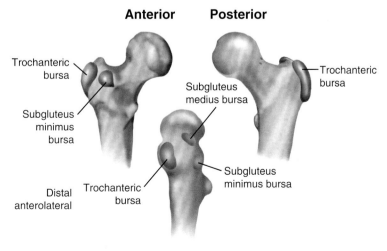

Figure 3C.1. The bursa surrounding the greater trochanter.

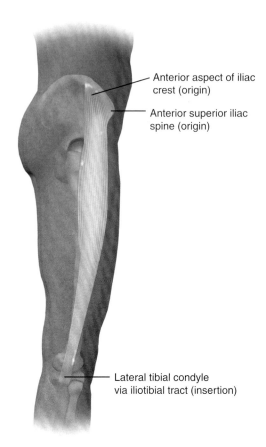

Anterior aspect of iliac crest (origin)

Anterior superior iliac spine (origin)

Lateral tibial condyle via iliotibial tract (insertion)

Figure 3C.2. Tensor fascia lata muscle (lateral aspect) showing the origin, insertion, action, and innervation.

- Alternative sources of lateral hip pain must be considered in unremitting cases, including spinal pathology (section 7), degenerative joint disease, meralgia paresthetica, gluteus medius or minimus tears (section 3E), external coxa saltans (section 3D), or intra-articular pathology
- Proximal IT band syndrome is a rare overuse injury most frequently seen in female runners or obese individuals[4,5]
  - Most patients present with gradually worsening lateral hip pain at the region of the proximal IT band enthesis along the iliac tubercle (Figure 3C.2)
  - First described by Sher et al[4] in 2011 after investigation of magnetic resonance imaging tests of 67 patients with lateral hip pain
    – Diagnosis made in 7 patients (4 female athletes, 3 obese nonathletes) who demonstrated a unique strain pattern at the proximal IT band enthesis along the iliac tubercle
  - Likely more common in females due to greater ratio between pelvic width and femoral length compared with males, which generates greater hip adductor movement and subsequent overload of lateral musculature to maintain pelvic balance[6]

PHYSICAL EXAMINATION

- In addition to the general hip examination described in the introduction section, the examiner should pay close attention to the following examination findings in a patient with suspected GTB or proximal IT band syndrome
  - Pain over the greater trochanter or IT band at the extremes of abduction and/or external rotation of the hip
  - Reduced range of motion, especially in abduction and/or external rotation of the hip
  - Leg length discrepancy may aggravate the greater trochanter bursa of the long extremity due to gait irregularity

- **Tenderness to Palpation** (Figure 3C.3)
  - **Maneuver**:
    - Patient lies on the examination table with affected side facing upward
    - The examiner palpates the region of the greater trochanter, using care to isolate the region directly adjacent to the most prominent area of the trochanter
    - The examiner also palpates along the iliac tubercle to assess the proximal enthesis of the IT band
  - **Limitations of Maneuver:**
    - May be difficult to palpate in obese patients. The greater trochanter is generally 20 cm below the pelvic brim in line with the iliac crest and the femur
    - Sensitive but not specific for any particular pathology

- **Ober Test** ▶ (Figure 3C.4)
  - First described in the literature in 1936 by Dr Frank R. Ober[7]
    - Initially developed to stretch the IT band and TFL in patients with low-back pain or sciatica
  - Modified by Kendall et al[8] in 1952 by extending the knee to 0° before the stretch
    - Both the original and modified Ober test have shown similar inter- and intraexaminer reliability[9-11]
  - **Maneuver**:
    - The examiner stands behind the patient in the lateral decubitus position with the affected side upward
    - The unaffected leg is placed in hip and knee flexion to eliminate lumbar lordosis
    - Place 1 hand on the iliac crest to support and stabilize the pelvis
    - The other hand supports underneath the knee, which is maintained at 90° of knee flexion
    - The examiner then brings the affected leg into hip abduction and extension until the leg is in line with the trunk

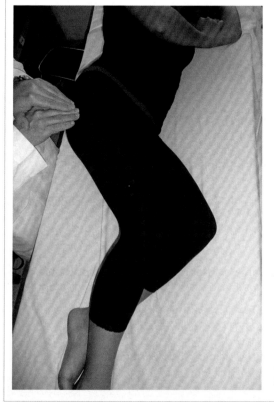

Figure 3C.3. Pain may be reproduced with palpation behind the tip of the greater trochanter. (Borrowed from Clohisy JC. *The Adult Hip: Hip Preservation Surgery*. Philadelphia: Wolters Kluwer; 2015.)

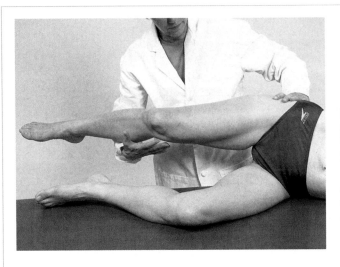

Figure 3C.4. Ober test. In a positive Ober test, adduction is limited when the hip is held in extension and neutral rotation. (From Oatis CA. *Kinesiology - The Mechanics and Pathomechanics of Human Movement*. Baltimore: Lippincott Williams & Wilkins; 2004.)

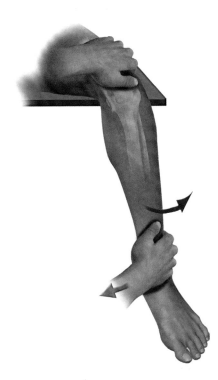

Figure 3C.5. Resisted internal rotation of the thigh test is performed when the patient actively resists the examiner (arrow) as an internal rotation force is applied to the leg.

- The leg is then lowered toward the table. Any limitation to the knee reaching the table is noted as a positive sign for IT band tightness
- Placing the examined leg in 0° of knee extension and then repeating the examination maneuver completes the modified Ober test
- **Limitations of Maneuver:**
  - Helps diagnose IT band tightness but rarely reproduces patient's symptoms
  - Performing test at higher knee flexion angles leads to less isolation of IT band

- **Resisted Internal Rotation of The Thigh Test** (Sensitivity: 0.88, Specificity: 0.97) (Figure 3C.5)
  - First described in the literature in 1961 by Gordon[12]
    - Performing a hip FABER maneuver elicited pain in 35 of 61 patients with a clinical diagnosis of GTB and abductor tendinopathy

- Modified by Bird et al[13] in 2001 to include resisted internal rotation (active external derotation) of a leg in neutral rotation
- Further modified by Lequesne et al[14] in 2008 to include resisted internal rotation of the hip with the hip and knee flexed to 90°
- **Maneuver:**
  - The examiner stands to the side of the patient in the supine position
  - The unaffected leg is relaxed in a neutral knee and hip position
  - The affected leg is brought to 90° of both hip and knee flexion followed by maximum external rotation
  - If lateral hip pain is elicited with complete external rotation, then it is decreased until there is no pain
  - The examiner then asks the patient to internally rotate the hip against resistance until it has returned to the neutral position while maintaining hip and knee in 90° of flexion
  - The test is considered positive if it reproduces spontaneous pain along the lateral hip
- **Limitations of Maneuver:**
  - Sensitive and specific for GTB and gluteus medius tendinopathy although it does not differentiate between the 2 entities
  - Can also be positive in individuals with snapping hip syndrome

IMAGING

Plain Radiographs

- Helpful in ruling out other pathologies, including hip degenerative joint disease, FAI, or hip dysplasia
- A greater trochanter protruding more lateral than the lateral border of the iliac crest has been shown to be a predisposing risk factor for GTB[15]
- Intrabursal calcification, calcific abductor tendinosis, and enthesophytes may be observed (Figure 3C.6)
  - Typically, peritrochanteric calcifications are nonspecific findings

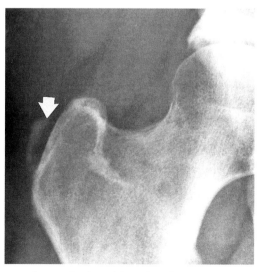

Figure 3C.6. Calcifying trochanteric bursitis. The faint amorphous calcification (arrow) separated from the lateral cortex of the greater trochanter coincides with the location of the trochanteric bursa. (From Pope TL, Harris JH, Harris JH. *Harris & Harris' Radiology of Emergency Medicine.* Wolters Kluwer; 2013.)

Computed Tomography

- Rarely beneficial for diagnosis of GTB or IT band pathology

Magnetic Resonance Imaging

- Gold standard for diagnosis of GTB, IT band pathology, and both intra- and extra-articular sources of lateral hip pain
- Usually reserved for patients with unremitting lateral hip pain without a complete diagnosis
- GTB diagnosed when inflammation and fluid collection is seen within the region of the greater trochanter bursa (Figure 3C.7)

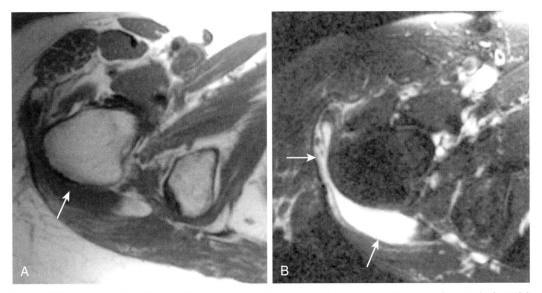

Figure 3C.7. Axial T1- (A) and T2-weighted (B) images demonstrating trochanteric bursitis (arrows). (Borrowed from Berquist TH, ed. *MRI of the Musculoskeletal System*. 6th ed. Philadelphia, PA: Wolters Kluwer; 2013)

Ultrasonography

- Very helpful modality becoming increasingly popular for diagnosis of lateral hip pain (Figure 3C.8)
- Dynamic component can help diagnose external snapping hip (section 3D) or isolate exact area of gluteal tendinopathy
- Long et al[1] reviewed 877 trochanteric sonograms in patients with lateral hip pain and found that 50% demonstrated gluteal tendinosis, 28.5% had a thickened IT band, 20% had GTB, and 0.5% had a gluteal tendon tear

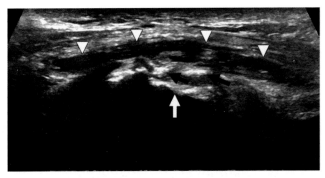

Figure 3C.8. Ultrasound image of the left lateral hip demonstrating linear echogenic foci with posterior acoustic shadowing (black arrows) in the expected position of the gluteus medius and minimus tendon insertions onto the greater trochanter (white arrow) in keeping with focal calcifications in the tendon. There is also a linear hypoechoic fluid collection (white arrowheads) between the gluteus maximus tendon and the gluteus medius tendon consistent with GTB. (From Chowdhury R, Naaseri S, Lee J, et al. Imaging and management of greater trochanteric pain syndrome. *Postgrad Med J.* 2014;90(1068):576-581.)

REFERENCES

1. Long SS, Surrey DE, Nazarian LN. Sonography of greater trochanteric pain syndrome and the rarity of primary bursitis. *AJR Am J Roentgenol.* 2013;201(5):1083-1086. doi:10.2214/AJR.12.10038.
2. Robertson WJ, Gardner MJ, Barker JU, Boraiah S, Lorich DG, Kelly BT. Anatomy and dimensions of the gluteus medius tendon insertion. *Arthroscopy.* 2008;24(2):130-136. doi:10.1016/j.arthro.2007.11.015.
3. Pfirrmann CW, Chung CB, Theumann NH, Trudell DJ, Resnick D. Greater trochanter of the hip: attachment of the abductor mechanism and a complex of three bursae–MR imaging and MR bursography in cadavers and MR imaging in asymptomatic volunteers. *Radiology.* 2001;221(2):469-477. doi:10.1148/radiol.2211001634.
4. Sher I, Umans H, Downie SA, Tobin K, Arora R, Olson TR. Proximal iliotibial band syndrome: what is it and where is it? *Skeletal Radiol.* 2011;40(12):1553-1556. doi:10.1007/s00256-011-1168-5.
5. Huang BK, Campos JC, Michael Peschka PG, et al. Injury of the gluteal aponeurotic fascia and proximal iliotibial band: anatomy, pathologic conditions, and MR imaging. *Radiographics.* 2013;33(5):1437-1452. doi:10.1148/rg.335125171.
6. Ferber R, Davis IM, Williams 3rd DS. Gender differences in lower extremity mechanics during running. *Clin Biomech.* 2003;18(4):350-357. doi:10.1016/S0268-0033(03)00025-1.
7. Ober F. The role of the iliotibial band and fascia lata as a factor in the causation of low-back disabilities and sciatica. *J Bone Joint Surg.* 1936;18:105-110.
8. Kendall H, Kendall F, Boynton D. *Posture and Pain.* Baltimore: Williams & Wilkins; 1952:135-138.
9. Gajdosik RL, Sandler MM, Marr HL. Influence of knee positions and gender on the ober test for length of the iliotibial band. *Clin Biomech.* 2003;18(1):77-79. doi:10.1016/S0268-0033(02)00168-7.
10. Melchione WE, Sullivan MS. Reliability of measurements obtained by use of an instrument designed to indirectly measure iliotibial band length. *J Orthop Sports Phys Ther.* 1993;18(3):511-515. doi:10.2519/jospt.1993.18.3.511.
11. Reese NB, Bandy WD. Use of an inclinometer to measure flexibility of the iliotibial band using the ober test and the modified ober test: differences in magnitude and reliability of measurements. *J Orthop Sports Phys Ther.* 2003;33(6):326-330. doi:10.2519/jospt.2003.33.6.326.
12. Gordon EJ. Trochanteric bursitis and tendinitis. *Clin Orthop.* 1961;20:193-202.
13. Bird PA, Oakley SP, Shnier R, Kirkham BW. Prospective evaluation of magnetic resonance imaging and physical examination findings in patients with greater trochanteric pain syndrome. *Arthritis Rheum.* 2001;44(9):2138-2145. doi:10.1002/1529-0131(200109)44:93.0.CO;2-M.
14. Lequesne M, Mathieu P, Vuillemin-Bodaghi V, Bard H, Djian P. Gluteal tendinopathy in refractory greater trochanter pain syndrome: diagnostic value of two clinical tests. *Arthritis Rheum.* 2008;59(2):241-246. doi:10.1002/art.23354.
15. Viradia NK, Berger AA, Dahners LE. Relationship between width of greater trochanters and width of iliac wings in tronchanteric bursitis. *Am J Orthop (Belle Mead NJ).* 2011;40(9):E159-E162.

SECTION D
Snapping Hip Syndrome (Coxa Saltans)

Samuel Evan Carstensen

HISTORY

- Occurring in 5% to 10% of the population, it is also referred to as coxa saltans or dancer's hip
  - 90% of elite ballet dancers found to have snapping hip syndrome (SHS)
    - 80% have symptoms bilaterally
- Two types based on location
  - External: usually caused by IT band, TFL, gluteus medius sliding across the greater trochanter
    - Also includes iliopsoas impinging medially on the hip capsule
  - Internal: iliopsoas tendon may slide across the lesser trochanter or iliopectineal ridge
- Often affects active individuals in the second or third decade of life

PHYSICAL EXAMINATION

- External: reproduction of external snapping hip by means of adduction and passive flexion
  - May be SEEN from across the room
- Internal: reproduction of internal snapping hip with hip initially flexed and externally rotated then passively extending and internally rotating the hip
  - May be HEARD from across the room
- Patients may have a tender area about the posterior aspect of the greater trochanter on the affected side

KEY EXAMINATION MANEUVERS

- Ober Test (Figure 3D.1)
  - First described in the literature in 1936 by Dr Frank R. Ober[3]
    - Initially developed to stretch the IT band and TFL in patients with low-back pain or sciatica
  - Modified by Kendall et al[8] in 1952 by extending the knee to 0° before the stretch
    - Both the original and modified Ober test have shown similar inter- and intraexaminer reliability
  - **Maneuver**:
    - The examiner stands behind the patient in the lateral decubitus position with the affected side upward
    - The unaffected leg is placed in hip and knee flexion to eliminate lumbar lordosis
    - Place 1 hand on the iliac crest to support and stabilize the pelvis
    - The other hand supports underneath the knee, which is maintained at 90° of knee flexion
    - The examiner then brings the affected leg into hip abduction and extension until the leg is in line with the trunk

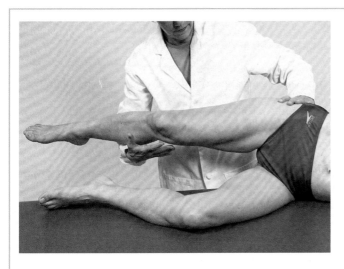

Figure 3D.1. Ober test. (From Oatis CA. *Kinesiology: The Mechanics and Pathomechanics of Human Movement*. 3rd ed. Philadelphia, Baltimore: Wolters Kluwer; 2017.)

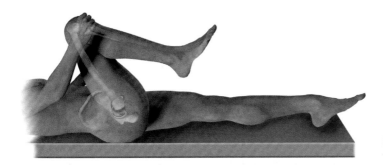

Figure 3D.2. Thomas test.

- The leg is then lowered toward the table. Any limitation to the knee reaching the table is noted as a positive sign for IT band tightness
- Placing the examined leg in 0° of knee extension and then repeating the examination maneuver completes the modified Ober test
- **Limitations of Maneuver:**
  - Helps diagnose IT band tightness but rarely reproduces patient's symptoms
  - Performing test at higher knee flexion angles leads to less isolation of IT band
  - Can also be positive in individuals with trochanteric bursitis

- Thomas Test (Sensitivity 0.89, Specificity 0.92) (Figure 3D.2)
  - First described by Hugh Owens Thomas in 1876[5]
  - This test was modified with the patient's legs hanging over the edge of the examination table in lieu of atop the table
    - Described by Ashton and colleagues in 1978[2]
  - **Maneuver:**
    - The examiner stands on the affected side with the patient supine
    - Both of the patient's hips are maximally flexed while their hands hold their knees to their chest
    - The affected hip is then passively extended back down toward neutral by the examiner
    - Stop passive extension once the pelvis begins to tilt anteriorly
    - Positive test: if the patients are unable to maintain their lower back and sacrum on the table due to contracture

IMAGING

Plain Radiographs

- AP view
  - Used to rule out other causes of hip pain, as no abnormalities are seen on the plain radiograph in coxa saltans
  - Review for any intra-articular loose bodies

Magnetic Resonance Imaging

- Useful by evaluating for intra-articular anomalies including loose bodies, labral tears, or bony abnormalities such as FAI (although this is better assessed on X-ray and CT)
- Thickening of the IT band, tendinitis, and/or bursal pathology may also be visualized

Ultrasonography

- Dynamic assessment of snapping hip syndrome (Figure 3D.3)
  - Gold standard for diagnosis
  - The femoral head and neck are the key structures identified initially
  - The patient is supine with both hips initially in a neutral position
    - External:
      - The probe placed about lateral aspect of the hip initially identifying the IT band
      - The hip is then passively flexed and extended permitting the IT band to move about the greater trochanter

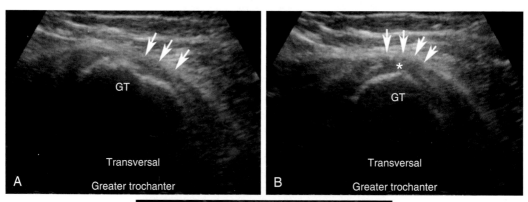

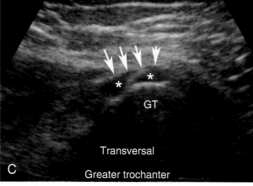

Figure 3D.3. A-C show the IT band in different positions due to the movement of the hip. GT, greater trochanter. Arrows are identifying the IT band. Asterisks identify the greater trochanteric bursa underlying the tendon. Dynamic assessment of snapping hip syndrome using ultrasonography. (From Clohisy JC. *The Adult Hip: Hip Preservation Surgery*. Philadelphia, Baltimore: Wolters Kluwer; 2015.)

  – Internal:
  • The probe is placed at the superior ilium in the oblique axial plane
  • The hip is moved from extension/adduction/internal rotation to flexion/abduction/external rotation

Hip Arthroscopy

- May be utilized to release the iliopsoas tendon in the setting of internal coxa saltans or IT band release with external coxa saltans (Figures 3D.4 and 3D.5)
- Both tendons may be surgically released, but nonoperative management should be trialed initially

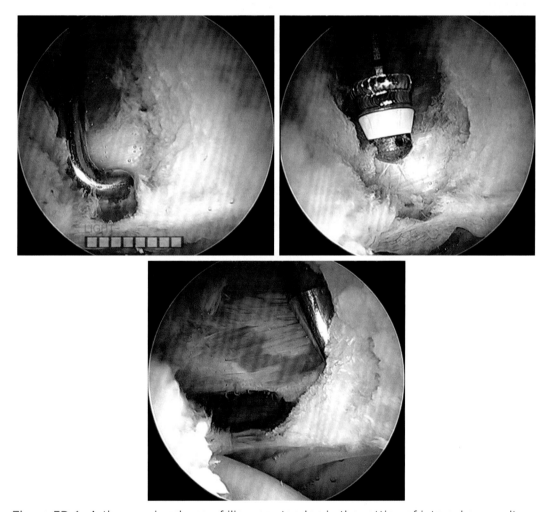

Figure 3D.4. Arthroscopic release of iliopsoas tendon in the setting of internal coxa saltans.

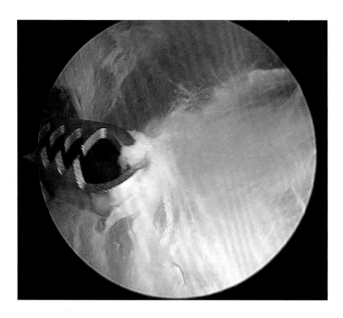

Figure 3D.5. Arthroscopic release of iliotibial band.

REFERENCES

1. Allen WC, Cope R. Coxa Saltans: the snapping hip revisited. *JAAOS*. 1995;3:303-308
2. Ashton BB, Pickles B, Roll JW. Reliability of goniometric measurements of hip motion in spastic cerebral palsy. *Dev Med Child Neurol*. 1978;20:87-94.
3. Ober FR. The role of low back disabilities and sciatica. *J Bone Joint Surg Am*. 1936;18:105-110.
4. Piechota M, Maczuch J, Skupiński J, Kukawska-Sysio K, Wawrzynek W. Internal snapping hip syndrome in dynamic ultrasonography. *J Ultrasonogr*. 2016;16(66):296-303.
5. Thomas HO. *Diseases of the Hip, Knee, and Ankle Joints and Their Deformities Treated by a New and Efficient Method*. Liverpool: T. Dobb & Co.; 1876:17-19.

SECTION E
Hip Abductor and Hamstring Injuries

Harrison S. Mahon

HISTORY

Piriformis Syndrome

- True injuries to the piriformis tendon are rare
- However, "piriformis syndrome" can be seen after a direct blow to the gluteal region
- Piriformis syndrome was initially described by Robinson as pain in the SI joint, greater sciatic notch, and piriformis muscle that extends down the limb[1]
- Pathophysiology is poorly described in the orthopedic literature; however, it is thought to be due to sciatic nerve entrapment beneath an inflamed piriformis tendon
- Owing to sciatic nerve irritation, pain can mimic radicular lumbar nerve root pain
- Pain is worsened by stooping or lifting, improved with traction on the affected limb while in the supine position[2]

Gluteus Medius/Minimus Pathology

- They form the primary hip abductor complex and are crucial for hip stability throughout the various stages of the gait cycle
- Pathology within the gluteus medius and minimus may fall anywhere on the spectrum between tendinosis and complete tear
- Gluteal tendinosis has been recognized as a cause of trochanteric bursitis or greater trochanter pain syndrome
- Three clinical scenarios of hip abductor tendon tear have been described[3]
  - Chronic, nontraumatic tear of anterior fibers of gluteus medius
  - Tears found coincidentally at the time of hip arthroplasty
  - Avulsion injuries after THA
- Chronic tear of gluteus medius coined "rotator cuff tear of the hip" by Bunker and Kagan[4,5]
- Patient usually presents with lateral hip pain and/or hip abduction weakness

Hamstring Injuries

- Hamstring injuries are one of the most common lower extremity injuries
- Muscle group includes biceps femoris (long and short heads), semimembranosus, and semitendinosus
- Injuries are generally either strain injuries or proximal avulsion injuries
- Injuries usually occur during eccentric contraction at the myotendinous junction
- Most patients describe acute sudden pain in the posterior thigh
- Can also be a more insidious, progressive tightness
- Commonly occurs in running, jumping, and kicking sports[6]

PHYSICAL EXAMINATION

- **Active Piriformis Test** (Sensitivity 0.78, Specificity 0.80)[7] (Figure 3E.1)
  - First described by Pace and Nagle in 1976 as pain and weakness with resisted abduction and external rotation of the affected thigh[8]
  - **Maneuver:**
    - The patient lies on the examination table in the lateral position with the affected side upward
    - The foot of the affected limb planted on the examination table
    - The examiner stands at the side of the table, facing the patient who is turned away from him/her
    - The examiner provides downward resistance at the knee level, as the patient abducts and externally rotates the hip

- **Piriformis Stretch Test** (Sensitivity 0.52, Specificity 0.90)[7] (Figure 3E.2)
  - Initially described in the literature in 1937 by Freiberg as pain with passive internal rotation of the hip[9]
  - **Maneuver:**
    - The patient in the seated position on the edge of the examination table
    - The examiner stands at the side of the table, 90° relative to the patient and facing the leg being tested
    - Greater sciatic notch is palpated
    - The knee is extended and the hip is flexed, adducted, and internally rotated to elicit pain symptoms

- **Lasègue Sign (Straight Leg Raise)** (Sensitivity 0.15, Specificity 0.95)[7] (Figure 3E.3)
  - First described in the literature in 1864 by Lasègue[10]
  - Found to be associated with piriformis syndrome in 1937 by Freiberg[9]
  - No recent modifications
  - **Maneuver:**
    - The patient lies supine on back
    - The examiner stands at the foot of the table
    - The straight leg is raised by the examiner
    - Radicular leg pain occurs between 30° and 70° of elevation

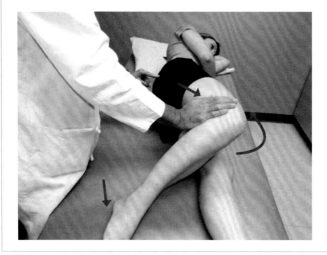

Figure 3E.1. Active piriformis test. (From Callaghan JJ. *The Adult Hip: Hip Arthroplasty Surgery*. Wolters Kluwer Health; 2016.)

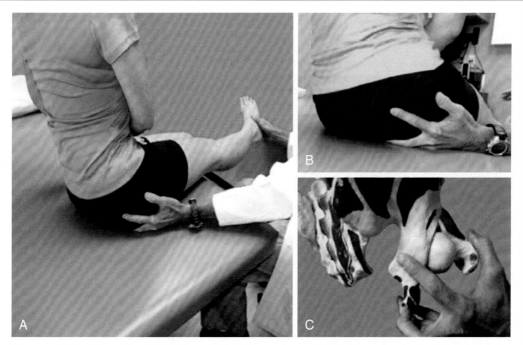

Figure 3E.2. Seated piriformis stretch test. A and B, The examiner palpating the piriformis muscle while adducting and internally rotating the lower extremity. C, The origin of the piriformis muscle. (From Callaghan JJ. *The Adult Hip: Hip Arthroplasty Surgery*. Wolters Kluwer Health; 2016.)

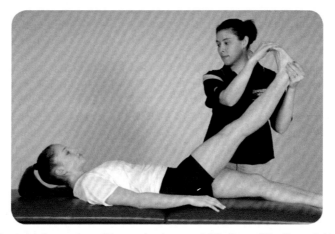

Figure 3E.3. Straight leg raise. (From Anderson MK, Parr GP. *Foundations of Athletic Training: Prevention, Assessment and Management*. Philadelphia: Lippincott Williams & Wilkins; 2013.)

KEY EXAMINATION MANEUVERS: GLUTEUS MEDIUS/MINIMUS

- **Trendelenburg Test** (Figure 3E.4)
  - Initially described by Friedrich Trendelenburg in 1897 to assess hip abductor function with specific reference to congenital hip dislocation and subsequent muscular atrophy[11]
  - The test generally suggests hip abductor weakness but is not specific to gluteus medius/minimus tears
  - Many variations but examined by Hardcastle in 1985[7] in an effort to normalize the test

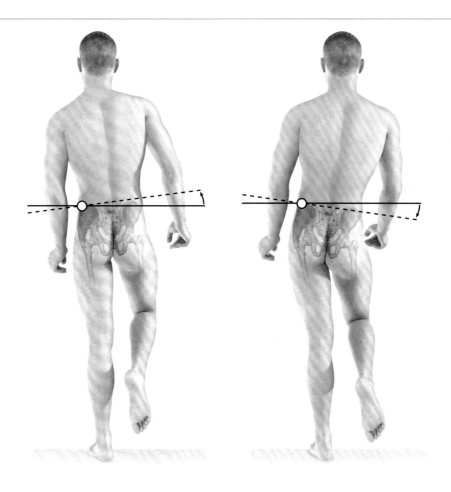

Trendelenberg sign is (−)
Patient can abduct pelvis on left femur

Trendelenberg sign is (+)
Patient unable to abduct pelvis on left
femur—right buttock droops

Figure 3E.4. Trendelenburg test. (From Pansky B, Gest TR. *Lippincott's Concise Illustrated Anatomy: Back, Upper Limb & Lower Limb*. Philadelphia: Wolters Kluwer/ Lippincott Williams & Wilkins Health; 2012.)

- **Maneuver:**
  - The examiner stands behind the patient
  - The patient raises the foot of the side not being tested; the hip is flexed to approximately 30°
  - The patient is then asked to elevate the nonstance side of the pelvis as high as possible while maintaining the spine alignment over the weight-bearing limb
  - The response is normal if the pelvis on the nonstance side can be elevated as high as hip abduction on the stance side will allow and the position can be held for 30 seconds
  - The response is abnormal if this cannot be done
- **Resisted Hip Abduction** (Figure 3E.5)
  - Not formally investigated in the literature but may also be used to assess hip abduction strength
  - **Maneuver:**
    - Usually tested in the lateral decubitus position
    - The patient lies on the table in the lateral decubitus position, facing away from the examiner

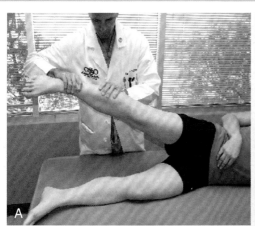
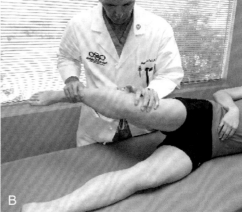
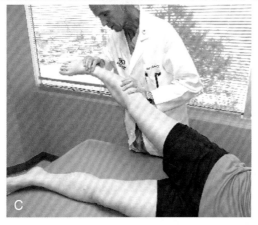

Figure 3E.5. Resisted hip abduction test. A flexed knee tests the gluteus medius (B), whereas an extended knee tests the gluteus maximus (A). Resistance may be provided (C) to detect subtle weakness. (From Callaghan JJ. *The Adult Hip: Hip Arthroplasty Surgery*. Wolters Kluwer Health; 2016.)

- The examiner stands at the side of the table behind the patient
- To test gluteus maximus, the patient keeps the knee extended while actively abducting the hip
- To test gluteus medius, the patient flexes the knee while actively abducting the hip
- The examiner may provide resistance to detect subtle weakness

KEY PHYSICAL EXAMINATION MANEUVERS: HAMSTRING

- **Puranen-Orava Test (Figure 3E.6) (Sensitivity 0.76, Specificity 0.82)**[12]
  - Described by Puranen and Orava in 1988[13]
  - **Maneuver:**
    - The patient stands beside a support just below the waist height (can be an examination table if the height is appropriate)
    - The patient flexes the hip to 90° and rests the heel on the table, keeping the knee extended
    - The knee is then actively and maximally extended
    - A positive test results in posterior thigh pain

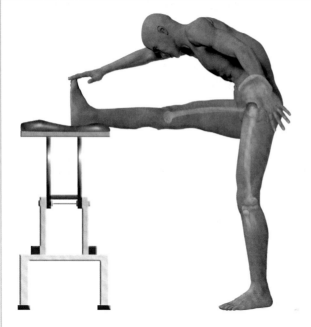

Figure 3E.6. Puranen-Orava test.

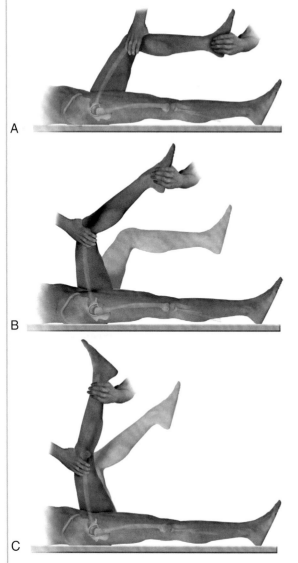

A

B

C

Figure 3E.7. Bent knee stretch test.

> • **Bent Knee Stretch Test (Figure 3E.7) (Sensitivity 0.84, Specificity 0.87)**[12]
>   • **Maneuver:**
>   – The patient lies on the table supine
>   – The hip and knee are maximally flexed
>   – The examiner stands at the side of the table, facing the leg being tested
>   – The knee is slowly and passively extended by the examiner
>   – A positive test results in posterior thigh pain
>   • **Modifications**
>   – The knee is rapidly straightened by the examiner after the hip and knee are maximally flexed

IMAGING

Piriformis

- **CT/MRI:** may reveal an enlarged piriformis or a mass causing pressure on the sciatic nerve in the area of the piriformis (Figure 3E.8)

Gluteus Medius/Minimus

- MRI
  - T1-weighted images with fat saturation and axial T2-weighted images with fast spin echo have been shown to accurately diagnose gluteal tendinopathy (Figure 3E.9)
  - Milwaukee classification system for abductor tears[14]
    – Four-part anatomic classification system based on the hours of a clock when then hip is viewed from a posterior surgical approach
    – Based on both MRI findings and surgical findings
    – In a right hip, the medius inserts between 11- and 3-o'clock positions
    – In a left hip, it inserts between 9- and 1-o'clock positions
    – Grade 1 corresponds to 1 hour involved, grade 2 with 2 hours, etc
- Hip Arthroscopy
  - Portals
    – Anterolateral, posterolateral, accessory distal lateral, and midanterior portals are used
  - Visualization
    – The accessory distal lateral portal is the primary viewing portal
    – Other portals may be used to perform a trochanteric bursectomy and place anchors if needed (**Figure 3E.10**)

Hamstring

- **X-ray**
  - Usually negative
  - May show an avulsion fracture from the ischial tuberosity
- **Ultrasonography**
  - Useful in the acute phase of injury and can be simultaneously paired with physical examination
  - May show fluid around the injured muscle or areas of echogenicity (Figure 3E.11)
- **MRI (Figure 3E.12)**
  - Most commonly used imaging modality for hamstring injuries
  - Can differentiate acute and chronic injuries

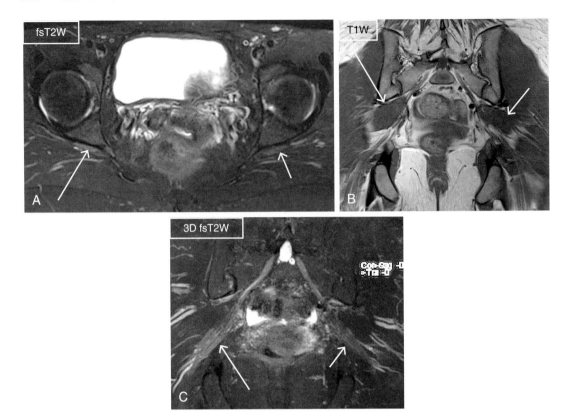

Figure 3E.8. Piriformis syndrome. The long arrows on axial (A) and coronal imaging (C) show increased size of the sciatic nerve relative to contralateral normal sciatic nerve (short arrow in C). Long arrow in B shows hypertrophy of the piriformis muscle compared with the normal side (short arrow). (From Chhabra A, Soldatos T. *Musculoskeletal MRI Structured Evaluation: How to Practically Fill the Reporting Checklist.* Wolters Kluwer Health; 2015.)

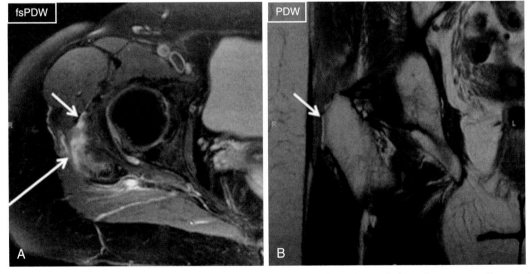

Figure 3E.9. Axial (A) and coronal (B) MRI show partial tearing of the gluteus medius and minimus tendons. Note the increased signal at their insertion on the greater trochanter, indicated by the white arrows in both images. (From Chhabra A, Soldatos T. *Musculoskeletal MRI Structured Evaluation: How to Practically Fill the Reporting Checklist.* Wolters Kluwer Health; 2015.)

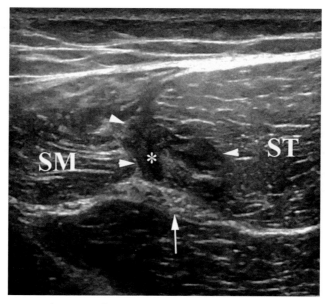

Figure 3E.10. Transverse ultrasound image shows hematoma (asterisk, with borders marked by arrowheads) in the semitendinosus (ST) near the semimembranosus (SM) margin. This can cause pressure on the sciatic nerve (arrow). (From Beggs I. *Musculoskeletal Ultrasound.* Philadelphia: Wolters Kluwer/Lippincott Williams & Wilkins Health; 2014.)

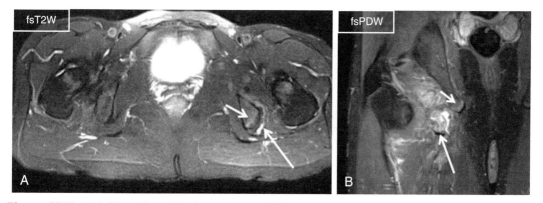

Figure 3E.11. Axial imaging (A) shows a partial hamstring avulsion (long arrow) and marrow edema (short arrow) at the attachment site. Coronal imaging in a different patient (B) shows a complete avulsion with several centimeters of retraction. (From Chhabra A, Soldatos T. *Musculoskeletal MRI Structured Evaluation: How to Practically Fill the Reporting Checklist.* Wolters Kluwer Health; 2015.)

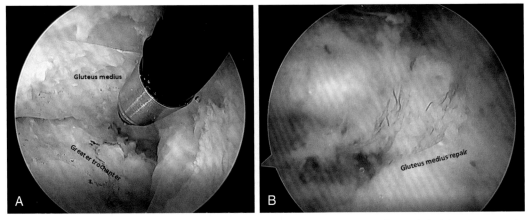

Figure 3E.12. A, An arthroscopic electrocautery tool being used to debride the greater trochanter and prepare the gluteus medius for repair. B, The final repair that was completed by placing suture anchors into the greater trochanter and passing the sutures through the medius tendon. (Credit: F. Gwathmey, MD.)

REFERENCES

1. Robinson DR. Pyriformis syndrome in relation to sciatic pain. *Am J Surg.* 1947;73(3):355-358.
2. Benson ER, Schutzer SF. Posttraumatic piriformis syndrome: diagnosis and results of operative treatment. *JBJS.* 1999;81(7):941-949.
3. Lachiewicz PF. Abductor tendon tears of the hip: evaluation and management. *J Am Acad Orthop Surg.* 2011;19(7):385-391.
4. Bunker TD, Esler CN, Leach WJ. Rotator-cuff tear of the hip. *J Bone Joint Surg Br.* 1997;79(4):618-620.
5. Kagan A. Rotator cuff tears of the hip. *Clin Orthop Relat Res.* 1999;(368):135-140.
6. Ahmad CS, Redler LH, Ciccotti MG, Maffulli N, Longo UG, Bradley J. Evaluation and management of hamstring injuries. *Am J Sports Med.* 2013;41(12):2933-2947. doi:10.1177/0363546513487063.
7. Martin HD, Kivlan BR, Palmer IJ, Martin RL. Diagnostic accuracy of clinical tests for sciatic nerve entrapment in the gluteal region. *Knee Surg Sports Traumatol Arthros.* 2014;22(4):882-888. doi:10.1007/s00167-013-2758-7.
8. Pace JB, Nagle D. Piriform syndrome. *West J Med.* 1976;124(6):435-439.
9. Freiberg A. Sciatic pain and its relief by operations on muscle and fascia. *Arch Surg.* 1937;34:337-350.
10. Kamath SU, Kamath SS. Lasègue's Sign. *J Clin Diagn Res.* 2017;11(5):RG01-RG02. doi:10.7860/JCDR/2017/24899.9794.
11. Hardcastle P, Nade S. The significance of the Trendelenburg test. *Bone Joint Lett J.* 1985;67(5):741-746.
12. Cacchio A, Borra F, Severini G, et al. Reliability and validity of three pain provocation tests used for the diagnosis of chronic proximal hamstring tendinopathy. *Br J Sports Med.* 2012;46(12):883-887. doi:10.1136/bjsports-2011-090325.
13. Puranen J, Orava S. The hamstring syndrome. A new diagnosis of gluteal sciatic pain. *Am J Sports Med.* 1988;16(5):517-521. doi:10.1177/036354658801600515.
14. Davies JF, Stiehl JB, Davies JA, Geiger PB. Surgical treatment of hip abductor tendon tears. *J Bone Joint Surg Am.* 2013;95(15):1420-1425. doi:10.2106/JBJS.L.00709.

SECTION F
Quadriceps Injury

Harrison S. Mahon

HISTORY

- Quadriceps muscle group consists of rectus femoris, vastus medialis, vastus intermedius, and vastus lateralis
- In athletes, injury usually occurs after forceful eccentric contraction of the quadriceps muscles
- Elderly or obese patients can sustain quadriceps injuries with lower energy mechanisms
- Injury is classically described as occurring in the distal aspect of the rectus femoris at the myotendinous junction[1]
- Injuries in the mid and proximal aspects of the rectus have also been described
- Classic triad of pain, inability to actively extend the knee, gap in rectus tendon proximal to the patella
- Pathology can range from tendinosis (jumper's knee) to partial rupture and complete rupture[2]

PHYSICAL EXAMINATION

General

- Visible or palpable defect may be observed within the quadriceps musculature
- Ecchymosis is also common starting 24 hours after the injury
- Hemarthrosis commonly accompanies the injury, making diagnosis difficult
- Diagnostic failure rates of 10% to 50% have been reported[3,4]

KEY EXAMINATION MANEUVERS

- Active Extension Test
  - No published information on origin or sensitivity/specificity
  - **Maneuver:**
    - The patient sits on the edge of the examination table
    - The examiner stands at the edge of the table, turned 90° relative to the patient and facing the leg that is being tested
    - The knee is actively extended and compared with well leg extension
    - If the patient can perform a full leg extension, the examiner places 1 hand on the patient's leg, just proximal to the knee. The other hand is placed on the ankle. The examiner then tries to flex the knee against the patient's best effort (Figure 3F.1)
    - Quadriceps injury will result in either complete inability to extend the knee, or an extensor lag, or a palpable defect in the quadriceps tendon, which indicates a positive result

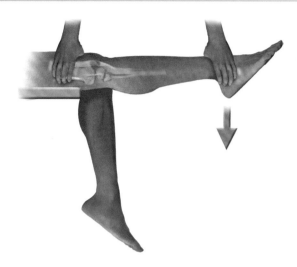

Figure 3F.1. Resisted active extension test.

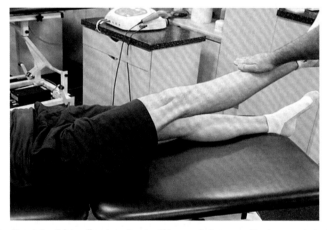

Figure 3F.2. Resisted hip flexion test. (From Johnson D, Amendola NA, Barber F. *Operative Arthroscopy*. Philadelphia: Wolters Kluwer; 2015.)

   – Quadriceps strains will result in subtle differences in strength between the injured and well leg

- **Hip Flexion Test**
  - No published information on origin or sensitivity/specificity
  - **Maneuver:**
    - The patient lies supine with the knee extended
    - The examiner stands beside the table, facing the leg that is being tested
    - The hip is flexed while maintaining the extended knee
    - Inability to perform the test, a palpable defect in the quadriceps tendon, or decreased strength compared with the well leg indicates a positive result (Figure 3F.2)
    - Useful when hemarthrosis may be limiting knee motion
    - However, an intact IT band or lateral patellar retinaculum can compensate for decreased quadriceps strength and give a false-negative test

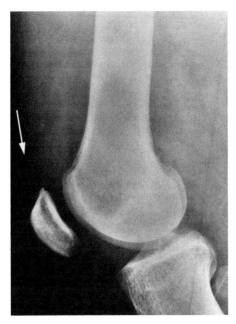

Figure 3F.3. Lateral radiograph of the knee shows a complete tear of the quadriceps tendon. Note the patella baja and lack of definition of the quadriceps tendon (arrow). (From Greenspan A. *Orthopedic Imaging: A Practical Approach*. 5th ed. Philadelphia, PA: Lippincott Williams & Wilkins; 2011:303.)

IMAGING

Plain Radiographs

- AP and lateral radiographs may show any of the following (Figure 3F.3):
  - Obliteration of the quadriceps shadow
  - Suprapatellar mass
  - Suprapatellar calcific densities
  - Patella baja

Ultrasonography

- Accuracy is operator-dependent but can be highly sensitive and specific
- Can differentiate complete rupture from partial rupture
- Rupture will appear as a hypoechoic gap (hematoma) between free ends of the tendon (Figure 3F.4)
- Also allows for imaging during active knee motion; in partial tears the gap will not widen with knee extension

Magnetic Resonance Imaging

- Most sensitive and specific imaging modality
- Can diagnose tendinosis and minor strains (Figure 3F.5)

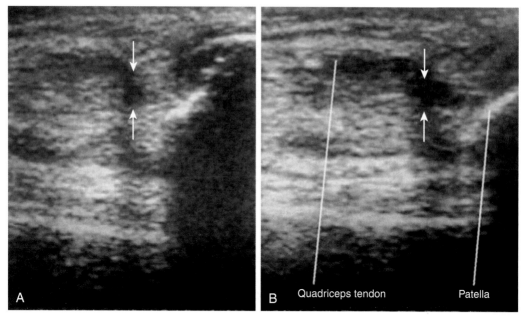

Figure 3F.4. Sagittal ultrasound image of a complete tear of the quadriceps tendon without (A) and with (B) manual distraction of the patella. Anechoic area (white arrows) represents the rupture site and hematoma. Note the increased gap with distraction of the patella. (From Bianchi S, Zwass A, Abdelwahab IF, et al. Diagnosis of tears of the quadriceps tendon of the knee: value of sonography. *AJR Am J Roentgenol.* 1994;162:1137-1140.)

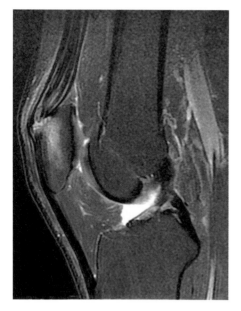

Figure 3F.5. MRI of tear of the quadriceps tendon. Sagittal T2-weighted fat-suppressed MRI shows a high-grade partial tear of the quadriceps tendon at its insertion to the patella. (From Greenspan A, Beltran J, Ovid Technologies I. *Orthopedic Imaging: A Practical Approach.* Philadelphia: Wolters Kluwer Health/Lippincott Williams & Wilkins; 2015.)

REFERENCES

1. Ilan DI, Tejwani N, Keschner M, Leibman M. Quadriceps tendon rupture. *J Am Acad Orthop Surg.* 2003;11(3):192-200.
2. Kary JM. Diagnosis and management of quadriceps strains and contusions. *Curr Rev Musculoskelet Med.* 2010;3(1-4):26-31. doi:10.1007/s12178-010-9064-5.
3. McGrory JE. Disruption of the extensor mechanism of the knee. *J Emerg Med.* 2003;24(2):163-168. doi:10.1016/S0736-4679(02)00719-9.
4. Siwek CW, Rao JP. Ruptures of the extensor mechanism of the knee joint. *JBJS.* 1981;63(6):932-937.

SECTION G
Hip Dislocation

Eric S. Larson

HISTORY

- The hip is an inherently stable joint due to contributions from the labrum, capsule, ligamentum teres, and bony anatomy[5]
- In native hips, dislocations are typically due to high-energy mechanisms such as motor vehicle accidents, when the femur is directed posteriorly through forceful contact of the knee with the dashboard (Figure 3G.1). As a result, the patient should be evaluated for other traumatic injuries in addition to the hip dislocation[2]
- In prosthetic hips, dislocation may often occur due to either malpositioning of the components or having the leg placed in a flexed, adducted, and internally rotated position

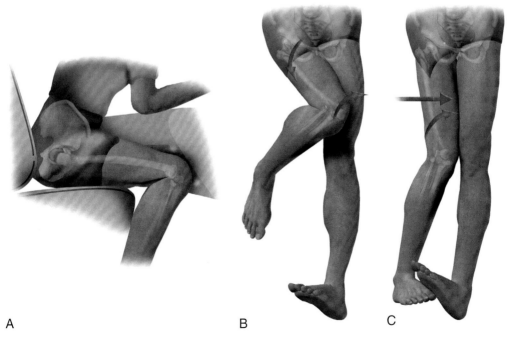

Figure 3G.1. Posterior dislocation of the hip. A, Mechanism of injury: The knee strikes the dashboard. The thigh is forced into flexion and adduction, and the femoral head is driven backward out of the acetabulum. B, Ischial dislocation: The hip (1) is flexed. The hip is markedly adducted, so that the knee of the affected limb lies on the opposite thigh. The limb is in extreme internal rotation. The greater trochanter and buttock on the affected side are unusually prominent. C, Iliac dislocation: As in B, the hip is flexed and is adducted.

PHYSICAL EXAMINATION

Observation

- Observe the affected leg for any leg length discrepancy when compared with the contralateral side, as a dislocated hip will make that leg appear shortened
- Observe the resting position of the affected leg while the patient is supine[1,3]
  - Posterior dislocations cause FADDIR of the affected leg
  - Anterior dislocations cause FABER of the affected leg
  - Ipsilateral leg trauma, however, may obscure these classic findings
- The presence of ipsilateral knee trauma—knee instability or transverse knee lacerations—may hint at dislocation of that hip[1,2]

KEY EXAMINATION MANEUVERS

- These maneuvers will elicit directional instability that may have led to a hip dislocation. They should not be used on a patient with a dislocated hip at presentation[6]

- Supine External Rotation Test[6] (Figure 3G.2)
  - **Maneuver:**
    - The patient is placed supine on the examination table
    - The examiner stands beside the examination table, with the patient's affected leg held in extension
    - The examiner then maximally externally rotates the patient's leg, feeling for a distinct endpoint
    - The contralateral leg is then assessed using the same maneuver
    - Positive test: increased external rotation of the affected leg, relative to the contralateral

- Axial Distraction Test[6] (Figure 3G.3)
  - **Maneuver:**
    - The patient is placed supine on the examination table
    - The examiner stands at the foot of the table, holding the ankle of the patient's affected extremity in 30° of flexion, 30° of abduction, and 15° of external rotation. The knee is extended
    - The examiner then applies axial traction
    - Positive test: increased distraction of the affected side relative to the contralateral side and a sense of pain and apprehension with traction

- Anterior Apprehension Test[6] (Figure 3G.4)
  - Also known as the hyperextension—external rotation test
  - **Maneuver:**
    - The patient is placed in the lateral decubitus position, on the unaffected extremity

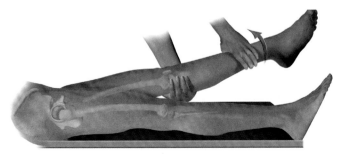

Figure 3G.2. Supine external rotation test. The examiner uses both hands to grasp the patient's affected leg and externally rotate it. An increase in external rotation relative to the unaffected side may indicate excessive hip laxity potentially leading to dislocation.

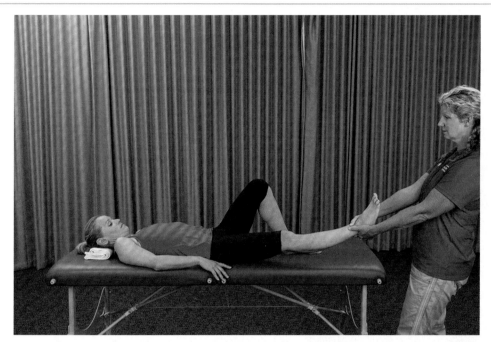

Figure 3G.3. Axial distraction test. The examiner stands at the foot of the examination table, grasping the ankle of the patient's affected extremity and applying axially directed traction. Increased joint distraction and/or a sense of pain or subluxation indicate(s) increased joint laxity. (From Brody LT, Hall CM. *Therapeutic Exercise: Moving toward Function*. Wolters Kluwer Health; 2018.)

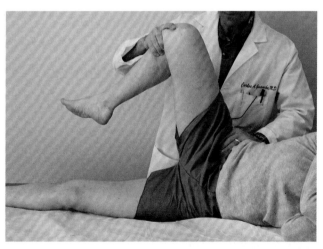

Figure 3G.4. Anterior apprehension test. The patient is placed in the lateral decubitus position on the unaffected side with the examiner standing behind the patient, supporting the affected extremity in an abducted and externally rotated position while applying an anteriorly directed force over the greater trochanter. This attempts to recreate an anterior dislocation. (From Guanche CA. *Hip and Pelvis Injuries in Sports Medicine*. Philadelphia: Wolters Kluwer/Lippincott Williams & Wilkin; 2010.)

- The examiner stands behind the patient, supporting the affected extremity in slight abduction with 1 hand and applying an anteriorly directed force over the posterior aspect of the greater trochanter with the other hand
- Positive test: reproduction of hip pain or a sensation of instability and subluxation

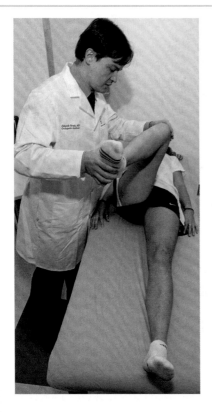

Figure 3G.5. Posterior apprehension test. The patient lies supine while the examiner flexes, adducts, and internally rotates the affected hip while applying an axially directed force down the shaft of the femur. This attempts to recreate a posterior dislocation. (From Barrack RL, Rosenberg AG. *Master Techniques in Orthopaedic Surgery: The Hip*. Wolters Kluwer Health, 2016.)

- Posterior Apprehension Test[6] (Figure 3G.5)
  - **Maneuver:**
    - The patient is placed supine on the examination table
    - The examiner flexes the affected hip to 90° while internally rotating and adducting the thigh
    - A posteriorly directed force is then placed axially on the flexed thigh
    - Positive test: reproduction of pain or sensation of subluxation is consistent with posterior hip instability[6]

IMAGING

Plain Radiographs

- The initial imaging modality of choice is an AP pelvis
- The AP pelvis will show a loss of articular congruence and parallelism between the head of the femur and the roof of the acetabulum
- Posterior hip dislocations (Figure 3G.6)
  - The head of the femur will appear smaller than the contralateral side
  - Because of the internal rotation associated with posterior dislocation, the lesser trochanter will either not be visible or have a smaller profile when compared with the contralateral side
    - This will also cause the femoral neck to be seen in a more profile view owing to its typical anteversion[3]
- Anterior hip dislocations (Figure 3G.7)
  - The head of the femur will appear larger than the contralateral side
  - Because of the external rotation associated with anterior dislocation, the profile of the lesser trochanter will be more pronounced when compared with the unaffected side

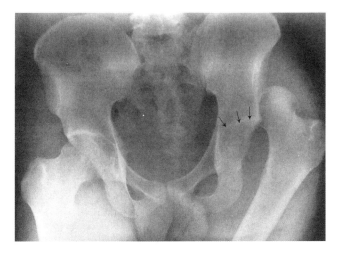

Figure 3G.6. Pelvis AP radiograph. Posterior dislocation of the left hip without fracture secondary to a motor vehicle accident. The left femoral head is displaced cephalad and lateral relative to the acetabulum (arrows). The right hip is normal and makes an excellent comparison. (From Smith WL, Farrell TA. *Radiology 101: The Basics and Fundamentals of Imaging.* Wolters Kluwer Health; 2014.)

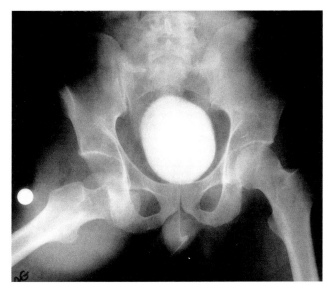

Figure 3G.7. Anterior dislocation of the right hip. Radiograph shows that the femoral head is inferior to the acetabulum. The femoral shaft is abducted and externally rotated, which can be appreciated by the increased profile of the lesser trochanter of the right femur when compared with the left one. There is also an associated right femoral head fracture. (From Mulholland MW, Ronald V, *Maier, et al. Greenfield's Surgery Scientific Principles and Practice.* 4th ed. Philadelphia: Lippincott Williams & Wilkins; 2006.)

- Associated injuries such as ipsilateral femoral neck fractures and pelvic ring fractures must be investigated, as they may necessitate open reduction of the hip[2,5]
- Following reduction, an AP of the pelvis should be repeated as well as Judet and inlet/outlet views

Computed Tomography

- Generally CT scans are delayed until after the hip has been reduced, unless there is question of an ipsilateral femoral neck fracture that is unable to be ruled out on plain radiographs[2]
- If the hip is unable to be reduced and open reduction is deemed necessary, a CT scan is useful to identify what structure is impeding reduction
- Following reduction, CT scan with 2 mm cuts is useful to identify any intra-articular fragments from an associated acetabular fracture or femoral head fracture as well as to evaluate for any femoral head impaction, thereby assisting with preoperative planning[3,4]

Magnetic Resonance Imaging

- The use of MRI in the setting of acute hip dislocation is not widespread
- MRI may be useful in the evaluation of a widened hip joint in the context of a normal CT, as the MRI may be able to evaluate soft tissue interposition in the joint

REFERENCES

1. Foulk DM, et al. Hip dislocation: evaluation and management. *J Am Acad Orthop Surg.* 2010;18(4):199-209.
2. Tornetta P, et al. Hip dislocation: current treatment regimens. *J Am Acad Orthop Surg.* 1997;5(1):27-36.
3. Kain MS, Tornetta P. Hip dislocations and fractures of the femoral head. In: Court-Brown CM, Heckman JD, McQueen MM, Ricci WM, Tornetta P, eds. *Rockwood & Green's Fractures in Adults.* 8th ed.; vol 2. Philadelphia: Wolters Kluwer Health; 2015:1983-2030.
4. Goulet JA. Hip dislocation. In: Browner BD, Jupiter JB, Krettek C, Anderson PA, eds. *Skeletal Trauma: Basic Science, Management, and Reconstruction.* 5th ed.; vol 2. Philadelphia: Saunders; 2015:1565-1595.
5. Kalisvaart MM, et al. Microinstability of the hip—it does exist: etiology, diagnosis, and treatment. *J Hip Preserv Surg.* 2015;2(2):123-135.
6. Guanche CA. Hip instability. In: Byrd T, Guanche CA, eds. The Hip. Philadelphia: Saunders Elsevier; 2010:107-120.

SECTION H
Sacroiliac Joint Dysfunction

Eric S. Larson

HISTORY

- SI joint dysfunction is thought to be responsible for 15% to 30% of lower back pain[1-4]
- Bimodal distribution
  - Young athletes may present with unilateral symptoms due to activities such as kicking that place unilateral force on the lower limbs
  - Elderly patients may present with bilateral symptoms due to age-related SI joint space narrowing and arthritis
- Females are 3 to 4 times more likely to be affected due to this condition's close association with pregnancy[4]
- Pain is often abrupt in onset, following a specific inciting event that patients are typically able to recall
- Patients will complain of pain just inferior to the posterior superior iliac spine (PSIS), in the area of the sacral sulcus[4]

PHYSICAL EXAMINATION

Observation

- The patient should be evaluated for any leg length discrepancy[4]
- The back should be examined for scoliosis and increased lumbar lordosis, as these abnormalities may shift the normal alignment of the SI joint
- Examine the patient's gait for any irregularity that may place increased force on the side of his/her lower back pain[3]

Palpation

- Pain elicited with palpation of the sacral sulcus has been shown to be 89% sensitive in the diagnosis of SI joint dysfunction. Unfortunately, this finding has poor specificity. The most common location of pain is illustrated in Figure 3H.1
- Pain with palpation over the PSIS or sacral sulcus in conjunction with maximal pain below L5 yields a 60% positive predictive value

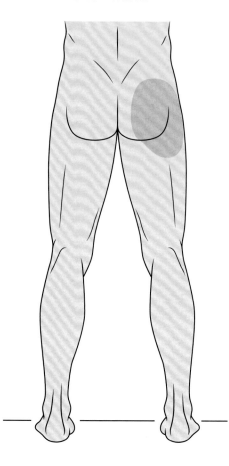

Figure 3H.1. Illustration of the typical pain pattern produced by the SI joint in the gluteal region, around the sacral sulcus. (From Rathmell JP, Nelson GJ. *Atlas of Image-Guided Intervention in Regional Anesthesia and Pain Medicine: Incl. Fully Searchable Text and Image Bank.* 2nd ed. Philadelphia: Wolters Kluwer, Lippincott Williams & Wilkins; 2012.)

KEY EXAMINATION MANEUVERS

- No single maneuver is particularly useful in the diagnosis of this condition; however, the presence of 3 of the following examination maneuvers has been shown to be 85% sensitive and 79% specific[4,5]

- Gaenslen Test[5] (Sensitivity 0.53-0.71, Specificity 0.26-0.77)[6] (Figure 3H.2)
  - First described by F. J. Gaenslen[7]
  - There have been no major modifications
  - **Maneuver:**
    - The patient is placed supine with the buttock of the affected side resting off of the edge of the examination table
    - The examiner hyperextends the affected hip off of the table while the contralateral hip is maximally flexed
    - Positive test: pain elicited in the region of the affected SI joint

- Distraction (Gapping) Test[5] (Sensitivity 0.60, Specificity 0.81)[6] (Figure 3H.3)
  - **Maneuver:**
    - The patient is placed supine with the examiner standing on the affected side
    - The examiner applies downward and laterally directed force to the bilateral anterior superior iliac spines (ASIS)
    - This maneuver distracts the ventral SI ligaments and compresses the dorsal ligaments
    - Positive test: pain elicited in the region of the affected SI joint

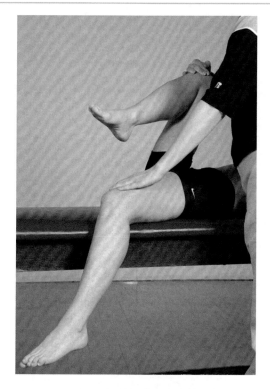

Figure 3H.2. Gaenslen sign. The patient is positioned so that the involved hip extends beyond the edge of the table. Both legs are drawn onto the chest, and then one is slowly lowered into extension. Increased pain may signal an ipsilateral sacroiliac joint lesion. (From Anderson MK, Parr GP. *Foundations of Athletic Training: Prevention, Assessment and Management.* Philadelphia: Lippincott Williams & Wilkins; 2013.)

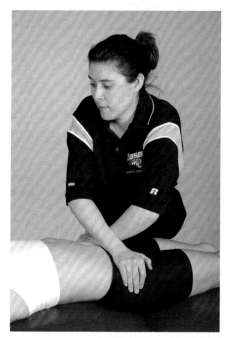

Figure 3H.3. Sacroiliac (SI) distraction test. The examiner applies a cross-arm pressure downward and outward to the anterior superior iliac spine with the thumbs. The action is repeated with pressure applied down through the anterior portion of the ilium, spreading the SI joint. Unilateral pain in the area of the SI joint may indicate joint dysfunction. (From Anderson MK, Parr GP. *Foundations of Athletic Training: Prevention, Assessment and Management.* Philadelphia: Lippincott Williams & Wilkins; 2013.)

- Compression Test[5] (Sensitivity 0.69, Specificity 0.69)[6] (Figure 3H.4)
  - **Maneuver:**
    - The patient is placed in the lateral position, resting on the unaffected side with the examiner standing behind the patient, placing downward-directed pressure over the iliac crest of the affected side
    - This maneuver is antagonistic to the distraction test; the ventral ligaments are compressed and the dorsal ligaments are distracted

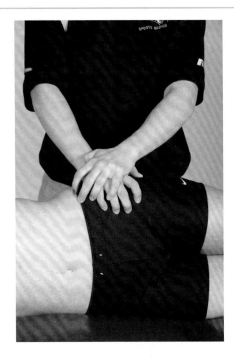

Figure 3H.4. Sacroiliac (SI) compression test. With the patient lying in the lateral position, the clinician applies a downward pressure over the iliac crest. Increased pain or feeling of pressure over the SI joints indicates possible sprain of the SI ligaments. (From Anderson MK, Barnum M. *Foundations of Athletic Training: Prevention, Assessment, and Management.* Wolters Kluwer Health; 2017.)

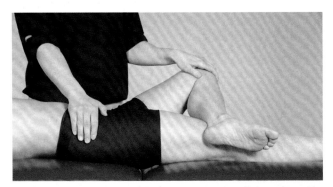

Figure 3H.5. Flexion-abduction-external rotation (FABER or Patrick) test. The foot and ankle of the involved leg are rested on the contralateral knee. Overpressure on the knee of the involved leg and the contralateral iliac crest may produce pain in the sacroiliac joint on the side of the involved leg, indicating pathology. (From Anderson MK, Barnum M. *Foundations of Athletic Training: Prevention, Assessment, and Management.* Wolters Kluwer Health; 2017.)

  – Positive test: recreation of pain in the affected SI joint[5]

● FABER Test or Patrick Test (Sensitivity 0.42-0.60, Specificity 0.18-0.75) (Figure 3H.5)
  • Also known as the Patrick test, it was first described by Hugh Talbot Patrick[8] in 1917
  • There have been no major modifications
  • **Maneuver:**
    – The patient lies supine with the examiner standing on the affected side
    – The patient's hip is fully flexed, abducted, and externally rotated
    – Positive test: recreation of symptoms of pain or impingement on the ipsilateral side, as the test is being performed upon
    – This test can also be positive for FAI or labral pathology

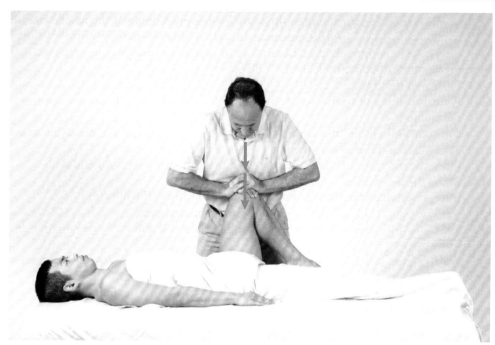

Figure 3H.6. Thigh thrust test. The patient lies supine with his/her affected hip flexed to 90°. The examiner applies an axially directed force through the shaft of the femur, which will reproduce the patient's pain in the sacroiliac joint. (From Muscolino JE. *Manual Therapy for the Low Back and Pelvis: A Clinical Orthopedic Approach.* Wolters Kluwer Health; 2015.)

- Thigh Thrust Test (Sensitivity 0.36-0.88, Specificity 0.50-0.69) (Figure 3H.6)
  - **Maneuver:**
    – The patient lies supine on the examination table with the hip of the affected side flexed to 90°
    – The examiner stands beside the patient, applying an axial force through the femur and into the hip
    – Positive test: reproduction of patient's pain in the area of the SI joint
- Pressure Over the Sacral Sulcus (Sensitivity 0.95, Specificity 0.09)
  - **Maneuver:**
    – As the name suggests, the examiner places steady, constant pressure over the sacral sulcus of the patient's affected side
    – Positive test: reproduction of patient's pain in the area of the SI joint

IMAGING

- Plain X-rays, CT scans, MRI scans, and bone scans are not particularly useful in the diagnosis of SI joint dysfunction. Their utility lies primarily in ruling out other pathology that may be responsible for the patient's lower back pain[3]
- Diagnostic SI joint injection[1-3]
  - This is the study of choice for diagnosing SI joint dysfunction
  - Technique:
    – Before injection, the patient's pain level should be assessed on a scale from 1 to 10
    – Then the patient is placed prone, and the skin overlying the SI joint is sterilely prepped and draped

- The soft tissue overlying the area of interest is anesthetized, and a small bore spinal needle is used to gain access to the joint. Proper positioning of the needle can be monitored with CT or MRI guidance, as well as ultrasonography; however, fluoroscopy is most commonly used because of its ease of use and inexpensive cost
    • Injections done without image guidance have been shown to enter the joint only 22% of the time
- A small volume of contrast material is injected into the joint to confirm proper positioning
- The joint is then injected with a combination of lidocaine and bupivacaine to confer immediate and longer term relief
- Once the injectate has had time to set in, the patient's pain is reevaluated
- Evaluation of the study
    - Interpretation of the study is based on pain relief from the injection
        • ≥75% pain relief is diagnostic of SI joint–mediated pain
        • 51% to 74% pain relief provides an equivocal result and further evaluation should be done
        • ≤50% pain relief is a negative result, and another source of lower back pain must be investigated
- This test may be further substantiated through a double-block technique in which 2 separate injections are given at different times
    - One injection contains a short-acting anesthetic and the other contains a longer acting anesthetic
    - The patient's ability to differentiate the timeline of action between these 2 injections helps to rule out a positive response due to placebo effect
- The diagnostic injection may be confounded by extravasation of injectate out of the joint and anesthetizing surrounding structures that may be the actual cause of the patient's symptoms, thereby providing a false-positive result
    - The risk of this may be decreased with fluoroscopic guidance and the injection of a small volume of anesthetic, as the SI joint may contain a maximum of 2.5 mL of fluid[1-3]

REFERENCES

1. Foley BS, et al. Sacroiliac joint pain. *Am J Phys Med Rehabil.* 2006;85(12):997-1006.
2. Rashbaum RF, et al. Sacroiliac joint pain and its treatment. *Clin Spine Surg.* 2016;29(2):42-48.
3. Dreyfuss P, et al. Sacroiliac joint pain. *J Am Acad Orthop Surg.* 2004;12(4):255-265.
4. Cohen SP, et al. Sacroiliac joint pain: a comprehensive review of epidemiology, diagnosis, and treatment. *Expert Rev Neurother.* 2013;13(1):99-116.
5. Isaac Z, Devine J. Sacroiliac joint dysfunction. In: Frontera WR, Silver JK, Rizzo TD, eds. *Essentials of Physical Medicine and Rehabilitation: Musculoskeletal Disorders, Pain, and Rehabilitation*, 2nd ed. Philadelphia: Saunders Elsevier; 2008:267-270.
6. Stuber KJ. Specificity, sensitivity, and predictive values of clinical tests of the sacroiliac joint: a systematic review of the literature. *J Can Chiropr Assoc.* 2007;51(1):30-41.
7. Gaenslen FJ. Sacroiliac arthrodesis: indications, author's technic and end-results. *JAMA.* 1927;89(24):2031-2035.

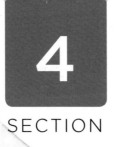

4
SECTION

The Elbow

Section Editor
Felix H. Savoie

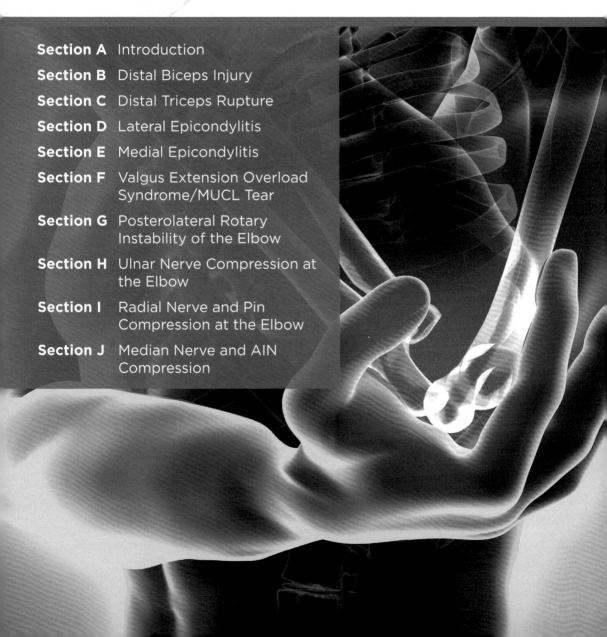

QUICK REFERENCE FLOW CHART

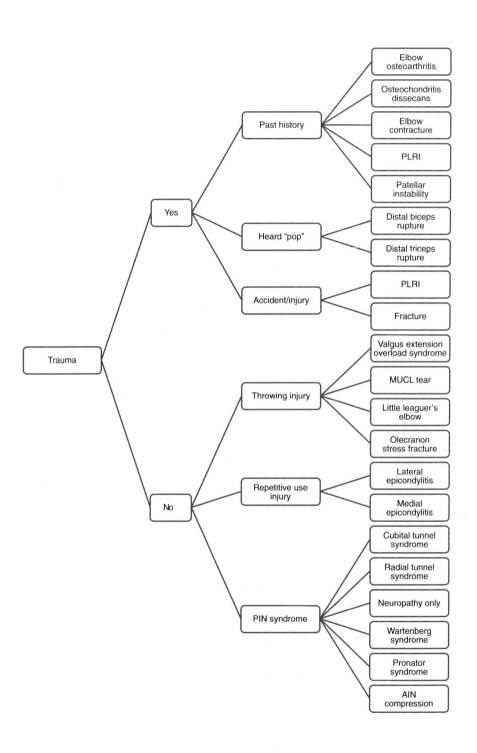

SECTION A
Introduction

Felix H. Savoie, Stephen G. Thon, and Mary K. Mulcahey

HISTORY

It is important to consider the following parameters when a patient presents to the clinic with an elbow complaint:

- Patient age
  - Younger patients are more likely to have trauma, a ligamentous injury, an acute tendon rupture, or an apophyseal injury
  - Older patients are more likely to have tendinopathy, neuropathy, osteoarthritis, or overuse injuries
- Chronicity of symptoms
  - Acute injuries generally involve fractures, ligamentous injuries, acute tendon ruptures, and dislocations
  - Chronic injuries can also involve ligamentous injuries from overuse, tendinopathies, neuropathies, or degenerative changes
- Mechanism of injury (if any)
  - Traumatic injury can lead to ligament tears, tendon ruptures, fractures, and/or dislocations
  - Repetitive motions/actions can lead to tendinopathies or neuropathies
  - Throwing or overhead activity can also lead to tendinopathies or ligamentous injuries
- Associated swelling (effusion)
  - Swelling is generally seen in acute traumatic injuries
  - Occasionally, swelling can be seen in the setting of tendinopathy
- Mechanical symptoms (locking, catching)
  - Usually associated with osteochondral lesions and osteoarthritis
- History of elbow injury
  - One must be concerned about reinjury
  - Evaluate range of motion. Deficits may indicate a contracture or possible heterotopic ossification
- History of elbow surgery
  - Critically analyze previous surgery. Obtain operative reports, intraoperative pictures (if available), and copies of relevant imaging
  - Check for heterotopic ossification (ie, X-rays, CT) with history of trauma or prior surgery
- Prior treatment
- Current medications

PHYSICAL EXAMINATION

Observation

- Observe the alignment of the patient's elbow in full extension and flexion
- In acute injuries, assess for swelling, ecchymosis, or erythema

Palpation

- Palpate all aspects of the elbow
  - An effusion can be appreciated in the "soft spot" at the lateral elbow or posteriorly in the olecranon fossa
  - Assess for an effusion directly over the olecranon
- Tenderness
  - Tenderness over the medial or lateral epicondyles can signify chronic tendinopathy
  - Assess the paths of the median, radial, and ulnar nerves for tenderness or hypersensitivity, which may indicate a neuropathy
  - Tenderness over the ulnar collateral ligament (UCL) may indicate a UCL injury
  - Tenderness over the insertion of the triceps or biceps tendons may signify a possible tendon injury
  - Deep tenderness may represent a fracture or bone bruise

Range of Motion

- Normal range of motion is typically in full extension from 0° to 150° of elbow flexion and 75° to 90° of pronation/supination
- Patients with generalized ligamentous laxity may show hyperextension of the elbow
  - If present, check for other signs of generalized ligamentous laxity using the Beighton-Horan scale for joint hypermobility (ie, hyper extension of the elbow, passive hyperextension of small fingers, passive abduction of thumbs to forearms)
- Loss of motion in any plane may be the result of contracture, heterotopic ossification, or prior injury

Muscular Strength

- Assess strength compared with the contralateral elbow in flexion, extension, pronation, and supination
  - Weakness or inability to extend the elbow may signify a triceps tendon injury
  - Weakness or inability to flex the elbow may signify a biceps tendon injury
  - Weakness or inability to supinate the forearm may indicate a biceps tendon injury
- Assess strength of the wrist flexion and extension, as deficits or pain may signal a tendinopathy or neuropathy
  - Pain/weakness in wrist extension may represent lateral epicondylitis or extensor tendinitis
  - Pain/weakness in wrist flexion may represent medial epicondylitis

Sensation

- Can be viewed as dermatomes C5-T1 or as peripheral nerves listed below (Figure 4A.1A and 4A.1B)
  - Lateral antebrachial cutaneous (C5-C6)
  - Medial antebrachial cutaneous (C8-T1)
  - Medial brachial cutaneous (T1-T2)
  - Radial nerve (C5-T1)
  - Ulnar nerve (C8-T1)
  - Median nerve (C5-T1)

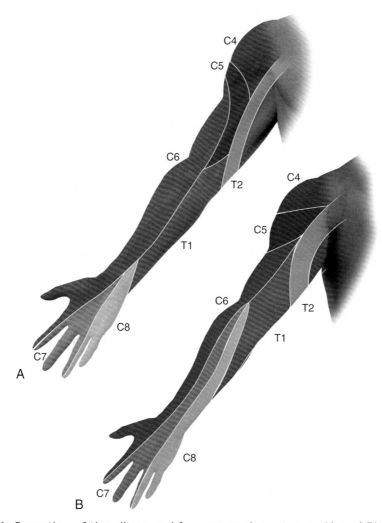

Figure 4A.1. Sensation of the elbow and forearm as dermatomes (A and B) and peripheral nerves (C). ((A and B) From Olinger AB. *Human Gross Anatomy*. Philadelphia: Wolters Kluwer; Wolters Kluwer Health; 2016 and (C) Agur AMR, Dalley AF. *Grant's Atlas of Anatomy*. Wolters Kluwer Health; 2017.)

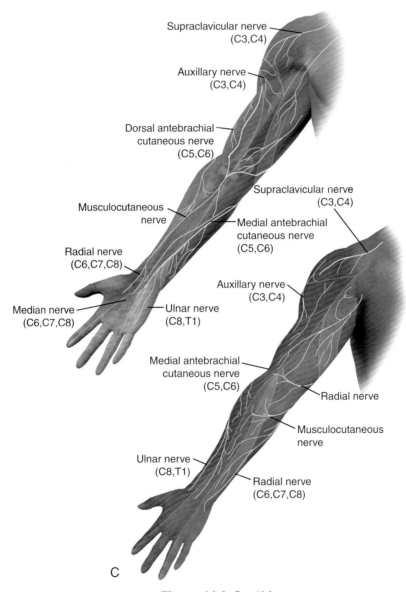

Supraclavicular nerve
(C3,C4)

Auxillary nerve
(C3,C4)

Dorsal antebrachial
cutaneous nerve
(C5,C6)

Supraclavicular nerve
(C3,C4)

Musculocutaneous
nerve

Medial antebrachial
cutaneous nerve
(C5,C6)

Radial nerve
(C6,C7,C8)

Auxillary nerve
(C3,C4)

Median nerve
(C6,C7,C8)

Ulnar nerve
(C8,T1)

Medial antebrachial
cutaneous nerve
(C5,C6)

Radial nerve

Musculocutaneous
nerve

Ulnar nerve
(C8,T1)

Radial nerve
(C6,C7,C8)

C

Figure 4A.1. Cont'd

KEY EXAMINATION MANEUVERS

- Distal Biceps rupture (Section B)
  - Hook test
  - Biceps crease interval (BCI) test
  - Ruland biceps squeeze test
  - Passive forearm pronation (PFP) test
  - Supination-pronation test

- Distal Triceps Rupture (Section C)
  - Modified Thompson squeeze test
  - Triceps stress test

- Lateral Epicondylitis (Section D)
  - Cozen test
  - Polk test
  - Maudsley test
  - Mill test
  - Grip strength

- Medial Epicondylitis (Section E)
  - Golfer's elbow test
  - Polk test
  - Resisted pronation test
  - Grip strength

- Valgus Extension Overload Syndrome/MUCL Tear (Section F)
  - Moving valgus stress test
  - Static valgus stress test
  - Milking maneuver

- Posterolateral Rotary Instability of the Elbow (PLRI) (Section G)
  - Table-top relocation test
  - Chair push-up test
  - Push-up test
  - Lateral pivot shift test

- Ulnar Nerve Compression about the Elbow (Section H)
  - Tinel sign
  - Elbow flexion test
  - Direct compression test
  - Combined elbow flexion test and direct compression test

- Radial Nerve and PIN Compression (Section I)
  - Maudsley test/resisted long finger extension test
  - Resisted supination test
  - Passive pronation with wrist flexion test
  - Radial tunnel injection
  - Resisted supination test
  - Ulnar-deviated wrist extension test
  - Wrist flexion, ulnar deviation, pronation test
  - Tinel sign
  - Finkelstein test

- Median Nerve and AIN Compression (Section J)
  - Pronator compression test
  - Resisted pronation and supination
  - Resisted flexion of PIP joint of long finger
  - Kiloh-Nevin sign/"OK" sign
  - Pinch grip test

IMAGING

Plain Radiographs

- AP view (Figure 4A.2)
- Lateral view (Figure 4A.2)
- Oblique view
- Valgus stress view

Magnetic Resonance Imaging

- Identify ligament or tendon injuries
- Evaluate for loose bodies

Computed Tomography

- Assess for bony injuries and heterotopic ossification

Ultrasonography

- Can be helpful in diagnosing tendinopathies, neuropathies, and ligamentous injuries
- Pros: inexpensive and easy to perform; can be done in office
- Cons: requires a skilled/trained technician

Elbow Arthroscopy (Figure 4A.3)

- Standard portals
  - Anteromedial
  - Anterolateral
  - Posterior
- Accessory portals
  - Direct lateral
  - Proximal anterolateral

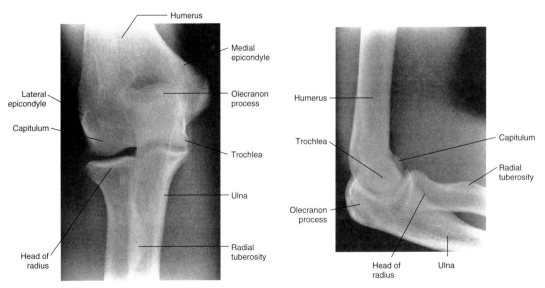

Figure 4A.2. Normal radiographic views of elbow. (From Dudek RW, Louis T. *High-Yield Gross Anatomy*. Wolters Kluwer Health; 2015.)

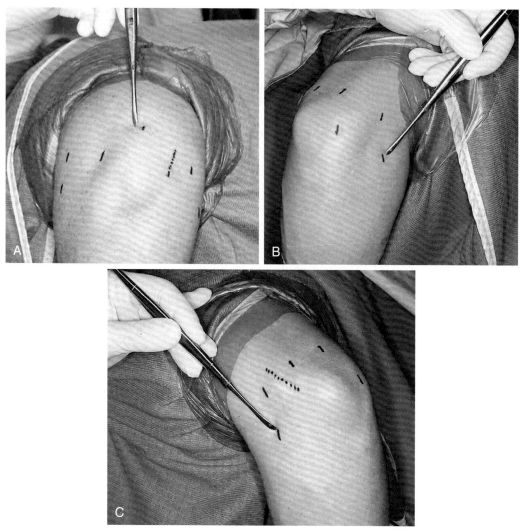

Figure 4A.3. Arthroscopic portals used in elbow arthroscopy as viewed from posterior (A), lateral (B), and medial (C). (From Steinmann SP. Elbow arthroscopy. *J Am Soc Surg Hand*. 2003;3:199-207; Figures 5-7, with permission.)

- Proximal anteromedial
- Posterolateral
- Visualization
  - Anteromedial: starting portal, radiocapitellar joint, proximal capsular insertion
  - Anterolateral: radial head, medial compartment, coronoid, trochlea
  - Posterior: olecranon, posteromedial compartment
  - Direct lateral: posterior compartment, capitellum, radial head, radioulnar joint
  - Proximal anterolateral: anterior radiohumeral and ulnohumeral joints
  - Proximal anteromedial: anterior compartment, radial head, capitellum, coronoid, trochlea
  - Posterolateral: posterior compartment, radiocapitellar joint, olecranon fossa

SECTION B
Distal Biceps Injury

Felix H. Savoie, Stephen G. Thon, and Mary K. Mulcahey

HISTORY

- Classically results from an eccentric contraction during flexion at the elbow
- Some patients report feeling or hearing a "pop" at the time of injury
- Weakness in the elbow flexion and forearm supination; supination > flexion
  - Significant weakness/pain with attempted resisted supination of forearm
- Most common in men, especially in the dominant arm
- Partial tears will present similar to complete tears
- Risk factors: anabolic steroids and smoking

PHYSICAL EXAMINATION

Common Physical Examination Findings

- Ecchymosis of the medial upper arm (Figure 4B.1A)
- "Reverse Popeye deformity" (Figure 4B.1B)
- Palpable defect at insertion of the biceps tendon

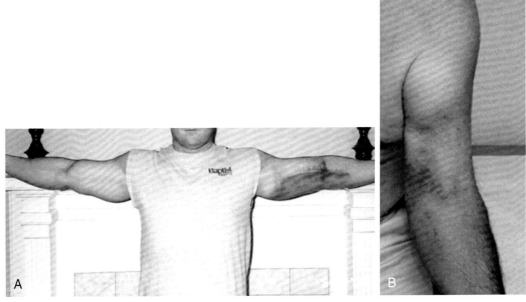

Figure 4B.1. Medial upper arm ecchymosis (A) and reverse "Popeye" deformity (B) of distal biceps rupture commonly found on physical examination. ((B) From Waldman SD, Lippincott Williams & Wilkins. *Waldman's Comprehensive Atlas of Diagnostic Ultrasound of Painful Conditions*. Wolters Kluwer Health; 2016.)

- **Hook Test** (Sensitivity: 1.00, Specificity: 1.00) (Figure 4B.2)
  - First described in the literature in 2007 by O'Driscoll[1]
  - **Maneuver**:
    - The patient flexes the elbow to 90° and fully supinates the forearm
    - The examiner uses the index finger to "hook" around insertion of the biceps tendon from medial to lateral
      - Absence of tendon signals complete tear
      - Palpation of cordlike structure signals the intact tendon or partial tear
    - Sensitivity and specificity are 1.0[1]

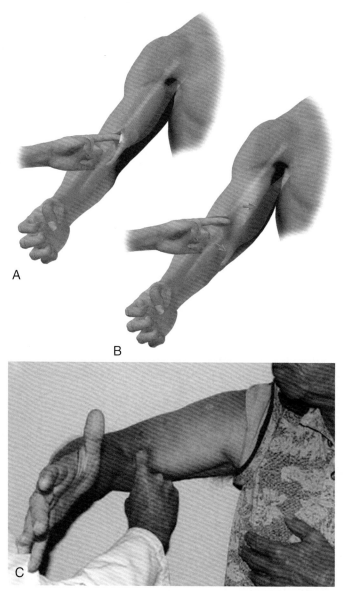

Figure 4B.2. Complete biceps avulsion. Abnormal hook test (A) compared with a normal result on the other side (B). The examiner's finger is unable to find a cordlike structure spanning the antecubital fossa behind which to hook. C, Four months postoperatively, the integrity of the repaired distal biceps tendon in the same patient can now be confirmed with an intact hook test. ((C) From Waldman SD, Lippincott Williams & Wilkins. *Waldman's Comprehensive Atlas of Diagnostic Ultrasound of Painful Conditions*. Wolters Kluwer Health; 2016.)

- **BCI Test** (Sensitivity: 0.92, Specificity: 1.00)
  - First described in the literature in 2008 by ElMaraghy and Devereaux[2]
  - **Maneuver**:
    - Find antecubital fossa crease with the arm flexed at 90° and trace with a pen or make a mark
    - Find the point that the curve of biceps begins to approach antecubital fossa and make another mark
    - Measure the distance between 2 marks down to the first decimal digit in centimeters
      - <5.0 cm = normal
      - >6.0 cm = positive finding for rupture
    - Compare to the opposite side
  - Limitations of Maneuver:
    - All subjective measuring by the examiner

- **Ruland Biceps Squeeze Test** (Sensitivity: 0.95, Specificity: 0.67)
  - First described in the literature in 2005 by Ruland[3]
  - **Maneuver**:
    - The patient is seated, with the elbow in ~70° of flexion and slightly pronated
    - The forearm resting on the table comfortably
    - The examiner places one hand on biceps tendon and the other on biceps muscle belly and squeezes BOTH the hands firmly
      - The test is considered positive when no supination of the forearm occurs or the patient experiences significant pain
      - Supination will be slight, even in intact tendon
      - Compare the test to the other side

- **Passive Forearm Pronation (PFP) Test** (Sensitivity: 0.95, Specificity: 1.00)
  - First described in the literature in 2005 by Harding[4]
  - **Maneuver**:
    - The examiner bends and supports the elbow in 90° of flexion, fully supinated
    - The examiner then passively supinates and pronates the forearm
    - Observe the motion of biceps muscle belly and compare with the intact side
      - Positive test: if there is no motion or significantly decreased motion to the contralateral side

- **Supination-Pronation Test** (Sensitivity: 1.00)
  - First described in the literature in 2015 by Metzman and Tivener[5]
  - **Maneuver**:
    - In a standing position, the patient abducts both shoulders to 90° and flexes both elbows to approximately 60° to 70°
    - Have the patient actively supinate and pronate the forearm
    - The examiner observes from the front of the patient and look for movement of biceps muscle belly
    - Lack of migration or decreased motion from the opposite arm is considered positive

IMAGING

Plain Radiographs

- Most commonly normal; may show small avulsion fracture of radial tuberosity

Magnetic Resonance Imaging

- Gold standard for diagnosis; can determine full versus partial tears and degree of retraction (Figure 4B.3)
- Holding the arm in abduction, the elbow in flexion, and the forearm in supination helps with sensitivity[6]

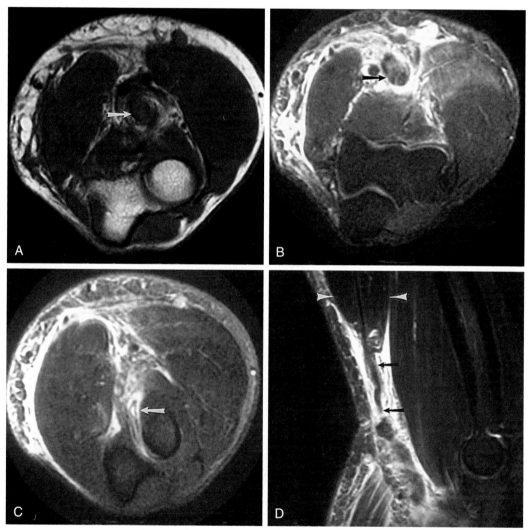

Figure 4B.3. Distal biceps tendon rupture. Axial T1-weighted (A) and T2-weighted (B) images display a markedly thickened distal biceps containing increased T2-weighted signal (arrow) proximal to the point of rupture. Increased T2-weighted fluid (hemorrhage) surrounds the tendon and extends throughout the deep fascial planes and the subcutaneous soft tissues. C, Axial T2-weighted image near the radial tuberosity demonstrates some frayed tendinous remnants (arrow) at the site of rupture. D, Sagittal FSE T2-weighted fat-saturated image displays the retracted biceps muscle (arrowheads) and the undulating ruptured biceps tendon (arrows). (From Berquist TH, ed. *MRI of the Musculoskeletal System*. 6th ed. Philadelphia, PA: Wolters Kluwer; 2013.)

REFERENCES

1. O'driscoll SW, Goncalves LB, Dietz P. The hook test for distal biceps tendon avulsion. *Am J Sports Med.* 2007;35(11):1865-1869.
2. Elmaraghy A, Devereaux M, Tsoi K. The biceps crease interval for diagnosing complete distal biceps tendon ruptures. *Clin Orthop Relat Res.* 2008;466(9):2255-2262.
3. Ruland RT, Dunbar RP, Bowen JD. The biceps squeeze test for diagnosis of distal biceps tendon ruptures. *Clin Orthop Relat Res.* 2005;(437):128-131.
4. Harding WG. A new clinical test for avulsion of the insertion of the biceps tendon. *Orthopedics.* 2005;28(1):27-29.
5. Metzman LS, Tivener KA. The supination-pronation test for distal biceps tendon rupture. *Am J Orthop.* 2015;44(10):E361-E364.
6. Devereaux MW, Elmaraghy AW. Improving the rapid and reliable diagnosis of complete distal biceps tendon rupture: a nuanced approach to the clinical examination. *Am J Sports Med.* 2013;41(9):1998-2004.

SECTION C
Distal Triceps Rupture

Felix H. Savoie, Stephen G. Thon, and Mary K. Mulcahey

HISTORY

- Sudden eccentric contraction of triceps (ie, weight lifting, fall, sports)[1]
  - May feel/hear an audible "pop"
- Can also be traumatic from direct blow or laceration (less common)
- Most commonly found at insertion on the olecranon or myotendinous junction
- Pain, swelling, and ecchymosis are common over posterior aspect of the elbow
- May have palpable defect just proximal to the olecranon[3]
- Inability or weakness to actively extend at the elbow
  - Complete loss of extension only seen in 20% of cases[2]
- Risk factors: anabolic steroids, local injections, fluoroquinolone use, chronic or infected olecranon bursitis

PHYSICAL EXAMINATION

KEY EXAMINATION MANEUVERS

- **Modified Thompson Squeeze Test** (Figure 4C.1)
  - First described in the literature in 1990 by Viegas[4]
  - **Maneuver**:
    - The patient lies prone with the elbow hanging over the edge of the examination table
    - The examiner firmly squeezes triceps muscle belly
    - Complete disruption will have no movement of the forearm
    - Positive findings are a lack of motion of the forearm with squeeze
  - **Limitations of Maneuver**:
    - The forearm is heavier and has a longer lever arm than the foot making the test in the triceps harder to elicit, even in an intact tendon
    - Sensitivity and specificity data have not been reported

- **Triceps Stress Test**
  - **Maneuver**:
    - The patient brings the shoulder into forward flexion of 90° and adduction
    - The examiner places the forearm in maximum flexion
    - The patient then attempts to actively extend against resistance while keeping the upper arm level with the floor
    - Positive finding if pain at the posterior elbow and/or inability to extend the forearm is found

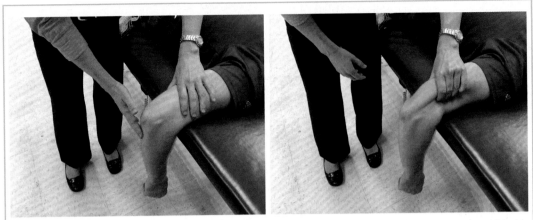

Figure 4C.1. Modified Thompson squeeze test. An intact triceps can be seen with its insertion into the elbow intact.

IMAGING

Plain Radiographs

- AP/lateral/oblique images of the affected elbow should be obtained
- The lateral image may show a "flake sign" of a small piece of olecranon that avulsed with the triceps tendon (Figure 4C.2)

Computed Tomography

- Helpful in ruling out other pathology, if suspected (eg, radial head fracture, olecranon fracture)

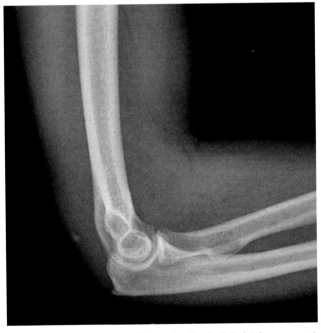

Figure 4C.2. Avulsion or "flake sign" of distal triceps rupture.

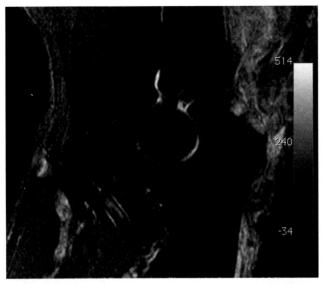

Figure 4C.3. Avulsion of distal triceps from olecranon. (From Iannotti JP, Williams GR, Miniaci A, Zuckerman JD. *Disorders of the Shoulder: Diagnosis & Management.* Wolters Kluwer; 2014.)

Magnetic Resonance Imaging (Figure 4C.3):

- Can determine partial versus complete ruptures
  - Partial ruptures: small fluid-filled defect with some intact tendon[6]
  - Complete ruptures: large fluid-filled defect and a measurable gap between the olecranon and distal tendon[6]
- Can determine the amount of retraction of tendon if present

Ultrasonography

- Can help differentiate between complete versus partial ruptures
  - In one series, the finding was 100% sensitive and 100% specific in identifying both complete and partial ruptures (but with limited patient numbers)[7]

Classic Arthroscopic Findings

- Utilizes a central posterior portal, a proximal posterior portal, and a distal posterior portal
  - The central portal is used for diagnostic arthroscopy
  - A camera is then placed in the distal posterior portal
  - The working portal is the proximal posterior portal
- After triceps bursectomy, the olecranon can be visualized with a bare spot at triceps insertion (Figure 4C.4) along with unattached distal aspect of the tendon[5]

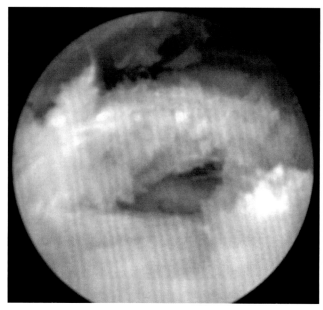

Figure 4C.4. Arthroscopic view from posterior portal of avulsion of distal triceps from olecranon.

REFERENCES

1. Yeh PC, Dodds SD, Smart LR, Mazzocca AD, Sethi PM. Distal triceps rupture. *J Am Acad Orthop Surg.* 2010;18(1):31-40.
2. Demirhan M, Ersen A. Distal triceps ruptures. *EFORT Open Rev.* 2016;1(6):255-259.
3. Thomas JR, Lawton JN. Biceps and triceps ruptures in athletes. *Hand Clin.* 2017;33(1):35-46.
4. Viegas SF. Avulsion of the triceps tendon. *Orthop Rev.* 1990;19:533-536
5. Ng T, Rush LN, Savoie FH. Arthroscopic distal triceps repair. *Arthrosc Tech.* 2016;5(4):e941-e945.
6. Kijowski R, Tuite M, Sanford M. Magnetic resonance imaging of the elbow. Part II: Abnormalities of the ligaments, tendons, and nerves. *Skeletal Radiol.* 2005;34(1):1-18.
7. Tagliafico A, Gandolfo N, Michaud J, Perez MM, Palmieri F, Martinoli C. Ultrasound demonstration of distal triceps tendon tears. *Eur J Radiol.* 2012;81(6):1207-1210.

SECTION D
Lateral Epicondylitis

Felix H. Savoie, Stephen G. Thon, and Mary K. Mulcahey

HISTORY:

- Commonly known as "tennis elbow"
- Classically an overuse injury, resulting from activities with repetitive wrist extension and pronation (ie, tennis backhand)
- More appropriately termed "tendinosis," as no inflammatory component is found
  - Most commonly affects the extensor carpi radialis brevis (ECRB) tendon origin
- Patients will complain of pain directly at or just anterior to the lateral epicondyle, especially after the offending activity (Figure 4D.1)

PHYSICAL EXAMINATION

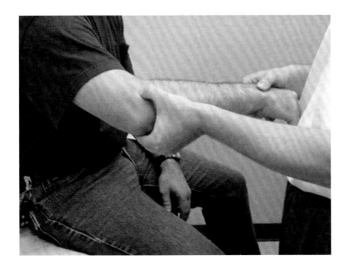

Figure 4D.1. Tenderness anterior to the lateral epicondyle.

KEY EXAMINATION MANEUVERS

- **Cozen Test** (Figure 4D.2)
  - **Maneuver**:
    - The patient in a seated position extends the elbow and puts the forearm into maximum pronation
    - The hand is made into a fist and deviated radially at the wrist
    - The examiner palpates the lateral epicondyle while the patient brings the wrist from extension to flexion
    - Pain at the lateral epicondyle is a positive test finding

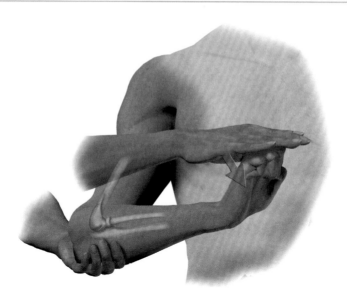

Figure 4D.2. Cozen test. (From Cipriano JJ. *Photographic Manual of Regional Orthopaedic and Neurological Tests*. 4th ed. Philadelphia: Lippincott Williams & Wilkins; 2003, with permission.)

- **Limitations of Maneuver**:
  - No sensitivity, specificity, or accuracy data have been reported
- **Polk Test**:
  - First described in the literature in 2002 by Polkinghorn[2]
  - **Maneuver**:
    - The patient is seated, with the elbow flexed slightly past 90° and the forearm in maximum pronation
    - The examiner hands the patient object between 5 to 10 lbs and asks him/her to hold in that position
    - Pain at the lateral epicondyle is a positive test finding
  - **Limitations of Maneuver**:
    - No sensitivity, specificity, or accuracy data have been reported

- **Maudsley Test** (Figure 4D.3)
  - First described in the literature in 1972 by Roles and Maudsley[4]
    - Also known as the middle finger resistance test
  - **Maneuver**:
    - The patient is seated with the elbow extended
    - The patient's forearms and palms are placed on the examination table
    - The examiner stabilizes the forearm on the table and then asks the patient to raise the long finger off the table while applying resistance
    - Pain at the lateral epicondyle is a positive test finding
  - **Limitations of Maneuver**:
    - No sensitivity, specificity, or accuracy data have been reported

- **Mill Test**
  - **Maneuver**:
    - The patient is seated with the elbow extended and forearm in maximum pronation
    - The examiner stabilizes the elbow, holds wrist, and passively moves wrist into flexion
    - Pain at the lateral epicondyle is a positive test finding

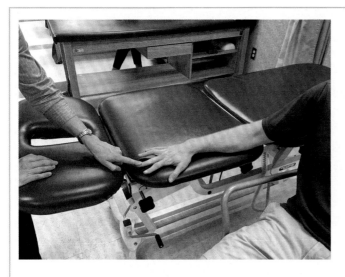

Figure 4D.3. "Maudsley test" or middle finger resistance test.

- **Limitations of Maneuver**:
  - No sensitivity, specificity, or accuracy data have been reported

- **Grip Strength**:
  - Sensitivity and specificity varied with changes in grip strength[1,5]
    - Loss of 5% strength = sensitivity: 0.83, specificity: 0.80
    - Loss of 8% strength = sensitivity: 0.80, specificity: 0.85
    - Loss of 10% strength = sensitivity: 0.78, specificity: 0.90
  - **Maneuver**:
    - The patient holds the shoulder in adduction, neutral rotation, with the elbow bent to 90° and the forearm and wrist placed in a neutral position
    - The patient squeezes the dynamometer as hard as possible; reading is recorded
    - Then ask the patient to extend the elbow fully and repeat
      - Repeat on the unaffected side and measure the difference in strength if necessary
    - Decrease in grip strength from flexion to extension signifies a positive test finding
  - **Limitations of Maneuver**:
    - Requires dynamometer and trained use

IMAGING (IF APPLICABLE)

Plain Radiographs

- AP, lateral, and oblique radiographs of the elbow are recommended to rule out other pathology
- Plain radiographs are often negative

Magnetic Resonance Imaging (Figure 4D.4)

- Will show tendinosis in ECRB origin
- Positive correlation of 0.92 between MRI findings and severity of lateral epicondylitis[3]

Ultrasonography (Figure 4D.5)

- Attenuation of the tendon at origin of extensor tendons
- Requires trained use and experienced technicians

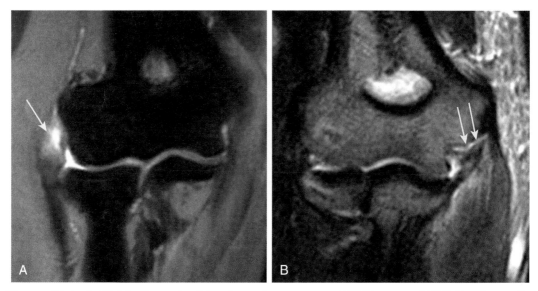

Figure 4D.4. A, Right elbow short tau inversion recovery (STIR) coronal MRI. Tendinopathy and partial tear of the common extensor tendon (arrow). This is sometimes mistakenly called lateral epicondylitis. B, Right elbow coronal fat-suppressed T2-weighted MRI of a tear of the humeral attachment of the ulnar collateral ligament (arrows). (From Smith WL, Farrell TA. *Radiology 101: The Basics and Fundamentals of Imaging*. Wolters Kluwer; 2014.)

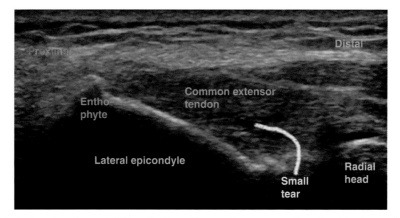

Figure 4D.5. Lateral epicondylitis of the elbow. Sonogram longitudinal to the common extensor tendons shows small tear of the common extensor tendon. Note enthesophyte of the lateral epicondyle, which is a classic finding of the tennis elbow. (From Waldman SD, *Waldman's Comprehensive Atlas of Diagnostic Ultrasound of Painful Conditions*. Lippincott Williams & Wilkins; 2016.)

REFERENCES

1. Dorf ER, Chhabra AB, Golish SR, Mcginty JL, Pannunzio ME. Effect of elbow position on grip strength in the evaluation of lateral epicondylitis. *J Hand Surg Am*. 2007;32(6):882-886.
2. Polkinghorn BS. A novel method for assessing elbow pain resulting from epicondylitis. *J Chiropr Med*. 2002;1(3):117-121.

3. Qi L, Zhang YD, Yu RB, Shi HB. Magnetic resonance imaging of patients with chronic lateral epicondylitis: is there a relationship between magnetic resonance imaging abnormalities of the common extensor tendon and the Patient's clinical symptom?. *Medicine (Baltimore)*. 2016;95(5):e2681.

4. Roles NC, Maudsley RH. Radial tunnel syndrome: resistant tennis elbow as a nerve entrapment. *J Bone Joint Surg Br*. 1972;54(3):499-508.

5. Bhargava AS, Eapen C, Kumar SP. Grip strength measurements at two different wrist extension positions in chronic lateral epicondylitis-comparison of involved vs. uninvolved side in athletes and non athletes: a case-control study. *Sports Med Arthrosc Rehabil Ther Technol*. 2010;2:22.

SECTION E
Medial Epicondylitis

Felix H. Savoie, Stephen G. Thon, and Mary K. Mulcahey

HISTORY

- Classically an overuse injury termed "Golfer elbow" in activities with the wrist flexion and pronation (ie, follow-through on golf swing or forehand in tennis)[4]
- More appropriately termed "tendinosis," as no inflammatory component is found[3]
  - Most commonly affects the pronator teres and flexor carpi radialis
- Patients will complain of pain directly at or just anterior to the medial epicondyle, especially after the offending activity
  - Most commonly 5 to 10 mm distal/anterior to the medial epicondyle
- More likely to require surgical intervention than the lateral counterpart
- ALWAYS check for signs and symptoms of ulnar neuropathy, highly associated with medial epicondylitis (up to 60%)[1]
  - See section H
- May also be associated with valgus stress to the elbow (ie, throwers)
  - See section F

PHYSICAL EXAMINATION

KEY EXAMINATION MANEUVERS

- **Golfer Elbow Test** (Figure 4E.1)
  - **Maneuver**:
    - The patient is seated, extends the elbow, and puts the forearm in maximum supination
    - The examiner stabilizes the patient's forearm and elbow
    - The patient flexes at the wrist against resistance
    - Pain at the medial epicondyle is a positive test finding
  - **Limitations of Maneuver**:
    - No sensitivity, specificity, or accuracy data have been reported
- **Polk Test**
  - First described in the literature in 2002 by Polkinghorn[6]
  - **Maneuver**:
    - The patient is seated, with the elbow flexed slightly past 90° and the forearm in maximum supination
    - The examiner hands the patient object between 5 to 10 lbs and asks him/her to flex at the wrist in that position
    - Pain at the medial epicondyle is a positive test finding

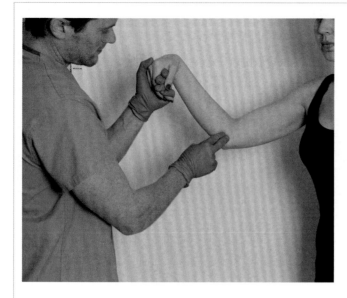

Figure 4E.1. "Golfer elbow test" with forearm supination and resisted wrist flexion. (From Waldman SD. *Comprehensive Atlas of Ultrasound-Guided Pain Management Injection Techniques*. Philadelphia: Wolters Kluwer Health/Lippincott Williams & Wilkins; 2014.)

- **Limitations of Maneuver**:
  - No sensitivity, specificity, or accuracy data have been reported

- **Resisted Pronation**:
  - Most sensitive maneuver for diagnosis[2]
  - **Maneuver**:
    - The patient flexes the elbow to 90°, with the arm at the side
    - The patient places the forearm into maximum supination
    - The examiner stabilizes the elbow with one hand and grips the forearm with the other
    - The patient is then asked to pronate the forearm against resistance
    - Pain at the medial epicondyle is a positive test finding
  - **Limitations of Maneuver**:
    - No sensitivity, specificity, or accuracy data have been reported

- **Mill test**
  - **Maneuver**:
    - The patient is seated with the elbow extended and the forearm in maximum pronation
    - The examiner stabilizes the elbow, holds the wrist, and passively moves the wrist into flexion
    - Pain at the medial epicondyle is a positive test finding
  - **Limitations of Maneuver**:
    - No sensitivity, specificity, or accuracy data have been reported

- **Grip Strength**
  - **Maneuver**:
    - The patient holds the shoulder in adduction, neutral rotation, with the elbow bent to 90°, wrist placed into a neutral position, and forearm fully supinated
    - The patient squeezes the dynamometer as hard as possible; reading is recorded
    - Repeat on the unaffected arm and compare the sides
    - Decrease in grip strength and pain during maneuver at the medial epicondyle signifies a positive finding
  - **Limitations of Maneuver**:
    - Requires a dynamometer and trained use

IMAGING (IF APPLICABLE)

Plain Radiographs

- AP, lateral, and oblique radiographs of the elbow are recommended to rule out other pathology
- May show calcification of the flexor pronator origin about the medial epicondyle
- Plain radiographs are often negative

Magnetic Resonance Imaging (Figure 4E.2)

- Will show tendinosis in flexor-pronator origin

Ultrasonography (Figure 4E.3)

- Attenuation of tendon at origin of flexors
- Sensitivity, specificity, accuracy, positive predictive value, negative predictive value all are >90% in one series[5]
- Requires trained use and experienced technicians

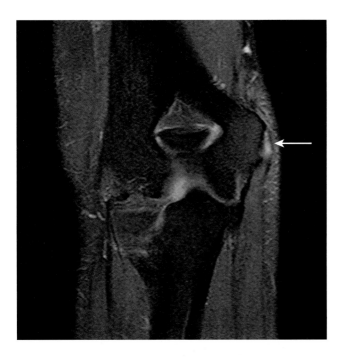

Figure 4E.2. MRI of medial epicondylitis. (From Dines JS. *Sports Medicine of Baseball*. Philadelphia: Wolters Kluwer Health/Lippincott Williams & Wilkins; 2012.)

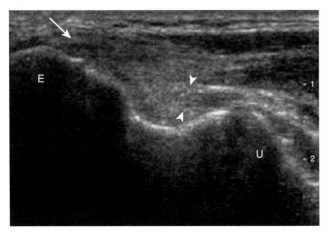

Figure 4E.3. Ultrasound of medial epicondylitis. Sonogram longitudinal to the common flexor tendons shows abnormal hypoechoic thickening. Note medial epicondyle (E), ulna (U), and ulnar collateral ligament (arrowheads). Arrow denotes area of epichoic signal within attachment of tendon to medial epicondyle.

REFERENCES

1. Kurvers H, Verhaar J. The results of operative treatment of medial epicondylitis. *J Bone Joint Surg Am.* 1995;77(9):1374-1379.
2. Gabel GT, Morrey BF. Operative treatment of medial epicondylitis. Influence of concomitant ulnar neuropathy at the elbow. *J Bone Joint Surg Am.* 1995;77(7):1065-1069.
3. Ciccotti MG, Ramani MN. Medial epicondylitis. *Tech Hand Up Extrem Surg.* 2003;7(4):190-196.
4. Pitzer ME, Seidenberg PH, Bader DA. Elbow tendinopathy. *Med Clin North Am.* 2014;98(4):833-849, xiii.
5. Park GY, Lee SM, Lee MY. Diagnostic value of ultrasonography for clinical medial epicondylitis. *Arch Phys Med Rehabil.* 2008;89(4):738-7342.
6. Polkinghorn BS. A novel method for assessing elbow pain resulting from epicondylitis. *J Chiropr Med.* 2002;1(3):117-121.

SECTION F
Valgus Extension Overload Syndrome/MUCL Tear

Felix H. Savoie, Stephen G. Thon, and Mary K. Mulcahey

HISTORY

- Common problem with ADULT overhead throwing athletes
  - Skeletally immature patients will alternatively have similar symptoms but usually have apophysitis or physeal injury of the medial epicondyle ("little leaguer's elbow")
- Acute injuries may present with an audible "pop"
- More commonly insidious or vague onset of medial elbow pain, especially in late cocking/early acceleration phase[2]
- Chronic valgus stress leads to attenuation/disruption/tearing of the anterior band of MUCL[4]
  - Poor throwing mechanics and scapular dyskinesis have been implicated[5]
- Associated with ulnar neuropathy, posteromedial impingement, and osteoarthritis of elbow

PHYSICAL EXAMINATION

KEY EXAMINATION MANEUVERS

- **Moving Valgus Stress Test** (Sensitivity: 1.00, Specificity: 0.75) (Figure 4F.1)
  - First described in the literature in 2005 by O'Driscoll[1]
  - Assesses the anterior band of MUCL
  - **Maneuver**:
    - The patient is seated upright, with the shoulder abducted to 90° and the elbow maximally flexed
    - Apply valgus pressure to the elbow until the shoulder has reached maximum external rotation
    - Quickly extend the elbow from the flexed position to 30°
    - A positive test is determined by reproduction of medial-sided elbow pain, apprehension, or guarding during maneuver
      - Pain should be maximal between 120° and 70°, referred to as the "shear angle"
  - **Limitations of Maneuver**:
    - Patients with concomitant shoulder pathology may not tolerate the procedure

- **Static Valgus Stress Test**
  - Sensitivity and specificity[1]
    - Pain with maneuver: sensitivity: 0.65, specificity: 0.50
    - Laxity with maneuver: sensitivity: 0.19, specificity: 0.100

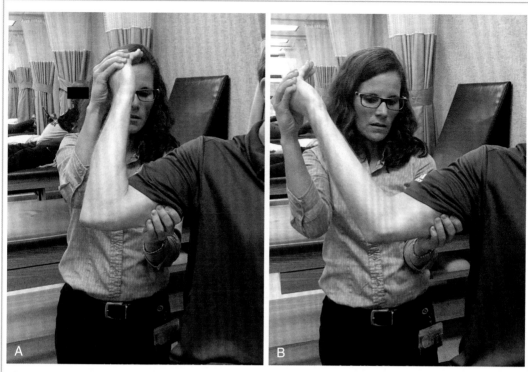

Figure 4F.1. Moving valgus stress test from flexion (A) to extension (B).

- **Maneuver**:
  - The patient is seated, with the elbow flexed to 70° and the forearm in maximum supination
  - The examiner holds the humerus and forearm, applies valgus stress across the forearm through the elbow
  - Pain or laxity at the medial elbow is a positive finding
    - For laxity, compare the results with the contralateral side
- **Limitations of Maneuver**:
  - Throwers generally have some laxity in the MUCL at baseline; therefore, the finding may be false positive

- **Milking Maneuver**
- Assesses the posterior band of MUCL
- **Maneuver**:
  - The patient is seated or supine, with the shoulder abducted to 90° and the forearm fully supinated (Figure 4F.2)
  - The elbow flexed to just past 90°
  - The examiner grabs the patient's thumb and pulls posteriorly until the shoulder reaches maximum external rotation (similar to moving valgus stress test)
    - This has also been described with the shoulder adducted and maximally rotated in 70° of flexion[3]
  - Positive test: if the patient has reproduction of pain, apprehension, or instability of the elbow during maneuver

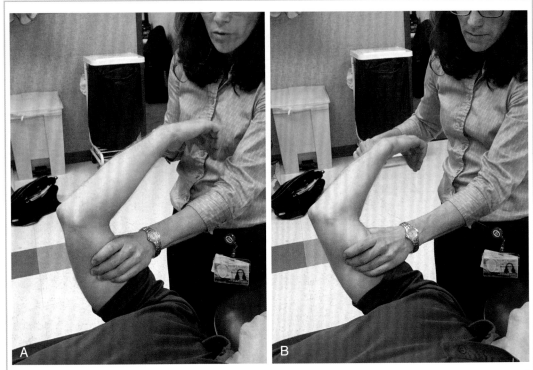

Figure 4F.2. Milking maneuver supine (A) placing the shoulder in maximum external rotation with valgus stress (B).

IMAGING

Plain Radiographs

- AP, lateral, and oblique radiographs of the elbow are recommended to rule out other pathology
  - May reveal avulsion fragment and calcification of MUCL
- Valgus stress radiographs are often helpful to determine the amount of laxity and to evaluate for ulnohumeral gapping

Computed Tomography

- CT arthrograms—sensitivity: 0.71 to 0.86, specificity: 0.91
  - Can show "T sign" in partial tears[3]

Magnetic Resonance Imaging

- Sensitivity: 0.57 to 0.79, specificity: 1.00 (Figure 4F.3)
- MR arthrograms—sensitivity: 0.97, specificity: 1.00
  - Will show fluid extravasation from the joint

Ultrasonography

- Rapid and can be performed in the office
- Will show discontinuity of MUCL
- Requires trained use and experienced technicians

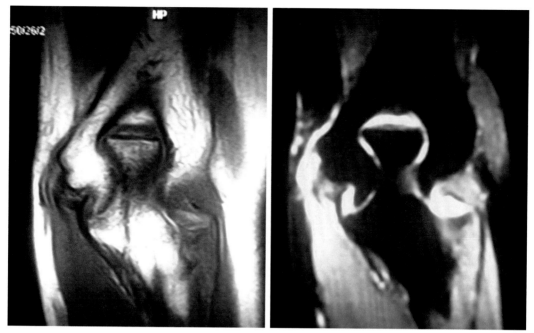

Figure 4F.3. MRI findings in MUCL rupture.

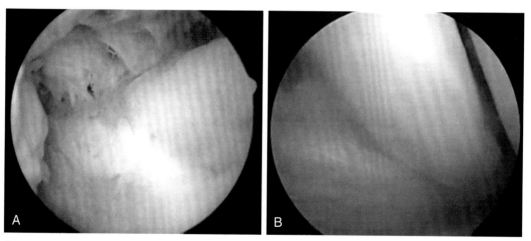

Figure 4F.4. Classic arthroscopic findings with acute avulsion (A) and gapping of the ulnohumeral joint (B).

Classic Arthroscopic Findings

- Best evaluated through the anterolateral portal (Figure 4F.4)
- Perform valgus stress test with the elbow at ~70° of flexion and the forearm pronated
  - Partial tears: 1 to 2 mm gapping
  - Complete tears: 4 to 10 mm gapping

REFERENCES

1. O'driscoll SW, Lawton RL, Smith AM. The "moving valgus stress test" for medial collateral ligament tears of the elbow. *Am J Sports Med*. 2005;33(2):231-239.
2. Dugas JR. Valgus extension overload: diagnosis and treatment. *Clin Sports Med*. 2010;29(4):645-654.

3. Hariri S, Safran MR. Ulnar collateral ligament injury in the overhead athlete. *Clin Sports Med.* 2010;29(4):619-644.
4. Daruwalla JH, Daly CA, Seiler JG. Medial elbow injuries in the throwing athlete. *Hand Clin.* 2017;33(1):47-62.
5. Nassab PF, Schickendantz MS. Evaluation and treatment of medial ulnar collateral ligament injuries in the throwing athlete. *Sports Med Arthrosc.* 2006;14(4):221-231.

SECTION G
Posterolateral Rotary Instability of the Elbow

Felix H. Savoie, Stephen G. Thon, and Mary K. Mulcahey

HISTORY

- Most common after trauma or dislocation of the supinated and flexed elbow[1]
  - Disruption of lateral collateral ligament complex (Figure 4G.1)
- Can be missed at the time of injury, as the elbow may spontaneously reduce
- Patients can present with "locking," "clicking," or "snapping" at the lateral elbow
- Pain usually noticed when the elbow is going from flexion to extension against resistance
  - Most commonly found at 40° to 50° of flexion
- Patients may guard or avoid offending actions

PHYSICAL EXAMINATION

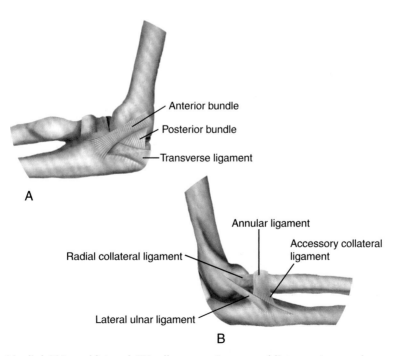

Figure 4G.1. Medial (A) and lateral (B) elbow anatomy and ligament complexes.

KEY EXAMINATION MANEUVERS

- **Table-top Relocation Test** (Sensitivity: 1.00) (Figure 4G.2)
  - First described in the literature in 2006 by Arvind[2]
  - **Maneuver**:
    - The patient stands in front of the examination table, the forearm is supinated, and the hand is placed on the edge of the table
    - The patient is then asked to lower the body toward the table
    - A positive finding is a feeling of apprehension, reproduction of pain, or instability noted at the lateral elbow
      - This usually occurs at ~40° to 50° of elbow flexion
    - Repeat the maneuver with examiner's elbow pressing on the lateral aspect of the patient's elbow over the radial head to help prevent subluxation
    - A positive finding is when application of pressure over the radial head prevents subluxation and feelings of pain
      - The examiner may release pressure when the patient's elbow is at 40° to 50° of flexion; return of pain and apprehension is also a positive finding
  - **Limitations of Maneuver**:
    - Per original authors, the test is sensitive but not specific (no data given on specificity)[2]

- **Chair Push-up Test** (Sensitivity: 0.88) (Figure 4G.3)
  - First described in the literature in 2006 by Regan and Lapner[4]
  - **Maneuver**:
    - The patient is seated, places hands on arm rests with the shoulder abducted and forearm in supination
    - Elbows bent to 90°
    - The patient is asked to rise from chair by pushing through elbows
    - A positive finding is pain or apprehension during rise

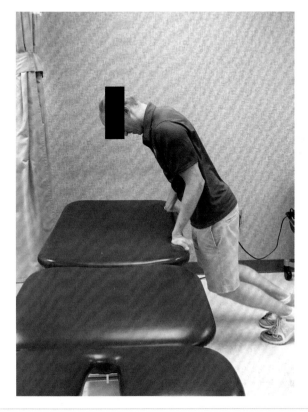

Figure 4G.2. Table-top test.

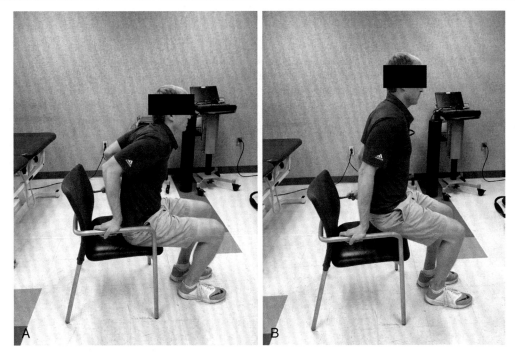

Figure 4G.3. Chair push-up test from seated (A) to upright (B). Note the supination of the forearms; the patient may need to move forward in seat to achieve adequate positioning.

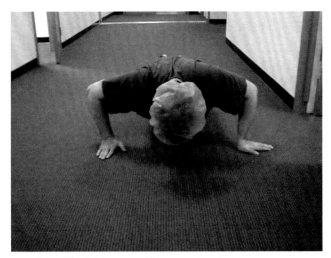

Figure 4G.4. Push-up test—another sign of PLRI is pain, apprehension, or inability to use one's hands to perform a push-up with one's arms supinated, shoulder width apart, and the elbows flexed. As the patient attempts to push up, he may have apprehension, pain, or clunking, which may be consistent with PLRI. (From Fu F, ed. *Master Techniques in Orthopaedic Surgery: Sports Medicine.* Philadelphia, PA: Wolters Kluwer; 2011.)

- **Push-up Test** (Sensitivity: 0.88) (Figure 4G.4)
  - First described in the literature in 2006 by Regan and Lapner[4]
  - **Maneuver**:
    - The patient is placed into push-up position on the floor
      - May be on knees if unable to support the full body weight

- Arms are placed into the abducted position greater than the shoulder width, with forearms supinated
- The patient lowers the body until elbows are in 90° of flexion and then he/she is asked to straighten the elbows, thereby raising the body back up
- Pain or apprehension at the lateral elbow over the radial head during elbow extension is considered a positive finding
  - The radial head may completely dislocate during this maneuver as well. The examiner can palpate the radial head during examination to assess for subluxation/dislocation
- **Limitations of Maneuver**:
  - The patient may not be able to perform push-ups or get into the push-up position
  - Requires the patient to get on the floor

- **Lateral Pivot Shift Test** (Video 4G.1)
  - First described in the literature in 1991 by O'Driscoll[5]
  - Best performed while the patient is under anesthesia
    - When awake: sensitivity: 0.38
    - Under anesthesia: sensitivity: 1.00
  - **Maneuver**:
    - The patient lies supine and the examiner stands behind the patient's head
    - The affected arm extended over the head with the shoulder in full external rotation
    - The examiner holds onto the wrist and the lateral forearm just distal to the elbow
    - The forearm is placed into maximum supination
    - The examiner slowly flexes the elbow while holding supination, applying the valgus force, and axial compression across the elbow
    - A positive finding is when the patient has pain, apprehension, or reproduction of symptoms
      - Usually happens at about 40° to 50° of elbow flexion

IMAGING

Plain Radiographs

- Obtain AP/lateral/oblique X-rays of the elbow
  - May show widening of the ulnohumeral joint or posterior displacement of the radial head

Computed Tomography

- Can help identify other injuries to bony structures (eg, coronoid, radial head fractures)
- Obtain after reduction of traumatic dislocation

Magnetic Resonance Imaging

- MRI utility is not always helpful in identifying injuries to LCL complex (may only identify 50% of injuries)[3]
- However, incongruity of radiocapitellar (>1.2 mm) and ulnohumeral (>0.7 mm) joints on MRI is highly suspicious of PLRI[6]
  - Sagittal plane (radiocapitellar joint)—1.2 mm incongruity: sensitivity 0.67, specificity 0.70
  - Axial plane (ulnohumeral joint)—0.7 mm incongruity: sensitivity 0.63, specificity 0.70

Classic Arthroscopic Findings

- Will see avulsion of LCL complex and gapping of the radiocapitellar joint on supination (Video 4G.2)
- Can also perform varus/valgus stress examinations of the elbow to assess for instability

REFERENCES

1. Mehta JA, Bain GI. Posterolateral rotatory instability of the elbow. *J Am Acad Orthop Surg.* 2004;12(6):405-415.
2. Arvind CH, Hargreaves DG. Tabletop relocation test: a new clinical test for posterolateral rotatory instability of the elbow. *J Shoulder Elbow Surg.* 2006;15(6):707-708.
3. Anakwenze OA, Kancherla VK, Iyengar J, Ahmad CS, Levine WN. Posterolateral rotatory instability of the elbow. *Am J Sports Med.* 2014;42(2):485-491.
4. Regan W, Lapner PC. Prospective evaluation of two diagnostic apprehension signs for posterolateral instability of the elbow. *J Shoulder Elbow Surg.* 2006;15(3):344-346.
5. O'Driscoll SW, Bell DF, Morrey BF. Posterolateral rotatory instability of the elbow. *J Bone Joint Surg Am.* 1991;73:440-446.
6. Hackl M, Wegmann K, Ries C, Leschinger T, Burkhart KJ, Müller LP. Reliability of Magnetic resonance imaging signs of posterolateral rotatory instability of the elbow. *J Hand Surg Am.* 2015;40(7):1428-1433.

SECTION H
Ulnar Nerve Compression at the Elbow

Felix H. Savoie, Stephen G. Thon, and Mary K. Mulcahey

HISTORY

- Ulnar nerve passes through the cubital tunnel on the medial side of the elbow and can be compressed through its course (ie, cubital tunnel syndrome)
  - Most common site of compression is between the 2 heads of the flexor carpi ulnaris[1]
  - Other sites of compression at the elbow include arcade of Struthers, Osborne ligament, medial head of triceps, medial epicondyle, or medial intermuscular septum
- Patients will present with paresthesias of the small finger and ulnar half of the ring finger
- Generally exacerbated by prolonged flexion at the elbow
- Late stages will show loss of motor to the intrinsic muscles of the hand (adductor pollicis, flexor pollicis brevis, interossei, and fourth and fifth lumbricals)
  - Leads to loss of grip strength, pinch strength, first web space atrophy
- Rarely do patients arrive complaining of pain
- Froment[5] sign: Loss of adductor pollicis leads to excessive IP joint flexion at the thumb during key pinch
- Jeanne sign[6]: Loss of flexor pollicis brevis leads to excessive MP joint hyperextension at the thumb during key pinch
- Wartenberg sign: inability to adduct the small finger due to weak third palmar interossei and fifth lumbrical
- Always palpate the full course of the ulnar nerve and assess for subluxation about the medial epicondyle (can be done while performing provocative maneuvers below)

PHYSICAL EXAMINATION

KEY EXAMINATION MANEUVERS

- **Tinel Sign** (Sensitivity: 0.70)[4]
  - **Maneuver**:
    - The examiner performs light percussion (a minimum of 1 min) over ulnar nerve, as it travels around the medial epicondyle
    - A positive finding is when percussion leads to exacerbation of pain, numbness, or tingling in ulnar nerve distribution
  - **Limitations of Maneuver**:
    - 24% false-positive rate[3]

- **Elbow Flexion Test** (Sensitivity: 0.32)[2,4]
  - First described in the literature in 1988 by Buehler and Thayer[3]

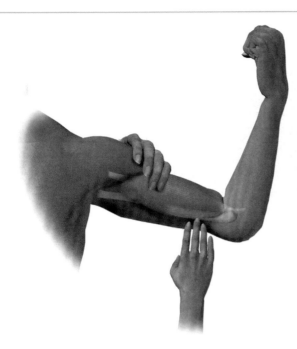

Figure 4H.1. Symptoms of ulnar nerve compression can be provoked by flexing the elbow and exerting pressure over the ulnar nerve just proximal to the cubital tunnel, which lies between the 2 heads of the flexor carpi ulnaris. Some prefer just to tap this area looking for the Tinel sign as evidence for a cubital tunnel entrapment neuropathy.

- **Maneuver**:
  - The examiner places the patient's affected elbow in full flexion and full extension of the wrist
  - This position is held for a minimum of 1 minute (can be held up to 3 min)
  - A positive finding is an exacerbation of pain, numbness, or tingling in ulnar nerve distribution
- **Limitations of Maneuver**:
  - 10% false-positive rate[4]

- **Direct Compression Test** (Sensitivity: 0.55)[4] (Figure 4H.1)
  - **Maneuver**:
    - The examiner places the index finger and long finger directly overlying the ulnar nerve behind the medial epicondyle
    - The examiner presses firmly to compress ulnar nerve at this site for a minimum of 1 minute
    - A positive finding is when direct compression leads to exacerbation of pain, numbness, or tingling in ulnar nerve distribution

- **Combined Elbow Flexion Test and Direct Compression Test** (Sensitivity: 0.91) (Figure 4H.2)
  - First described in the literature in 1994 by Novak et al[4]
  - Most sensitive examination maneuver
  - **Maneuver**:
    - The examiner performs an elbow flexion test (as above) while simultaneously performing a direct compression test with the examiner's other hand
    - This position is held for a minimum of 30 seconds
    - A positive finding is an exacerbation of pain, numbness, or tingling in ulnar nerve distribution

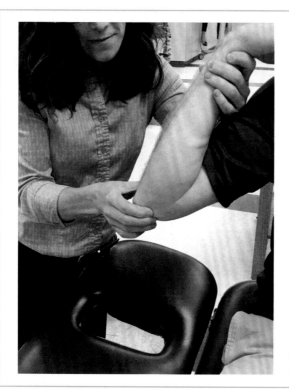

Figure 4H.2. Combined elbow flexion test and direct compression test.

IMAGING

Plain Radiographs

- AP, lateral, and oblique X-rays of the elbow are often normal and used to rule out bony deformity or abnormality
- May show calcifications at the medial epicondyle

Electromyography/Nerve Conduction Velocity

- Decreased amplitudes
- Decreased conduction velocity
- Increased latency
- Muscle fibrillations in late stages

REFERENCES

1. Chimenti PC, Hammert WC. Ulnar neuropathy at the elbow: an evidence-based algorithm. *Hand Clin.* 2013;29(3):435-442.
2. Rayan GM, Jensen C, Duke J. Elbow flexion test in the normal population. *J Hand Surg Am.* 1992;17:86-89.
3. Buehler MJ, Thayer DT. The elbow flexion test. A clinical test for the cubital tunnel syndrome. *Clin Orthop Relat Res.* 1988;(233):213-216.
4. Novak CB, Lee GW, Mackinnon SE, Lay L. Provocative testing for cubital tunnel syndrome. *J Hand Surg Am.* 1994;19(5):817-820.
5. Froment J. La prehension dans les paralysies, du nerf cubital et la signe du ponce. *Presse Med.* 1915;23:409.
6. Jeanne M. La deformation du ponce la paralysie cubitale. *Bul Mem Soc Chir Paris.* 1915;41:703-719.

SECTION I
Radial Nerve and Pin Compression at the Elbow

Felix H. Savoie, Stephen G. Thon, and Mary K. Mulcahey

HISTORY

- Radial nerve compression at the elbow/forearm manifests itself as 3 different syndromes
  - Radial tunnel syndrome: pain ONLY; no motor/sensory component[2]
  - Posterior interosseous nerve (PIN) compression syndrome: motor loss ONLY; pain with motor weakness in wrist, finger, and thumb extension
  - Wartenberg syndrome: sensory loss ONLY; pain with sensory changes in superficial radial nerve (SRN) distribution
- Radial nerve compressed at the leash of Henry, medial side of ECRB, arcade of Frohse, and distal supinator (Figure 4I.1)
  - Radial tunnel syndrome: arcade of Frohse is the most common site of compression

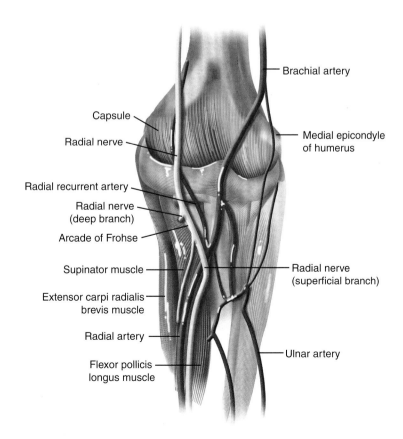

Figure 4I.1. Anatomy of radial nerve.

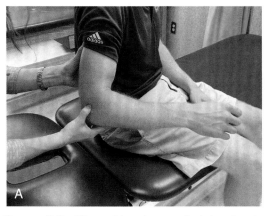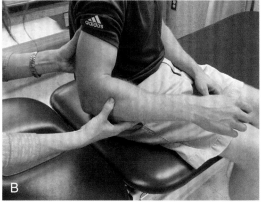

Figure 4I.2. Sites of tenderness in lateral epicondylitis (A) vs radial tunnel (B).

- SRN compressed between the brachioradialis and ECRL tendon during pronation
- Radial tunnel syndrome: deep aching pain in dorsal forearm, tender over mobile wad, worse with forearm activities
  - Pain is more distal than in lateral epicondylitis (Figure 4I.2)
- PIN compression: weakness in the forearm, wrist, and finger extensors, late-stage muscle atrophy of extensor compartment[3]
- Wartenberg syndrome: pain over the distal dorsal portion of the forearm/wrist, paresthesias in the same area, aggravated by repetitive wrist flexion and ulnar deviation

PHYSICAL EXAMINATION

RADIAL TUNNEL KEY EXAMINATION MANEUVERS

- **Maudsley Test/Resisted Long Finger Extension Test** (Figure 4I.3)
  - First described in the literature in 1972 by Roles and Maudsley[1]
    - Also known as the middle finger resistance test
  - **Maneuver:**
    - The patient is seated with the elbow extended
    - The patient's forearms and palms are placed on the examination table
      - The examiner stabilizes the forearm on the table and then asks the patient to raise the long finger off the table while applying resistance
      - Pain just DISTAL to the lateral epicondyle is a positive test finding
      - Pain at the lateral epicondyle may be a sign of lateral epicondylitis
  - **Limitations of Maneuver:**
    - No sensitivity, specificity, or accuracy data have been reported
    - Can be confounding with lateral epicondylitis

- **Resisted Supination Test**
  - **Maneuver:**
    - Both the elbow and wrist of the patient are in full extension
    - The forearm is in pronation
    - The patient is then asked to supinate the forearm against resistance
    - A positive finding is pain at the radial tunnel (3-5 cm distal to the lateral epicondyle)

- **Passive Pronation with Wrist Flexion Test**
  - **Maneuver:**
    - The examiner holds the patient's wrist in maximal flexion and maximum supination with the elbow at the side and flexed to 90°

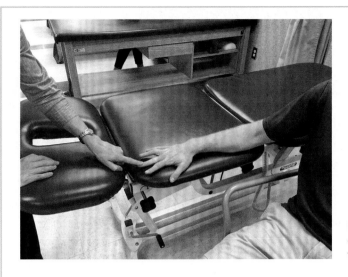

Figure 41.3. "Maudsley test" or middle finger resistance test.

- The examiner then passively pronates the supinated forearm until at maximum pronation
  - This puts the extensors and radial tunnel on maximum stretch
- A positive finding is pain at the radial tunnel (3-5 cm distal to the lateral epicondyle)

- **Radial Tunnel Injection Test** (Figure 41.1)
- **Maneuver**:
  - The point of maximum tenderness along the radial tunnel is palpated
  - Injection of anesthetic directly into this area at the point of maximum tenderness
  - The same point is palpated after anesthetic application
  - A positive finding is a relief of pain at the point of maximum tenderness at the radial tunnel (3-5 cm distal to the lateral epicondyle)
- **Limitations of Maneuver**:
  - Invasive test

PIN COMPRESSION KEY EXAMINATION MANEUVERS

- **Resisted Supination Test**
- **Maneuver**:
  - The patient flexes the elbow to 90° and the forearm in maximum pronation
  - The examiner stabilizes the patient's elbow and applies resistance to the forearm, as the patient attempts to supinate the forearm
  - A positive finding is pain and/or weakness overlying PIN (3-5 cm distal to the lateral epicondyle)
- **Limitations of Maneuver**:
  - No sensitivity or specificity data have been reported

- **Ulnar-deviated Wrist Extension Test**
- **Maneuver**:
  - The examiner ulnarly deviates the patient's wrist and stabilizes the patient's elbow
  - The patient is then asked to extend the wrist with ulnar deviation
  - A positive finding is weakness of wrist extension with ulnar deviation and pain overlying PIN
    - The patient will still be able to extend at the wrist in radial deviation because of ECRL

● **Wrist Flexion, Ulnar Deviation, Pronation Test**
  • **Maneuver**:
    – The examiner places the patient's wrist in maximum flexion, ulnar deviation, and pronation (hold the position for a minimum of 1 min)
    – A positive finding is exacerbation of symptoms in SRN distribution
      • The maneuver places the nerve on maximum stretch

● **Tinel Sign**
  • Most common physical examination finding
  • **Maneuver**:
    – The examiner performs direct percussion over the course of the SRN
    – The point of contact is most commonly 9 cm proximal to the radial styloid
    – A positive finding is exacerbation of symptoms in SRN distribution
  • **Limitations of Maneuver**:
    – No sensitivity or specificity data have been reported

● **Finkelstein Test**
  • Traditionally used for the diagnosis of de Quervain tenosynovitis
  • **Maneuver**:
    – The examiner grasps the thumb of the patient and ulnarly deviates the hand
    – A positive finding will be reproduction of pain or exacerbation of symptoms in SRN distribution
  • **Limitations of Maneuver**:
    – Can often be confounding for de Quervain tenosynovitis

IMAGING

Plain Radiographs

● Not usually helpful in diagnosis
● Can help rule out other potential causes of elbow pain

Magnetic Resonance Imaging

● Radial tunnel: 52% will show denervation, edema, or atrophy of supinator/extensor muscles[3]

Electromyography/Nerve Conduction Velocity

● Can be supportive of diagnosis, but often lacks specific findings

REFERENCES

1. Roles NC, Maudsley RH. Radial tunnel syndrome: resistant tennis elbow as a nerve entrapment. *J Bone Joint Surg Br.* 1972;54(3):499-508.
2. Sarhadi NS, Korday SN, Bainbridge LC. Radial tunnel syndrome: diagnosis and management. *J Hand Surg Br.* 1998;23:617-619
3. Naam NH, Nemani S. Radial tunnel syndrome. *Orthop Clin North Am.* 2012;43(4):529-536.
4. Huisstede BM, Miedema HS, Van opstal T, et al. Interventions for treating the posterior interosseus nerve syndrome: a systematic review of observational studies. *J Peripher Nerv Syst.* 2006;11(2):101-110.
5. Jacobson JA, Fessell DP, Lobo Lda G, Yang LJ. Entrapment neuropathies I: upper limb (carpal tunnel excluded). *Semin Musculoskelet Radiol.* 2010;14(5):473-486.
6. Plate AM, Green SM. Compressive radial neuropathies. *Instr Course Lect.* 2000;49:295-304.
7. Knutsen EJ, Calfee RP. Uncommon upper extremity compression neuropathies. *Hand Clin.* 2013;29(3):443-453.

SECTION J
Median Nerve and AIN Compression

Felix H. Savoie, Stephen G. Thon, and Mary K. Mulcahey

HISTORY

- Median nerve compression about the elbow manifests itself in 2 patterns
  - Pronator syndrome
  - Anterior interosseous nerve (AIN) compression syndrome
- Both will have vague proximal volar forearm pain
- Pronator syndrome: motor and a sensory component
  - Median nerve paresthesias (can present similar to carpal tunnel syndrome)
  - Will also have paresthesias in the proximal forearm in distribution of the palmar cutaneous branch of the median nerve (PCBMN)—differentiates from carpal tunnel syndrome
- AIN contains no sensory fibers; therefore, true AIN compression will lack sensory deficits
  - Arises 4 cm distal to the medial epicondyle on dorsal and radial aspects of the median nerve
  - Weakness of FPL function is the most pronounced physical examination finding/complaint
- Motor examination should focus on muscles innervated by AIN and median nerve (ie, pronator teres, flexor carpi radialis, palmaris longus, flexor digitorum superficialis, flexor pollicis longus, FDP of index and long fingers, and pronator quadratus)
- Always perform simultaneous carpal tunnel examination to rule out other causes of median nerve compression

PHYSICAL EXAMINATION

PRONATOR SYNDROME KEY EXAMINATION MANEUVERS

- **Pronator Compression Test** (Figure 4J.1)
  - Most common sign of pronator syndrome
  - **Maneuver**:
    - The examiner applies direct pressure just proximal and lateral to the edge of the pronator teres muscle belly on the volar forearm (hold for a minimum of 1 min)
    - A positive finding is the reproduction or exacerbation of pain/symptoms

- **Resisted Pronation and Supination**
  - **Maneuver**:
    - The patient places the shoulder in adduction, the elbow in 90°of flexion, the forearm in maximum supination
    - The examiner stabilizes the elbow and asks the patient to pronate against resistance
    - A positive finding is pain at the pronator teres
      - Repeat the examination with the forearm in supination

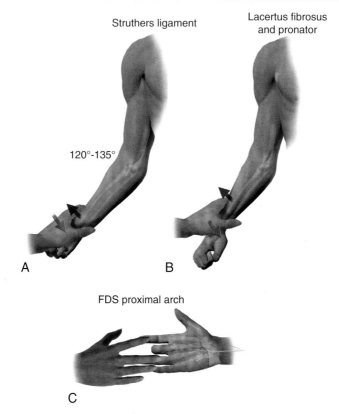

Figure 4J.1. Pronator compression test. A, Test for presence of ligament of Struthers. B, Test for lacertus fibrosus and pronator teres muscle compression. C, Test for median nerve compression by a fibrous tissue arch in the FDS of the middle finger.

- **Resisted Flexion of PIP Joint of the Long Finger**
  - **Maneuver**:
    - The examiner stabilizes the long finger just proximal to the PIP joint with the finger in full extension
    - The patient is then asked to flex the long finger at the PIP joint against resistance
      - If possible, have the patient hold sustained flexion for at least 30 seconds
    - A positive finding is pain at the pronator teres or exacerbation of symptoms
  - **Limitations of Maneuver**:
    - The maneuver is also positive in carpal tunnel syndrome

AIN COMPRESSION KEY EXAMINATION MANEUVERS

- **Kiloh-Nevin Sign/"OK" Sign** (Figure 4J.2)
  - First described in the literature in 1952 by Kiloh and Nevin[3]
  - **Maneuver**:
    - The patient is asked to bring tips of the thumb and index finger together
    - A positive finding is the inability of the thumb to flex at the IP joint (loss of FPL) and inability of the index finger to flex at the DIP joint (loss of FDP)

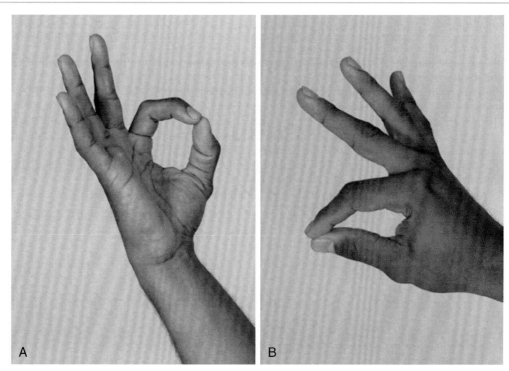

Figure 4J.2. Kiloh-Nevin sign. The clinician instructs the patient to make an "O" with the thumb and forefinger. A, Normal tip-to-tip. B, Abnormal pulp-to-pulp, which signifies entrapment of the interior interosseous nerve. (From Anderson MK, Barnum M. *Foundations of Athletic Training: Prevention, Assessment, and Management.* Wolters Kluwer Health; 2017.)

- **Pinch Grip Test**
  - **Maneuver**:
    - The patient is asked to pinch a piece of paper using only the finger tips of thumb and index finger
    - The examiner then attempts to remove the piece of paper from the grip of the patient
    - A positive finding is weakness with pinch grip and/or inability to flex the IP joint of the thumb and DIP joint of the index finger

IMAGING

Plain Radiographs

- AP, lateral, and oblique views: usually negative

Electromyography/Nerve Conduction Velocity

- Pronator syndrome: predominantly normal, but may be helpful to rule out other causes of pain (eg, carpal tunnel syndrome)
- AIN compression: affected muscles will show fibrillation, sharp waves, and increased latency

REFERENCES

1. Hartz CR, Linscheid RL, Gramse RR, Daube JR. The pronator teres syndrome: compressive neuropathy of the median nerve. *J Bone Joint Surg Am.* 1981;63(6):885-890.
2. Olehnik WK, Manske PR, Szerzinski J. Median nerve compression in the proximal forearm. *J Hand Surg Am.* 1994;19(1):121-126.
3. Kiloh LG, Nevin S. Isolated neuritis of the anterior interosseous nerve. *Br Med J.* 1952;1(4763):850-851.
4. Knutsen EJ, Calfee RP. Uncommon upper extremity compression neuropathies. *Hand Clin.* 2013;29(3):443-453.
5. Strohl AB, Zelouf DS. Ulnar tunnel syndrome, radial tunnel syndrome, anterior interosseous nerve syndrome, and pronator syndrome. *J Am Acad Orthop Surg.* 2017;25(1):e1-e10.
6. Rodner CM, Tinsley BA, O'malley MP. Pronator syndrome and anterior interosseous nerve syndrome. *J Am Acad Orthop Surg.* 2013;21(5):268-275.
7. Ponnappan RK, Khan M, Matzon JL, et al. Clinical differentiation of upper extremity pain etiologies. *J Am Acad Orthop Surg.* 2015;23(8):492-500.

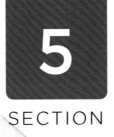

5

SECTION

Wrist/Hand

Section Editor
A. Rashard Dacus

QUICK REFERENCE CHART

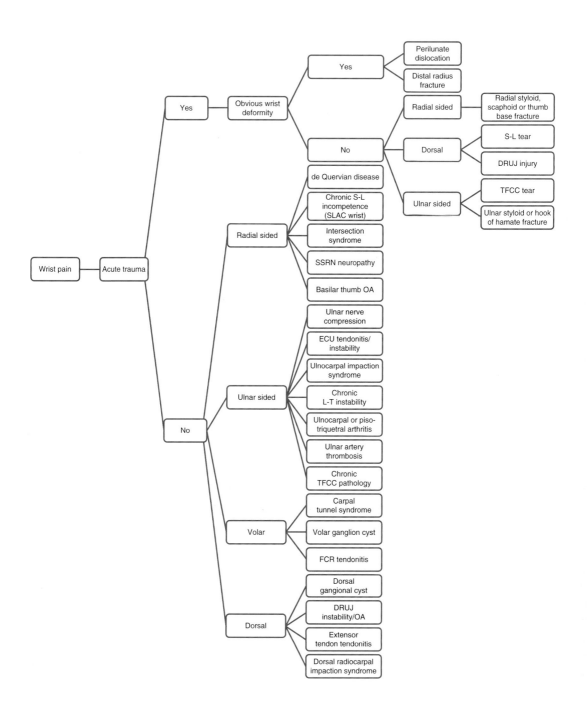

SECTION A
Introduction

Jeffrey D. Boatright

HISTORY

It is important to consider the following parameters when a patient presents to the clinic with a wrist or hand complaint[1]:

- Patient age
  - Younger patients are more likely to have an acute traumatic injury
    - Note, however, that hand and wrist complaints are the most common initial presentation of rheumatoid arthritis
  - Older patients are more likely to have osteoarthritis and/or other degenerative conditions of joints and tendons
- Hand dominance
- Occupation
  - Acute injuries and overuse syndromes are common in manual laborers
    - Appropriate level of suspicion should be maintained for potential secondary gain in patients whose symptoms, mechanism of injury, complaints, and examination do not appropriately align
- Chronicity of symptoms
  - Acute injuries may involve fractures, ligamentous injuries, dislocations, tendon ruptures, triangular fibrocartilage complex (TFCC) tears, lacerations of tendons, arteries, nerves, or various tendinopathies
  - Chronic injuries may represent untreated or unrecognized ligament injures and their degenerative sequelae, osteoarthritis, joint contractures, erosive changes secondary to untreated inflammatory or crystalline arthropathies, and maladaptive changes secondary to untreated injuries or malunited fractures
- Mechanism of injury (if any)
  - Fall on an outstretched hand is a common mechanism of injury for distal radius fracture, scaphoid fracture, scapholunate ligament injury
  - "Jammed finger" is a common mechanism for IP joint dislocations, volar plate injuries, mallet finger, or other extensor tendon rupture
  - Absence of a history of trauma suggests a degenerative condition
- Associated swelling (effusion)
  - Common in the acute setting after a fracture or other acute injury
  - Also associated with osteoarthritis and inflammatory/crystalline arthropathies in the chronic setting
- Progressive deformity
  - Development of a swan neck or boutonniere deformity can represent delayed presentation of finger tendon or ligament injury
  - Progressive MCP and IP joint contracture is common with Dupuytren disease
- Mechanical symptoms (locking, catching)
  - Commonly associated TFCC tears, distal radioulnar joint (DRUJ) injury

- History of trauma
  - One must be concerned about reinjury versus maladaptive derangement or posttraumatic arthritis
- History of surgery
  - Critical to gain an understanding of the technical aspects of the prior intervention; therefore, evaluate critically for technical errors, misdiagnosis, and concurrent conditions
    - Pre- and postoperative images, preoperative electrodiagnostic studies, operative reports, outside physician's clinical notes, etc, are all important
- Prior treatment
- Current medications
- Aggravating or alleviating factors
- Medical and family history
  - Especially applicable for Dupuytren disease and inflammatory arthropathies as well as atypical infections
- One-finger test: Ask patients to point, with 1 finger, to the area where it hurts (they often cannot do so, but it can be helpful)

PHYSICAL EXAMINATION

Observation

- Observe how the patient uses or guards the affected hand/wrist
  - If the right hand/wrist is of interest, do they shake hands with the opposite side?
- Always compare with the contralateral hand/wrist
- Observe the resting posture of the hand and wrist
  - This is an extremely important component of the physical examination
  - Resting posture represents an equilibrium point between the resting tone of the flexors versus the resting tone of the extensors
  - Disruption of a flexor or extensor tendon will alter this equilibrium, resulting in abnormal resting posture relative to the uninjured digits **(see section E, Figure 5E.3)**
    - Flexor tendon injury will result in a relative extension resting posture
    - Extensor tendon injury will result in a relative flexion resting posture
- Observe the cascade of the fingers **(Figure 5A.1)**
  - Abnormal cascade often indicates either an acute or malunited metacarpal or phalangeal fracture with malrotation
- Observe the tenodesis effect
  - Observe the behavior of the fingers while passively flexing and extending the wrist
    - See section E for details related to performing and interpreting the tenodesis effect **(see section E, Figure 5E.4)**

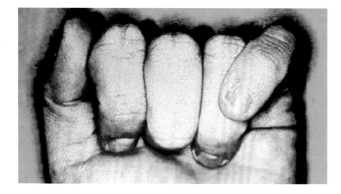

Figure 5A.1. With the MCP and PIP joints flexed, the tips of the fingers should converge to point toward the scaphoid tuberosity. Alteration of this cascade, as seen with the small finger here, can indicate a rotational deformity of the metacarpal or phalanx. (Picture courtesy of Ghazi Rayan MD.)

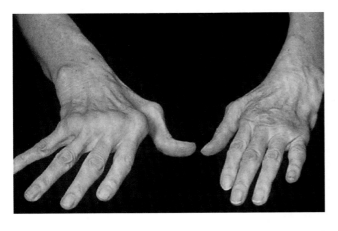

Figure 5A.2. Classic ulnar deviation of the fingers at the MCP joint seen in rheumatoid arthritis. (From Hinkle JL, Cheever KH. *Brunner & Suddarth's Textbook of Medical-Surgical Nursing.* Wolters Kluwer; 2014.)

- Also inspect for
  - Alignment of the wrist and fingers
    – Ulnar deviation can be a classic rheumatoid arthritis presentation **(Figure 5A.2)**
  - Rotational deformity
    – Could indicate metacarpal or phalangeal fracture
  - Heberden and Bouchard nodes **(Figure 5A.3)**
    – Common with osteoarthritis
  - Gouty tophi **(Figure 5A.4)**
  - Dupuytren cords **(Figure 5A.5)**
  - Static contractures or other deformities
    – Swan neck and boutonniere deformities **(Figure 5A.6)**
  - Shoulder sign **(Figure 5A.7)**
    – Can be indicative of thumb CMC arthritis
  - Dorsal prominence of the distal ulna
    – Could indicate DRUJ injury or caput ulna in rheumatoid patients
  - Diminished MCP "knuckle" prominence dorsally **(Figure 5A.8)**
    – Could indicate a metacarpal neck fracture
  - Clawing and/or intrinsic hand muscular atrophy **(Figure 5A.9)**
    – Indicative of an ulnar nerve palsy
  - Lacerations, scars, callouses, lesions
  - Evaluate the nails for pigmented lesions, evidence of poor perfusion, and other deformities such as clubbing, hook nails, and paronychial infection

Palpation

- Tenderness
  - Radial styloid
  - Anatomic snuffbox dorsally (interval between extensor pollicis longus [EPL] and extensor pollicis brevis [EPB]/abductor pollicis longus [APL] at the dorsoradial thumb base) **(Figure 5A.10)**
  - Scaphoid tubercle volarly
    – Tenderness at either of these locations in the setting of an acute injury should raise suspicion for a scaphoid fracture, even if radiographs are negative
  - Thumb CMC joint
  - First dorsal compartment (EPB and APL tendons)
    – Tenderness here may indicate de Quervain tenosynovitis
  - Second dorsal compartment (extensor carpi radialis longus [ECRL] and extensor carpi radialis brevis [ECRB] tendons)
    – Pain here, especially approximately 5 cm proximal to the joint line may indicate intersection syndrome

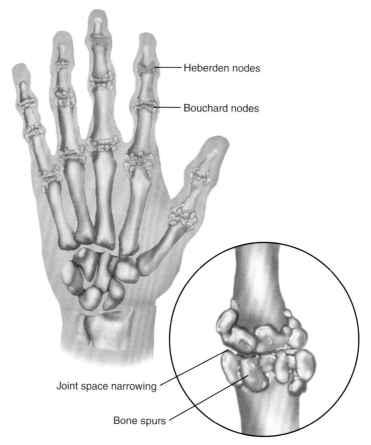

Heberden nodes

Bouchard nodes

Joint space narrowing

Bone spurs

Figure 5A.3. Development of osteophytes as a result of osteoarthritis at the DIP and PIP joints leads to a swollen nodular clinical appearance of the fingers, often referred to as Heberden and Bouchard nodes, respectively.

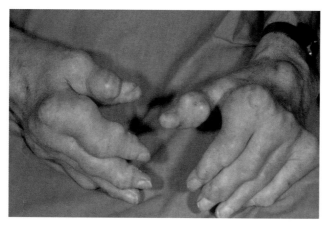

Figure 5A.4. Classic clinical appearance of hands with gouty tophi. (From Rubin E, Farber JL. *Pathology*. 3rd ed. Philadelphia: Lippincott Williams & Wilkins; 1999.)

- Dorsal wrist "soft spot"
  - Pain here may indicate scapholunate ligament pathology
- DRUJ
- Ulnar styloid

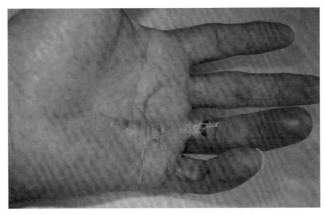

Figure 5A.5. Classic appearance of a Dupuytren cord in the palm. (Image provided by Stedman's.)

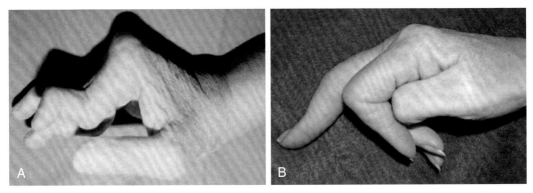

Figure 5A.6. Classic appearance of a swan neck (A) and boutonniere (B) deformity. (From Hunt TRI, Wiesel SW. *Operative Techniques in Hand, Wrist, and Elbow Surgery.* Wolters Kluwer; 2016.)

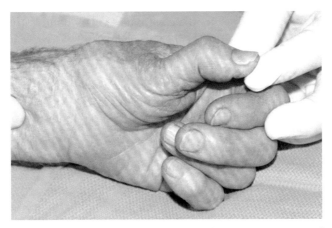

Figure 5A.7. Radial prominence at the base of the thumb CMC joint often seen in thumb CMC arthritis is referred to as the shoulder sign. Note the commonly seen compensatory MCP hyperextension deformity as well. (From Maschke SD, Graham TJ, Evans PJ. *Master Techniques in Orthopaedic Surgery: The Hand.* Wolters Kluwer; 2016.)

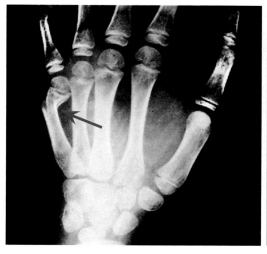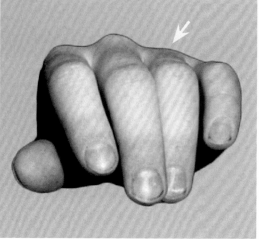

Figure 5A.8. Note the loss of the dorsal "knuckle" prominence of the ring finger (arrows) as the result of an angulated metacarpal neck fracture. (From Staheli LT. *Fundamentals of Pediatric Orthopedics*. 5th ed. Philadelphia: Wolters Kluwer; 2016.)

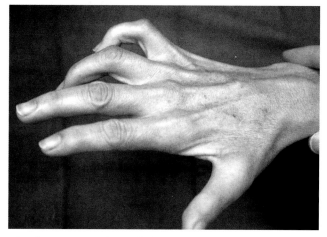

Figure 5A.9. Note the hyperextension of the MCP joints and associated flexion at the IP joints in the small and ring fingers seen in a classic ulnar claw hand. Intrinsic hand muscular atrophy is also apparent in this image. (From McCall RE, Tankersley CM. *Phlebotomy Exam Review*. Wolters Kluwer; 2016.)

- Fovea
  - Bordered by the ulnar styloid, flexor carpi ulnaris (FCU) tendon, ulnar head, and pisiform
    - Pain here can indicate TFCC or ulnotriquetral (U-T) ligament pathology
- Pisiform and FCU tendon
- Hook of the hamate
  - Can be difficult to palpate in muscular hands but can be found in a line volarly from the pisiform to the second metacarpal head
- Palpation along the digits, MCP, and IP joints

Range of Motion

- Should always compare all with the contralateral side
  - Wrist ROM
    - Normal
      - 80° flexion, 70° extension, 30° ulnar deviation, 20° radial deviation
      - Supination and pronation (see section 4, The Elbow)

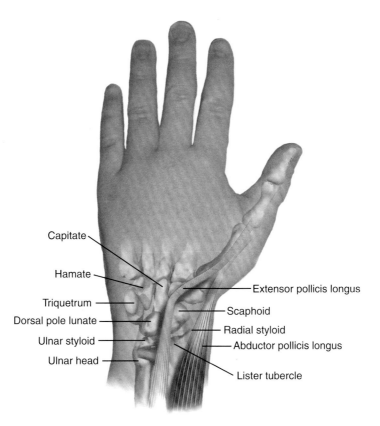

Capitate
Hamate
Triquetrum
Dorsal pole lunate
Ulnar styloid
Ulnar head

Extensor pollicis longus
Scaphoid
Radial styloid
Abductor pollicis longus
Lister tubercle

Figure 5A.10. Illustration depicting the region known as the anatomic snuffbox.

- Also evaluate tendons crossing the wrist joint during active range of motion for pathology—such as snapping extensor carpi ulnaris (ECU) tendon
- Finger ROM[9]
  - Evaluate the flexor and extensor tendons during active range of motion of the digits
    - Volar pain or catching over the A1 pulley can indicate trigger finger
    - Bowstringing of the flexor tendons can indicate a pulley rupture
    - Subluxation of the extensor tendons can indicate a sagittal band rupture
  - Normal
    - MCP (second to fifth)
      - 30° to 45° extension, 90° flexion
    - PIP (second to fifth)
      - 0° extension, 100° flexion
    - DIP (second to fifth)
      - 20° extension, 90° flexion
    - Thumb
      - MCP
        - 0° extension, 50° flexion
      - IP
        - 20° extension, 90° flexion
    - Palmar abduction 70°
    - Radial abduction 50°
    - Opposition
      - Should be able to oppose the thumb tip to the tip of all other digits and the palmar digital crease of the small finger

Muscular Strength

- Normally graded 1 to 5 (see section 1, The Knee, introduction for strength grading details)
- Important to understand the functions and innervations of the intrinsic and extrinsic hand and wrist musculature
- Median nerve/AIN
  - Wrist flexors/pronators
    - FCR, palmaris, pronator teres, pronator quadratus
  - Extrinsic finger flexors
    - Flexor digitorum superficialis (FDS), flexor digitorum profundus (FDP) (dually innervated; radial half-AIN, ulnar half-ulnar nerve), flexor pollicis longus (FPL) (AIN)
  - Intrinsic hand muscles (recurrent motor branch of median nerve)
    - First and second lumbricals, opponens pollicis, abductor pollicis brevis, flexor pollicis brevis (dually innervated; superficial head-recurrent motor branch of median nerve, deep head-ulnar nerve)
- Radial nerve/posterior interosseous nerve (PIN)
  - Wrist and finger extensors
    - ECRL, ECRB (PIN), EPL (PIN), EIP (PIN), extensor digitorum communis (EDC) (PIN), extensor digiti minimi (PIN), APL (PIN), EPB (PIN)
- Ulnar nerve
  - Wrist flexors/extensors
    - FCU, ECU
  - Extrinsic finger flexors
    - FDP (dually innervated; radial half-AIN, ulnar half-ulnar nerve)
  - Intrinsic hand muscles
  - Third and fourth lumbricals, palmar and dorsal interossei, flexor pollicis brevis (dually innervated; superficial head-recurrent motor branch of median nerve, deep head-ulnar nerve), adductor pollicis, abductor digiti minimi, flexor digiti minimi, opponens digiti minimi
- Remember that motor and/or sensory anastomoses in the forearm or hand can confound examination
  - Martin-Gruber anastomosis is a median to ulnar nerve interconnection in the forearm
  - Riche-Cannieu anastomosis is a deep branch of ulnar nerve to recurrent branch of median nerve interconnection in the hand
  - There are many anatomic variations of these upper extremity nerve anastomoses, and they are not uncommon
- Test finger flexor tendon integrity and strength as follows:
  - FDS
    - Assess by extending all other digits (other than the one being tested) flush on a table and asking the patient to flex the PIP joint **(see section E, Figure 5E.6B)**
      - Of note, FDS to the small finger is absent in 6% to 25% of individuals, which can confound the examination
        - Can be absent unilaterally or bilaterally
  - FDP
    - Examine by holding the finger in question flush on a table with the MCP and PIP joints held in extension while asking the patient to flex the DIP joint **(see section E, Figure 5E.6A)**
- Wrist/hand extensor weakness
  - Can be due to tendon rupture/tendonitis, PIN/radial nerve injury, or compression neuropathy
    - Also remember to evaluate for cervical spine pathology

- Wrist/hand flexor weakness
  - Can be due to tendon rupture/tendonitis, median nerve/AIN or ulnar nerve injury, or compression neuropathy
    – Also remember to evaluate for cervical spine pathology
    – Also consider neuralgic amyotrophy (Parsonage-Turner syndrome)
      - Idiopathic, mostly self-limiting, brachial neuritis likely related to viral infection or autoimmune response
      - Can be patchy and involve virtually any upper extremity nerve distribution. AIN or radial nerve involvement is not uncommon

Sensation (Figure 5A.11)

- Can be viewed as dermatomes C5-T1 or as peripheral nerves listed below:
  - Median
  - Ulnar
  - Radial
  - Medial antebrachial cutaneous
  - Lateral antebrachial cutaneous

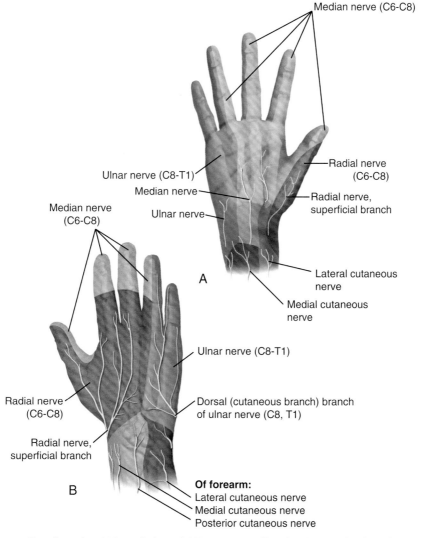

Figure 5A.11. Classic volar (A) and dorsal (B) sensory distribution in the hand.

KEY EXAMINATION MANEUVERS

- **Carpal Instability**
  - S-L ligament
    - Watson test
    - Resisted extension test
    - S-L ballottement test
  - L-T ligament
  - L-T ballottement test
  - Derby test
  - Midcarpal instability
    - Midcarpal shift test

- **ECU Pathology, TFCC Injuries, and Ulnar Impaction**
  - ECU synergy test
  - Snapping ECU test
  - Fovea sign
  - Ulnar stress test

- **de Quervain Tenosynovitis**
  - Eichhoff test
  - Finkelstein test
  - Wrist hyperflexion and abduction of thumb (WHAT)
  - Brunelli test
  - EBP entrapment test

- **Flexor and Extensor Tendon Injuries**
  - Elson test
  - Resting posture
  - Tenodesis effect

- **Ligamentous Injury to the Thumb**
  - Valgus and varus stress test in 0° and 30° flexion

- **Dupuytren Disease**
  - Hueston tabletop test

- **Ulnar Nerve Compression at the Wrist**
  - Froment sign
  - Tinel sign
  - Allen test
  - Wartenberg sign

- **Wartenberg Syndrome**
  - Tinel sign
  - Pronation, flexion, and ulnar deviation test

- **Carpal Tunnel Syndrome (CTS)**
  - Tinel sign
  - Phalen wrist flexion test
  - Durkan compression test

- **Hand Infections**
  - Kanavel signs

IMAGING

- Standard wrist series includes PA, lateral, +/− oblique radiographs
  - Additional views such as clenched fist AP and scaphoid view can be useful
- Standard hand series includes PA and lateral views
  - 30° supination oblique can be helpful in evaluating radial-sided injuries such as index finger CMC dislocation
  - 30° pronation oblique can be helpful in evaluating ulnar-sided injuries such as ring and small finger CMC dislocation
- Standard finger series includes AP, lateral, and oblique radiographs
- MRI, CT, and ultrasonography are useful adjuncts on a case-by-case basis, and their indications are discussed in the appropriate sections

Wrist Arthroscopy (Figure 5A.12)

- Standard dorsal wrist arthroscopy portals are illustrated in Figure 5A.12

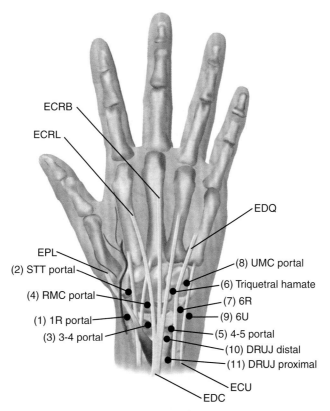

Figure 5A.12. Illustration depicting the many options for wrist arthroscopy portals. These are mostly by convention labeled relative to their location in respect to the dorsal extensor compartments. The most commonly used portals are the 3-4, 4-5, 6R, 6U, and radial (RMC) and ulnar (UMC) midcarpal portals.

REFERENCES

1. Green DP. In: Wolfe SW, Pederson WC, Hotchkiss RN, Kozin SH, eds. *Green's Operative Hand Surgery.* 6th ed. Philadelphia, PA: Elsevier Churchill Livingstone; 2011:3-24.
2. Hoppenfeld S. *Physical Exam of the Spine & Extremities.* Norwalk, CT: Appleton & Lange; 1976.

SECTION B
Carpal Instability

Jeffrey D. Boatright

HISTORY

- Carpal instability is a broad diagnosis, incorporating many separate entities, ranging from acute traumatic injuries to chronic degenerative conditions
- Four main categories[1] (Figure 5B.1):
  - Carpal instability dissociative (CID)—instability within a carpal row, involves intrinsic wrist ligament pathology
    - Scapholunate (S-L) injury leads to dorsal intercalated segment instability (DISI)— scaphoid flexes, lunate extends **(Figure 5B.1C)**
      - Acute—typically presents with acute-onset dorsoradial wrist pain after a fall most commonly with the wrist in extension, ulnar deviation, and carpal supination
      - 10% to 30% of intra-articular distal radius fractures involve S-L ligament injury
      - Chronic—insidious onset dorsoradial wrist pain
      - 50% of patients >80 years of age have chronic S-L injury
    - Lunotriquetral (L-T) injury leads to volar intercalated segment instability (VISI)— lunate flexes, triquetrum extends **(Figure 5B.1D)**
      - Less common than DISI
      - Typically presents after a wrist hyperextension-radial deviation injury
      - Ulnar-sided wrist pain worses with pronation and ulnar deviation, weakness with power grip
  - Carpal instability nondissociative (CIND)—instability between carpal rows, involves extrinsic wrist ligaments
    - Typical presenting complaints of either painless or painful wrist instability ("giving way")
    - Radiocarpal—typically associated with high-energy injury
      - Can be associated with distal radius malunion
  - Midcarpal—typically associated with no history of trauma
  - Carpal instability complex (CIC)—instability within and between rows
    - Involves elements of CID and CIND, history varies as such
  - Carpal instability adaptive (CIA)—instability secondary to pathology or anatomic variants either proximal or distal to the carpus
    - Rare, variable history, those associated with malunion of prior fracture will report remote history of injury
  - Predisposing factors include wrist trauma, prior wrist surgery, and inflammatory arthropathies

PHYSICAL EXAMINATION

Inspection

- Often no gross deformity
- Radiocarpal CIND, CIC, and CIA may show resting subluxation of the carpus or evidence of malalignment or prior nonunion

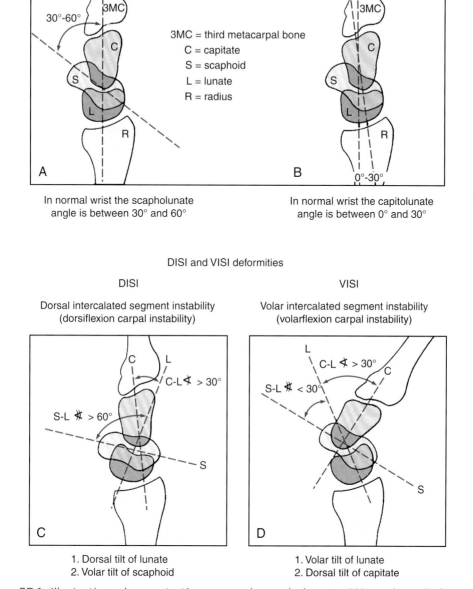

Figure 5B.1. Illustration demonstrating normal scapholunate (A) and capitolunate (B) alignment. In DISI (dorsal intercalated segment instability) deformity (C), there is either an S-L ligament injury or scaphoid fracture, which allows the scaphoid to flex and lunate to extend increasing the S-L and C-L angles. In VISI (volar intercalated segment instability) deformity (D), there is injury to the L-T ligament, which causes the lunate to flex with the scaphoid, thus decreasing the S-L angle, whereas the capitate extends, thereby increasing the capitolunate angle.

Palpation

- Highly variable depending on the type of carpal instability and ligaments involved
- Acute S-L ligament injury will be tender to palpation over the dorsoradial wrist in the "soft spot" between the wrist extensors and common digital extensors 1 cm distal to Lister tubercle
- Acute L-T ligament injury may be tender to palpation over either the volar or dorsal ulnar side of the wrist

Range of Motion

● Motion may be preserved or diminished in any form of carpal instability

Strength

● Loss of grip strength to varying degrees accompanies all forms of carpal instability

Sensation

● Typically preserved; an exception is perhaps carpal instability associated with a missed perilunate dislocation, which may present with diminished sensation in a median nerve distribution

---

KEY EXAMINATION MANEUVERS

● **S-L Ligament Injury**
  • **Watson Test (scaphoid shift test)** 🔊 **(Sensitivity 0.69, Specificity 0.66) (Figure 5B.2)**
    – First described by Watson[2] in 1988
    – **Maneuver:**
      • The examiner places 4 fingers on the dorsum of the distal radius and applies pressure using the thumb to the scaphoid tuberosity volarly
      • The examiner's other hand is used to bring the wrist passively from ulnar deviation to radial deviation
      • Pressure on the scaphoid tuberosity (from the examiner's thumb) prevents the scaphoid from flexing, as it is moved into radial deviation, which causes the proximal pole to subluxate dorsally over the dorsal lip of the distal radius
      • The examiner's thumb is then removed, which elicits a palpable clunk as the scaphoid reduces
      • A positive test elicits a palpable painful clunk
    – **Limitations of Maneuver:**
      • Very technique-dependent. Experience with the test is imperative
      • Generalized ligamentous laxity in the absence of an S-L ligament injury can lead to a painless clunk. Comparison with the contralateral side can be helpful in distinguishing the 2
  • **Resisted Extension Test**
    – Also described by Watson
    – **Maneuver:**
      • Resisted index and middle finger extension with the wrist in partial flexion elicits pain in the dorsal S-L ligament region
      • Useful for detecting dynamic or predynamic S-L instability
    – **Limitations of Maneuver:**
      • Sensitive but not specific
  • **Scapholunate Ballottement Test**
    – **Maneuver:**
      • The examiner uses his/her thumb and index finger of one hand to stabilize the patient's lunate both volarly and dorsally, while the same is performed on the patient's scaphoid with the examiner's other hand
      • The examiner then translates the patient's scaphoid dorsally and volarly
      • Excessive translation and/or pain indicates a positive test

● **L-T Ligament Injury**
  • **L-T Ballottement Test** 🔊 (Sensitivity 0.64, Specificity 0.44)[3] **(Figure 5B.3)**
    – Described by Reagan[4] in 1984
    – Modified by Kleinman (shear test)

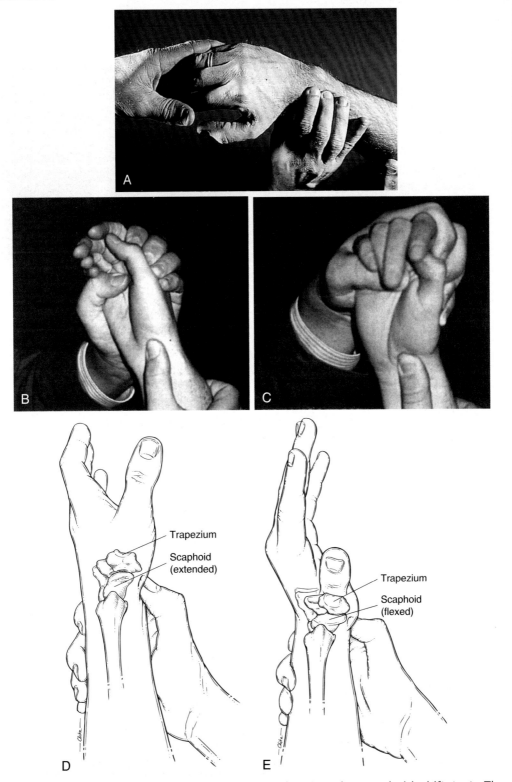

Figure 5B.2. A-C, Clinical photographs of performing the scaphoid shift test. The wrist is brought passively from ulnar deviation to radial deviation with the examiner's thumb on the scaphoid tuberosity preventing flexion of the scaphoid, which causes the proximal pole to sublux over the dorsal lip of the radius. When the thumb is removed, the scaphoid flexes, which reduced the proximal pole back into the scaphoid facet. D and E, The behavior of the scaphoid during this test. ((A-C) From Cooney WP. *The Wrist Diagnosis and Operative Treatment.* London: Lippincott Williams and Wilkins; 2010.)

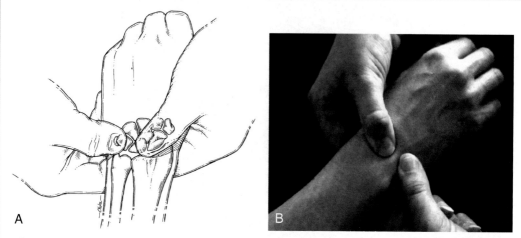

A
B

Figure 5B.3. Illustration (A) and clinical photograph (B) of the L-T ballottement test. (From Cooney WP. *The Wrist Diagnosis and Operative Treatment*. London: Lippincott Williams and Wilkins; 2010.)

- **Maneuver:**
  - The patient's lunate is stabilized by the examiner's thumb and index finger of one hand both volarly and dorsally while the same is performed on the patient's triquetrum/pisiform complex with the examiner's other hand
  - The patient's triquetrum/pisiform is translated dorsally and volarly by the examiner
  - Excessive translation and/or pain indicate a positive test
  - **Kleinman Modification (shear test)**
    - The patient's lunate is stabilized in the same fashion by the examiner
    - Dorsally directed pressure on the pisiform by the examiner creates shear between the triquetrum and lunate, which elicits pain
- **Derby Test**
  - Described by Christodoulou and Bainbridge[5] in 1999
  - **Maneuver**:
    - Similar maneuver to the shear test; however, radial deviation of the wrist decreases pain and instability and increases grip strength as long as pressure over the pisiform is maintained by the examiner
    - Radial deviation with pressure over the pisiform anatomically aligns the L-T joint
  - **Limitations of Maneuver:**
    - All these maneuvers are sensitive but not specific. Other causes of ulnar-sided wrist pain remain in the differential

- **CIND—Midcarpal Instability**
  - **Midcarpal Shift Test** 🔘
    - Described by Lichtman[6] in 1981
    - **Maneuver:**
      - The examiner applies a volarly directed force to the patient's carpus in an ulnar, which is placed in an ulnar-deviated and pronated position
      - Graded I (most subtle) to V (most severe) based on how much resistance is required by the examiner to keep the patient's carpus volarly subluxed in this position

- CIC and CIA do not have any commonly accepted special tests

IMAGING

- Static radiographs are routine early in the workup for patients with suspected carpal instability
  - Gross S-L injury will show scapholunate interval widening (Terry Thomas sign) **(Figure 5B.4)**
  - A clenched fist view will stress this interval and reveal dynamic widening, which may not be apparent on a static nonstressed radiograph
  - A classic perilunate dislocation will show disruption of the carpal row intervals (Gilula lines) and "piece of pie" sign on the AP, and an "empty tea cup" sign on the lateral **(Figure 5B.5)**
- Dynamic radiographs or cineradiography can be very helpful in gaining an understanding for the type and degree of instability
- Advanced imaging such as MRI can be useful in some cases; however, the sensitivity of MRI for most intrinsic wrist ligament injuries is relatively low

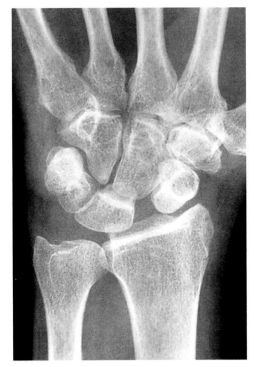

Figure 5B.4. PA wrist radiograph showing significant widening of the S-L interval (Terry Thomas sign). (From Greenspan A, Beltran J, Ovid Technologies I. *Orthopedic Imaging: A Practical Approach*. Philadelphia: Wolters Kluwer Health/Lippincott Williams & Wilkins; 2015.)

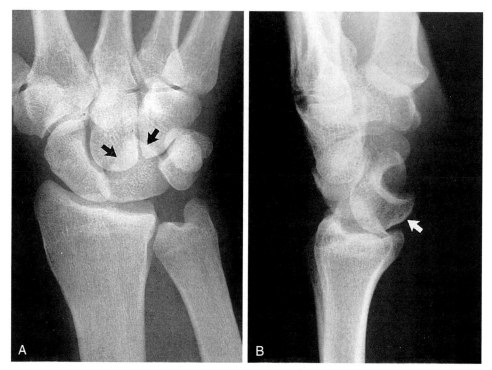

Figure 5B.5. AP (A) and lateral (B) radiographs showing classic findings of a perilunate dislocation. On the AP radiograph, disruption of Gilula lines and the "piece of pie" sign of the lunate (black arrows) are apparent. The lateral radiograph shows the classic appearance of the lunate, the so-called "empty tea cup" sign (white arrow). (From Yochum TR, Rowe LJ. *Yochum and Rowe's Essentials of Skeletal Radiology*. 3rd ed. Philadelphia, PA: Lippincott Williams & Wilkins; 2004.)

REFERENCES

1. Garcia-Elias M, Geissler WB. *Carpal Instability*. In: Green DP, Hotchkiss RN, Pederson WC, Wolfe SW, eds. *Green's Operative Hand Surgery*. 5th ed. Philadelphia: Elsevier Churchill Livingstone; 2005:535-604.
2. Watson HK, Ashmead IV D, Makhlouf MV. Examination of the scaphoid. *J Hand Surg Am*. 1988;13(5):657-660.
3. LaStayo P, Howell J. Clinical provocative tests used in evaluating wrist pain: a descriptive study. *J Hand Ther*. 1995;8:10-17.
4. Reagan DS, Linscheid RL, Dobyns JH. Lunotriquetral sprains. *J Hand Surg Am*. 1984;9(4):502-514.
5. Christodoulou L, Bainbridge LC. Clinical diagnosis of triquetrolunate ligament injuries. *J Hand Surg Br*. 1999;24(5):598-600.
6. Lichtman DM, Schneider JR, Swafford AR, Mack GR. Ulnar midcarpal instability—clinical and laboratory analysis. *J Hand Surg*. 1981;6:515-523.

SECTION C
ECU Pathology, TFCC Injuries, Ulnar Impaction (Ulnar-Sided Wrist Pain)

Daniel E. Hess

HISTORY

- Ulnar-sided wrist pain is a common complaint seen in the clinic and can be from various etiologies. The following items in a patient's clinical history are common for ulnar-sided wrist pain:
  - Patients will often report a specific injury to which they can relate the start of their pain. This will often be some variation of a fall on an outstretched hand
  - Patients with chronic symptoms may not be able to recount a traumatic event but may relate it to their occupation or hobbies
    - Sports or occupations requiring repeated pronation/supination, radial/ulnar deviation, and axial loading predispose to ulnar-sided wrist problems[1,9]
  - It is important to determine the history of treatment modalities for new patients and their response to the various treatment modalities. These include bracing (ask about the type of brace), NSAIDs, and injections (as about the location of the injection)

PHYSICAL EXAMINATION

General Examination

- **Inspection**
  - Look for any swelling or deformity. Compare with the uninjured side
- **Palpation**
  - Determine the point of maximal tenderness
- **Range of motion**
  - Determine if there are any limitations or block to motion
  - Describe what motion is painful
  - Note any snapping (typically the ECU dorsally) that occurs with range of motion

---

KEY EXAMINATION MANEUVERS

- **ECU Synergy Test** (Figure 5C.1)
  - First described in the literature in 2008 by Ruland and Hogan[6] in the Journal of Hand Surgery
  - Help differentiate ECU pathology from other intra-articular diagnoses
  - **Maneuver:**
    - The patient's arm is resting on the examination table with the elbow at 90° and the wrist in supination
    - The patient radially abducts the thumb against resistance
    - Reproduction of pain in the ECU tendon is a positive test

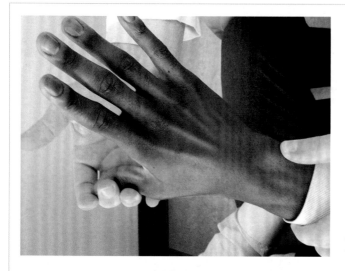

Figure 5C.1. Extensor carpi ulnaris (ECU) synergy test. A positive test is a reproduction of pain in the ECU tendon near the examiner's left thumb.

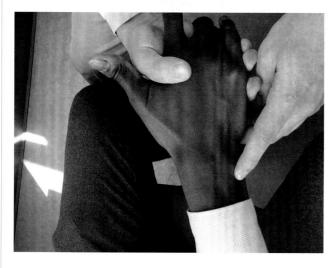

Figure 5C.2. Resisted extension and supination will cause instability and "snapping" of the extensor carpi ulnaris (ECU) tendon out of its groove when the tendon subsheath has been injured.

- **Limitations of Maneuver:**
  - It is based on the theory that there is isometric contraction of the ECU during resisted thumb abduction. The test is difficult to perform if there is any concurrent injury to the thumb or radial wrist. Sensitivity and specificity are not known

- **ECU Snapping** 🔘 (Figure 5C.2)
  - Help to distinguish ECU instability secondary to subsheath tears, which can lead to tendonitis, pain, and attritional rupture
  - **Maneuver:**
    - The examiner is sitting across from the patient
    - The patient's arm is resting on the table with the elbow at 90°
    - Extension and supination of the wrist elicit and dislodge the ECU tendon, as it runs over the dorsal distal ulna
    - ECU tendon reduces with pronation
    - Painful snapping over the dorsal ulnar wrist is a positive sign
  - **Limitations of Maneuver:**
    - Painless instability can be due to congenital flattening of the ECU groove and possible attenuation of subsheath

- **Fovea Sign** 🔘 (Figure 5C.3) (Sensitivity 0.95, Specificity 0.865)
  - First described in the literature in 2007 by Dr. Richard Berger of The Mayo Clinic.
  - Useful technique to detect foveal disruptions of the TFCC and U-T ligament injuries

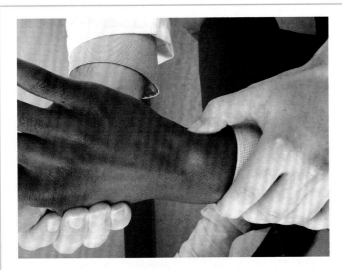

Figure 5C.3. The examiner is demonstrating the maneuver to elicit the fovea sign in patients with triangular fibrocartilage complex (TFCC) injuries.

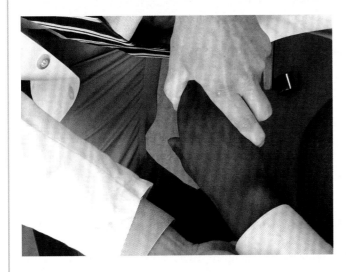

Figure 5C.4. Ulnar stress test. A positive result is reproduction of the patient's pain.

- **Maneuver:**
  - The patient's arm is resting on table with the elbow at 90° to 110° with the arm relaxed and wrist in neutral rotation, supported by the examiner, who is sitting across from the patient
  - The examiner's thumb is pressed deep and in a distal trajectory in the interval soft spot between the ulna styloid, FCU, and pisiform
  - The test is positive when exquisite tenderness is elicited compared with the contralateral side
- **Limitations of Maneuver:**
  - Distinction should be made clinically between central foveal disruption and U-T ligament disruption, which can both produce positive fovea signs. The DRUJ is typically unstable with a foveal tear and stable with a U-T ligament tear

- **Ulnar Stress Test** (Figure 5C.4)
  - Helps diagnose ulnar impaction syndrome[2]
  - **Maneuver:**
    - The patient's arm is resting on the table with the elbow at 90°
    - The examiner, sitting across from the patient, uses one hand to support the elbow and the other hand to grab the carpal bones and bring the wrist into ulnar deviation

- With the patient's wrist in maximal ulnar deviation, provide axial stress with passive supination and pronation
- A positive test is reproduction of patient's pain
- An audible click is not necessarily a positive test
- **Limitations of Maneuver:**
  - Unknown sensitivity and specificity

IMAGING

Plain Radiographs

- Often noncontributory
- Can assess ulnar variance, shape, and length of ulnar styloid. Ulnar positive variance and a long ulnar styloid are at higher risk for ulnar impaction and degenerative tears of the TFCC. The more ulnar-positive the wrist is, the more weight-bearing force the ulna is going through. Comparison views with the contralateral side can be helpful
- Ulnar styloid fractures can be a source of pain and can be a sign of TFCC injury
- Gapping between the distal radius and distal ulna suggests DRUJ instability

Computed Tomography

- Not typically obtained

Magnetic Resonance Imaging

- In general: static imaging, typically highly sensitive for pathology but may have incidental findings, and important to correlate clinically
- ECU pathology
  - Tenosynovitis and tendinopathy will show increased signal intensity although the clinical relevance of this has come into question[3]
  - Can assess the integrity of the extensor retinaculum, ECU subsheath, and ECU tendon position
  - The position of the tendon, however, is highly dependent on the position of the wrist in the MRI, and it is recommended that imaging studies be taken in both pronation and supination
- TFCC injuries (Figure 5C.5)
  - Most commonly used imaging modality to assess TFCC pathology
  - Sensitivity ranges from 67% to 100%, and specificity, from 60% to 100%[4]
  - Helpful in determining location of tear (peripheral vs central) and degenerative vs acute appearing
  - Pathology may be found in asymptomatic patients and is relatively common in patients older than 50 years
  - Increased sensitivity and specificity with magnetic resonance arthrography (MRA) and high-resolution MRI (8-T)
  - Controversial reports in literature about routine MRI for ulnar-sided wrist pain

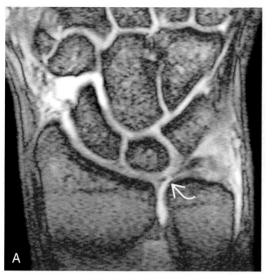
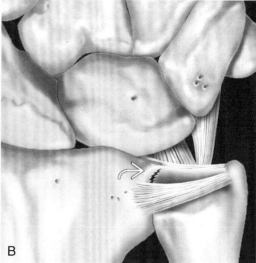

Figure 5C.5. A, T2-weighted MRI arthrogram of a wrist demonstrating a central triangular fibrocartilage complex (TFCC) tear (white arrow) with extravasation of contrast into the distal radioulnar joint. B, Diagram depicting a similar central TFCC tear (white arrow) to what is seen on the MRI with relevant surrounding anatomy.

Ultrasonography

- In general: cost-effective, easily accessible, and can be performed dynamically and compared with the contralateral side. It is, however, highly operator-dependent
- ECU pathology
  - Dynamic evaluation in different wrist/forearm positions is very helpful and can be performed in the clinic. Can assess inflammatory changes as well
  - Up to 50% of volar displacement with maximum supination, ulnar deviation, and flexion of the wrist may be a normal finding[5]
  - Up to 75% of asymptomatic wrists have been shown to demonstrate some mild tendinosis on ultrasonography. Patient education of findings and clinical correlation to symptoms is very important[5]
- TFCC injuries
  - Dynamic ultrasonography while stressing the DRUJ and comparing it with the contralateral side has a reported 88% sensitivity and 81% specificity for determining DRUJ instability

Classic Arthroscopic Findings (Figures 5C.6 and 5C.7)

- Arthroscopy remains the gold standard for diagnosis of TFCC pathology
  - Central tears lack sufficient vascularity to heal and often appear frayed. These are treated with debridement to a stable edge[7]
  - Disruption of the foveal attachment may lead to DRUJ instability and should be surgically repaired
  - Peripheral TFCC tears have adequate vascularization and can benefit from a repair if conservative management has failed

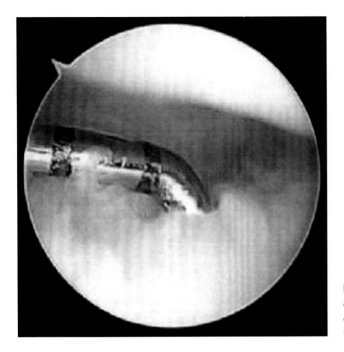

Figure 5C.6. Arthroscopic image of an arthroscopic probe identifying a triangular fibrocartilage complex (TFCC) tear.

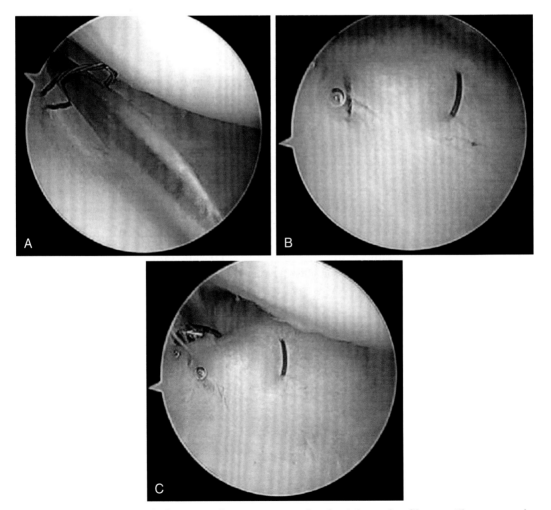

Figure 5C.7. Arthroscopic images of a suture repair of a triangular fibrocartilage complex (TFCC) tear (A and B). The probe is then reinserted and the repair is tested to confirm that it is complete (C).

REFERENCES

1. Montalvan B, Parier J, Brasseur JL, Le Viet D, Drape JL. Extensor carpi ulnaris injuries in tennis players: a study of 28 cases. *Br J Sports Med.* 2006;40(5):424-429 [discussion 429]. doi:10.1136/bjsm.2005.023275.
2. Harley BJ, Pereria ML, Werner FW, Kinney DA, Sutton LG. Force variations in the distal radius and ulna: effect of ulnar variance and forearm motion. *J Hand Surg Am.* 2015;40(2):211-216. doi:10.1016/j.jhsa.2014.10.001.
3. Kuntz MT, Janssen SJ, Ring D. Incidental signal changes in the extensor carpi ulnaris on MRI. *Hand (N Y).* 2015;10(4):750-755. doi:10.1007/s11552-015-9764-9.
4. Lee YH, Choi YR, Kim S, Song H-T, Suh J-S. Intrinsic ligament and triangular fibrocartilage complex (TFCC) tears of the wrist: comparison of isovolumetric 3D-THRIVE sequence MR arthrography and conventional MR image at 3 T. *Magn Reson Imaging.* 2013;31(2):221-226. doi:10.1016/j.mri.2012.06.024.
5. Sole JS, Wisniewski SJ, Newcomer KL, Maida E, Smith J. Sonographic evaluation of the extensor carpi ulnaris in asymptomatic tennis players. *PM R.* 2015;7(3):255-263. doi:10.1016/j.pmrj.2014.08.951.
6. Ruland RT, Hogan CJ. The ECU synergy test: an aid to diagnose ECU tendonitis. *J Hand Surg Am.* 2008;33(10):1777-1782. doi:10.1016/j.jhsa.2008.08.018.
7. Bednar MS, Arnoczky SP, Weiland AJ. The microvasculature of the triangular fibrocartilage complex: its clinical significance. *J Hand Surg Am.* 1991;16(6):1101-1105.
8. Tay SC, Tomita K, Berger RA. The "ulnar fovea sign" for defining ulnar wrist pain: an analysis of sensitivity and specificity. *J Hand Surg Am.* 2007;32(4):438-444. doi:10.1016/j.jhsa.2007.01.022.
9. Pang EQ, Yao J. Ulnar-sided wrist pain in the athlete (TFCC/DRUJ/ECU). *Curr Rev Musculoskelet Med.* 2017;10(1):53-61. doi:10.1007/s12178-017-9384-9.

SECTION D
de Quervain Tenosynovitis

Trenton Gause

HISTORY

- de Quervain disease is a stenosing tenosynovitis of the first dorsal extensor compartment of the wrist
  - Involves APL and EPB tendons **(Figure 5D.1)**
- First described by Swiss physician Fritz de Quervain in 1895[6]
- Patients note insidious onset of pain or tenderness localized along the radial side of the wrist
  - Usually in dominant hand
  - Oftentimes pain is increased by activities such as grasping, thumb abduction, or ulnar deviation of wrist
  - Pain is worsening with repetitive actions with the thumb
  - Usually better with activity avoidance, rest, or immobilization
  - Lack of neurologic symptoms, ie, paresthesias
- Predisposing factors include
  - Female sex (M:F is approximately 1:6), middle age
  - Occupations involving repetitive lifting and typing tasks
  - Historically, daily household chores of homemakers were a precipitant of the disease
  - A subgroup of patients commonly cited in the literature are pregnant or newly postpartum females due to carrying the infant and frequent breastfeeding[10]
  - Anatomic variations are also thought to be a major inciting factor in the development of the disease
    - Several studies have linked septation between the APL and EBP within the first dorsal compartment as a risk factor[1]
    - Bahm et al[3] found that 60% of symptomatic patients has some degree of septation, either partial or complete

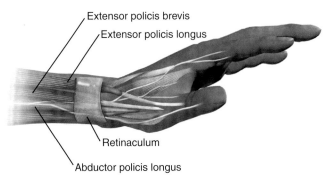

Figure 5D.1. Anatomy of the first dorsal compartment consisting of the abductor pollicis longus (APL) and the extensor pollicis brevis (EPB) with insertion sites. Also demonstrated is the third dorsal compartment of the extensor pollicis longus (EPL), which, along with the first dorsal compartment, forms the border of the anatomic snuff box.

PHYSICAL EXAMINATION

- **Eichhoff Test** (Sensitivity 0.89, Specificity 0.14) **(Figure 5D.2)**
  - First described in 1927 by Eichhoff[11]
  - There have been no significant modifications
  - Often mistakenly called the Finkelstein test[7]
  - **Maneuver:**
    - The examiner sits in front of the patient and grasps the affected wrist with one hand
    - The patient should clench the thumb into a fist
    - The physician then places the other hand on the fist with the patient's wrist in neutral pronation-supination
    - Supporting the wrist with one hand, the physician then quickly ulnarly deviates the wrist
    - Pain is considered a positive test
    - May be performed standing or sitting
  - **Limitations of Maneuver:**
    - Low specificity
    - Basal arthritis of the thumb (or Wartenberg syndrome) intersection syndrome, radial neuritis (Wartenberg syndrome), radial styloid fracture, scaphoid fracture, and radioscaphoid arthritis may all produce pain
    - Passive examination
      - Relies on skill of the examiner to provoke pain

- **Finkelstein Test** 🔘 **(Figure 5D.3)**
  - First described in 1930 by Finkelstein[8]
  - Classic maneuver, considered pathognomonic for the disease
  - There have been no recent modifications
  - **Maneuver:**
    - The examiner sits or stands in front of the patient
    - With one hand, the physician grasps the wrist of the patient on the affected side

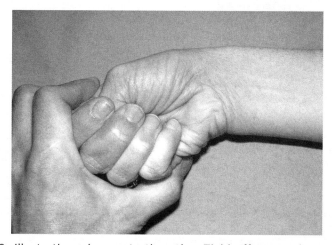

Figure 5D.2. Illustration demonstrating the Eichhoff test where the patient clenches the thumb in a fist with ulnar deviation of the wrist. (From Frassica FJ. *The 5-Minute Orthopaedic Consult.* Philadelphia: Lippincott Williams & Wilkins; 2007.)

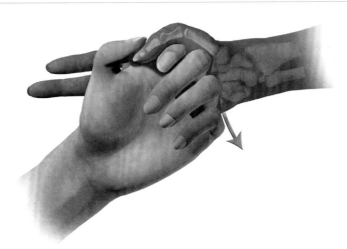

Figure 5D.3. Illustration depicting the Finkelstein test as described in the original article, where the physician grasps the patient's thumb and ulnarly deviates the hand and wrist.

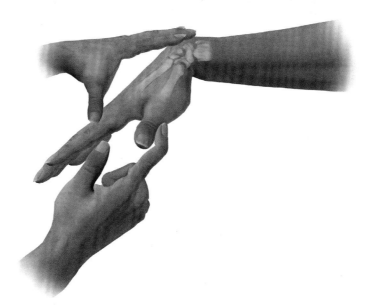

Figure 5D.4. WHAT test demonstration with wrist hyperflexion and thumb abduction, which is thought to increase shear forces of the synovial lining of the first compartment.

- – The physician then grips the patient's thumb with the free hand
- – Pulling slight longitudinal traction on the affected thumb, the physician then deviates the wrist and thumb ulnarly
- Pain renders the test positive but again may be confused with underlying arthritis or other disease entities
- **Limitations of Maneuver:**
  - – Similar to limitations of Eichhoff test

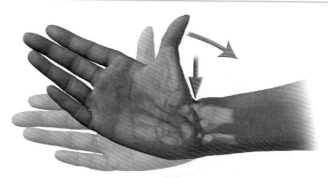

Figure 5D.5. Illustration demonstrating the Brunelli examination with thumb abduction with the wrist in radial deviation, which theoretically would produce irritation of the first dorsal compartment tendons against their corresponding pulleys.

- **Wrist Hyperflexion and Abduction of Thumb (WHAT) Test** (Sensitivity 0.99, Specificity 0.29) **(Figure 5D.4)**
  - Described in 2014 by Goubau et al[9]
  - Purported to demonstrate higher sensitivity and specificity than the gold-standard Eichhoff test
  - Solely tests the tendons of the first compartment
  - **Maneuver:**
    - The patient is asked to fully flex the affected wrist
    - The patient is then asked to abduct and extend the affected thumb
    - Standing in front of the patient, the physician may use one hand to brace the dorsum of the patient's hand for stabilization as depicted
    - With the free hand, the physician then applies increasing resistance to abduction of the patient's thumb
    - The patient is free to release the abduction and extension force if they experience pain
    - Pain on resistance is considered a positive result
  - **Limitations of Maneuver:**
    - Active test; therefore, patient must be able to understand and follow commands

- **Brunelli Test (Figure 5D.5)**
  - Put into practice in 2003 by Brunelli et al[5]
  - Thought to irritate tendons against the pulley in the corresponding compartment
  - No recent modifications
  - **Maneuver:**
    - The patient is asked to strongly abduct the affected thumb with the wrist in radial deviation and neutral pronosupination
  - **Limitations of Maneuver:**
    - Active test, thus depending on the patient's ability and willingness to participate
    - Not well studied in the literature

- **EBP Entrapment Test (Figure 5D.6)**
  - Examination is detailed in the paper by Alexander et al[2] in 2002
  - Two-part test, slightly more complex but believed to isolate de Quervain caused by separate APL and EPB compartments (sensitivity of 0.81 and specificity of 0.5 in identifying patients requiring surgery with separate compartments)
  - No recent modifications

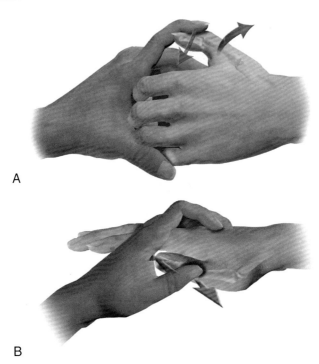

Figure 5D.6. Illustration depicting the EPB entrapment test. It is a 2-part test. A, The physician resists extension at the affected thumb MCP joint. B, The physician resists palmar abduction of the affected thumb. If the pain is greater in extension than that in abduction, the test is considered positive.

- **Maneuver:**
  - The patient stabilizes the arm on a table in neutral supination-pronation
  - Standing or sitting in front of the patient, the examiner first asks the patient to extend the affected thumb at its MCP joint
  - The patient and physician then relax, and the patient is then asked to place the affected thumb in palmar abduction while the physician resists again
  - If pain in extension is greater than pain in abduction, the test is considered positive
- **Limitations of Maneuver:**
  - Utility in the literature largely limits it to identifying cases of de Quervain requiring surgery and the presence of a separated first dorsal compartment
  - Slightly more complex than other tests
- Corticosteroid Injection
  - 80% of patients respond to corticosteroid injections of the first dorsal compartment after only 1 to 2 injections, rendering this a valuable therapeutic and diagnostic tool[4]
  - Of those that continue to experience pain after corticosteroid injections, studies have shown that up to 78% of corticosteroid resistant patients had a separate compartment for EPB causing stenosis

IMAGING

- Not routinely indicated in diagnosis of de Quervain disease, clinical presentation and examination should suffice
- May pursue wrist imaging if concomitant scaphoid or styloid fracture is suspected

- Thumb/hand X-ray images may be helpful in discerning if a patient's symptoms may result from underlying arthritis; however, as previously mentioned, the 2 diseases can occur concomitantly
- Occasional bony lesions or spurs on the distal radius may be identified as a source of compression on the first dorsal compartment
- In difficult cases, advanced imaging modalities such as ultrasonography or MRI may be used to further characterize swelling or irritation of the tendon but are not commonly used if presentation is clear

REFERENCES

1. Adams JE, Habbu R. Tendinopathies of the hand and wrist. *J Am Acad Orthop Surg.* 2015;23(12):741-750.
2. Alexander RD, Catalano LW, Barron OA, Glickel SZ. The extensor pollicis brevis entrapment test in the treatment of de Quervain's disease. *J Hand Surg.* 2002;27(5):813-816.
3. Bahm J, Szabo Z, Foucher G. The anatomy of de Quervain's disease. *Int Orthop.* 1995;19(4):209-211.
4. Blood TD, Morrell NT, Weiss AP. Tenosynovitis of the hand and wrist. *JBJS Rev.* 2016;4(3):e7.
5. Brunelli G. Finkelstein's versus Brunelli's test in De Quervain tenosynovitis. *Chir Main.* 2003;22(1):43.
6. de Quervain F. On a form of chronic tendovaginitis by Dr. Fritz de Quervain in la Chaux-de-Fonds. 1895. *Am J Orthop (Belle Mead NJ).* 1997;26(9):641-644.
7. Elliott BG. Finkelstein's test: a descriptive error that can produce a false positive. *J Hand Surg Br.* 1992;17(4):481-482.
8. Finkelstein H. Stenosing tendovaginitis at the radial styloid process. *J Bone Joint Surg Am.* 1930;12(3):509-540.
9. Goubau JF, Goubau L, Van Tongel A, et al. The wrist hyperflexion and abduction of the thumb (what) test: a more specific and sensitive test to diagnose de Quervain tenosynovitis than the Eichhoff's test. *J Hand Surg Eur Vol.* 2014;39(3):286-292.
10. Ilyas AM, Ast M, Schaffer AA, et al. De Quervain tenosynovitis of the wrist. *J Am Acad Orthop Surg.* 2007;15(12):757-764.
11. Eichhoff E. Zur pathogenese der tendovaginitis stenosans. *Bruns' Beitrage Z Klin Chir.* 1927:746-55.

SECTION E
Flexor and Extensor Tendon Injuries

Jeffrey D. Boatright

HISTORY

- Broad range of injuries and mechanisms affecting either the flexor or extensor tendons within the hand and wrist
  - Many, especially zone II flexor tendon injuries, have historically poor outcomes
    - While advances in repair techniques and rehabilitation have improved outcomes, these still remain a challenge
- Both the flexor and extensor tendons are divided into zones
  - Facilitates easy communication and description of the location of injury
  - Treatment and often prognosis vary, at least partially, based on the zone of injury
  - Commonly associated injuries also vary based on the zone of injury
- Flexor zones **(Figure 5E.1)**
- Extensor zones **(Figure 5E.2)**

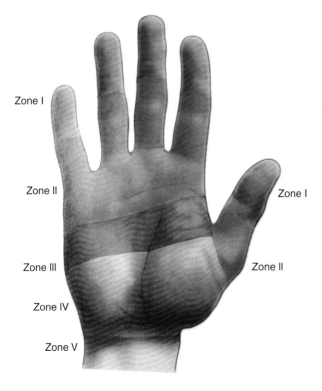

Zone I
Zone II
Zone III
Zone IV
Zone V
Zone I
Zone II

Figure 5E.1. Depicted are the flexor tendon zones in the hand and wrist. Zone I—distal to flexor digitorum superficialis (FDS) insertion. Zone II—FDS insertion to distal palmar crease. Both tendons reside within the fibro-osseous sheath in the finger. Zone III—distal palmar crease to distal edge of transverse carpal ligament. Concurrent neurovascular injury is common in this zone. Zone IV—spans the carpal tunnel. Zone V—proximal edge of the transverse carpal ligament extending proximally into the forearm. (From Malone KJ, Trumble T. Chapter 56: Staged digital flexor tendon reconstruction. In: Wiesel SW, ed. *Operative Techniques in Orthopaedic Surgery*. Vol 3. Philadelphia: Wolters Kluwer, Lippincott Williams & Wilkins; 2011:2570.)

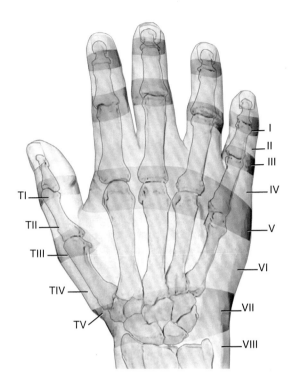

Figure 5E.2. Depicted are the extensor tendon zones within the hand and wrist. Easy to recall if you keep in mind that they run in ascending order from distal to proximal with the odd-numbered zones over the joints and even-numbered zones of the bony diaphyses. (From Hunt TRI, Wiesel SW. *Operative Techniques in Hand, Wrist, and Elbow Surgery*. 2016.)

- History varies dramatically based on flexor versus extensor involvement as well as zone of injury
  - Present with pain, weakness, or complete inability to flex or extend 1 or more joints within a digit
  - Closed injuries are often avulsion mechanisms with or without associated fracture and present with a history of a sudden eccentrically directed external force against maximal flexion or extension of a digit
  - Tendon lacerations present with a history of sharp penetrating trauma, often from an accidental self-inflicted knife injury
    - Laceration injuries also frequently present with numbness or paresthesias in the affected digit secondary to concurrent nerve injury

PHYSICAL EXAMINATION

- General examination considerations for flexor or extensor tendon injury
  - Resting position
    - Important to inspect the resting position of each digit relative to one another
    - Resting position is a point of equilibrium between the resting tone of the flexors vs the resting tone of the extensors
    - Disruption of a flexor or extensor tendon will alter this equilibrium, resulting in an abnormal resting posture relative to the uninjured digits **(Figure 5E.3)**
      - Flexor tendon injury will result in a relative extension resting posture
      - Extensor tendon injury will result in a relative flexion resting posture
  - Tenodesis effect **(Figure 5E.4)**
    - Very useful tool in helping to diagnose flexor and extensor tendon injuries in the hand
    - Passive wrist extension and flexion alters the tension of the finger flexor and extensor tendons

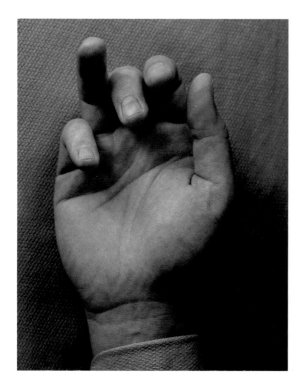

Figure 5E.3. Resting posture of the hand is a key physical examination component, which is the equilibrium point resulting from the sum of the finger flexor and extensor resting tones. Disruption results in a disturbance of this equilibrium point. In this photograph, the patient has a ring finger FDP (flexor digitorum profundus) rupture, resulting in an abnormal flexion cascade compared with the other digits. (From Dines JS, Ovid Technologies I. *Sports Medicine of Baseball*. Philadelphia: Wolters Kluwer Health/Lippincott Williams & Wilkins; 2012.)

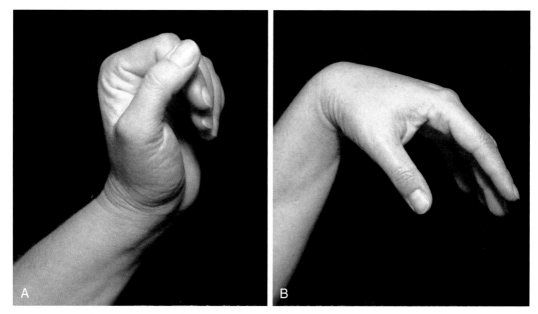

Figure 5E.4. The tenodesis effect is another key physical examination component. Passive wrist extension results in increased tension on the flexors and decreased tension on the extensors, causing the MCP, PIP, and DIP joints to flex (A). The converse is true with passive wrist flexion (B). An injury to a flexor or extensor tendon will alter the tenodesis effect. (From Radomski MV, Latham CAT. *Occupational Therapy for Physical Dysfunction*. 2014.)

– Under normal circumstances:
  • Passive wrist extension puts greater tension on the finger flexors and less tension on the finger extensors resulting in MCP, PIP, and DIP flexion
  • Passive wrist flexion puts greater tension on the finger extensors and less tension on the finger flexors resulting in MCP, PIP, and DIP extension

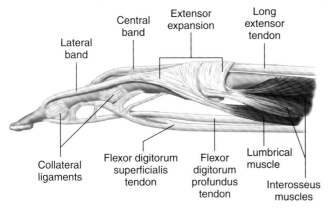

A   **Lateral view**

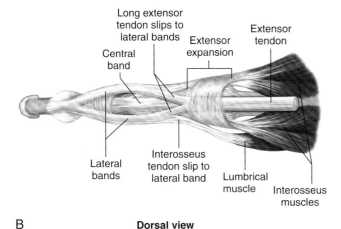

B   **Dorsal view**

Figure 5E.5. A and B, The intricate anatomy of the flexor and extensor anatomy in the finger and palm from the lateral and dorsal views, respectively. (From Beggs I. *Musculoskeletal Ultrasound.* Wolters Kluwer Health/Lippincott Williams & Wilkins; 2014.)

- Injury to a finger flexor or extensor tendon will alter the tenodesis effect relative to the uninjured fingers
- Skin and neurovascular examination are critical in tendon injuries of the hand because a large number are related to lacerations
  - Inspect for retained foreign bodies and arthrotomy
- Rotational deformity can indicate concurrent fracture or collateral ligament injury
- Active motion
  - Important to understand the anatomy of the finger flexors and extensors to appropriately interpret motion deficits **(Figure 5E.5)**
  - Motion of each joint should be examined in isolation
    - FDS
      - Individual muscle bellies in the forearm
      - Insert on the volar surface of the base of the middle phalanx
      - Flex PIP joint and assist with MCP flexion
      - Assess by extending all other digits (other than the one being tested) flush on a table and asking the patient to flex the PIP joint **(Figure 5E.6B)**
        - Extension of other digits takes the FDP out of the equation
        - Of note, FDS to the small finger is absent in 6% to 25% of individuals, which can confound the examination
          - Can be absent unilaterally or bilaterally
    - FDP
      - Share a common muscle belly in forearm
        - Thus extension of other digits prevents flexion of any single DIP joint

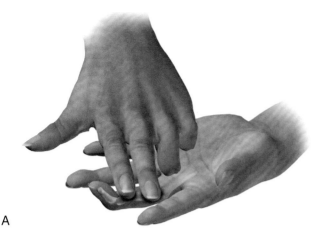

A

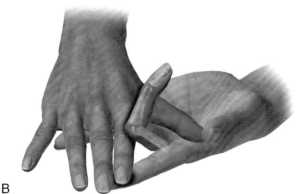

B

Figure 5E.6. Active FDP (flexor digitorum profundus) function is tested by holding the PIP joint in extension while asking the patient to flex the DIP joint (A). Active FDS (flexor digitorum superficialis) function is tested by holding the adjacent fingers in extension while asking the patient to flex the PIP joint of the isolated digit (B).

- Insert on the volar surface of the base of the distal phalanx
- Examine by holding the finger in question flush on a table with the MCP and PIP joints held in extension **(Figure 5E.6A)**
- Ask the patient to flex the DIP joint
- Finger extensor mechanism will be discussed in a zone-specific fashion below, as it relates to the various common extensor tendon injuries
- Extensor tendon injuries
  - Zone V extensor tendon injury—sagittal band rupture aka "boxer's knuckle," "flea-flicker injury"
    - EDC contributes to MCP extension via the lasso effect due from its connections to the sagittal bands
    - Presents with pain over the dorsum of the MCP joint and extensor tendon subluxation after forceful resisted MCP extension or a direct blow to the dorsal MCP joint
      - Can also occur as the result of an inflammatory arthropathy
    - Inability to initiate extension due to EDC subluxation, "pseudotriggering"
      - Sagittal band acts to centralize the tendon directly over the MCP joint
        - Radial sagittal band rupture causes ulnar subluxation of tendon
          - Nine times more common than ulnar sagittal band rupture
    - Active MCP flexion against resistance with the wrist flexed accentuates the subluxation and pain
    - May see bowstringing of the extensor tendon with MCP hyperextension
  - Zone III extensor tendon injury—central slip injury
    - The central slip is a portion of the finger extensor mechanism, which inserts onto the proximal dorsal base of the middle phalanx and helps extend the PIP joint

– Typically presents with pain over the PIP joint after a direct blow "jammed finger" or volar PIP dislocation
  • Causes central slip avulsion +/– piece of bone
– PIP joint extensor lag +/– DIP hyperextension

KEY EXAMINATION MANEUVERS

- **Elson Test** 🎥 **(Figure 5E.7)**
  - Described by Elson in 1986[3]
  - Used to test central slip injuries
  - **Maneuver:**
    - The examiner passively flexes the patient's PIP joint over the edge of the table top
    - The examiner applies a flexion force to the dorsal middle phalanx while asking the patient to extend the PIP joint against resistance while assessing both the PIP extension force and DIP joint rigidity (which is assessed with the examiner's contralateral hand)
    - A central slip injury will result in PIP extension weakness and obligatory DIP extension or hyperextension, which manifests as DIP rigidity
      - DIP rigidity occurs secondary to extension force transmission across the DIP joint via the lateral bands when the central slip has been injured

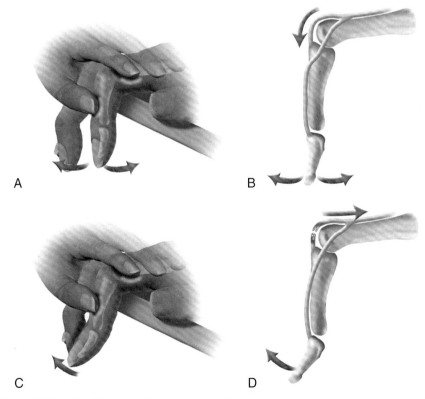

A

B

C

D

Figure 5E.7. The Elson test is performed to evaluate for a central slip injury. The finger is flexed to 90° over the edge of a table. The patient is asked to extend the PIP joint against resistance while the examiner assesses both middle phalanx extension force and DIP rigidity. With an intact central slip, the examiner will appreciate active extension force at the middle phalanx and a flaccid DIP joint (A and B). In the presence of a central slip rupture, there will be no active middle phalanx extension force, and the DIP joint will become rigid (C and D).

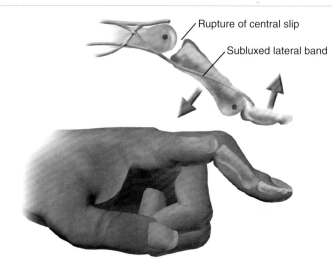

Rupture of central slip

Subluxed lateral band

Figure 5E.8. Typically, over 2 to 3 wk, a central slip injury will lead to a classic boutonniere deformity with PIP joint flexion and DIP joint extension. This occurs as the triangular ligament attenuates, causing the lateral bands to drift volar to the PIP joint axis of rotation, which turns the hand intrinsics into PIP joint flexors while hyperextending the DIP joint.

- In the acute setting, a digital block before the Elson test can be a useful adjunct, as it eliminates associated pain as a potential confounding variable

- If diagnosis is delayed greater than 2 to 3 weeks, a boutonniere deformity will become evident on examination **(Figure 5E.8)**

- Fixed flexion of the PIP joint with hyperextension of the DIP joint
  - This occurs, as the triangular ligament distally attenuates causing the lateral bands to drift volar to the PIP joint axis of rotation turning the hand intrinsics into PIP joint flexors
    - Zone I extensor tendon injury—terminal extensor tendon injury aka "mallet finger"

- Terminal extensor tendon inserts on the proximal dorsal base of the distal phalanx and helps with DIP extension

- Typically presents as pain and swelling over the DIP joint after an impaction injury "jammed finger" or forceful flexion of a fully extended DIP joint often occurring in ball sports

- May be either a purely tendinous or a bony avulsion injury

- Results in an abnormal resting posture with the DIP joint in ~45° of flexion and inability to extend the DIP joint **(Figure 5E.9)**

- Associated PIP hyperextension may result in swan neck deformity **(Figure 5E.10)**
  - This occurs, as the volar plate of the PIP attenuates, the lateral bands migrate dorsally, and the triangular ligament develops contracture

- Flexor Tendon Injuries 🔘
  - Zone I flexor tendon injury—FDP injury aka "jersey finger" **(Figure 5E.11)**
    - 75% involves the ring finger
    - Most frequently present with pain and inability to flex the DIP joint after a forcible extension moment exerted on a maximally flexed finger
      - Patients often report a mechanism of getting a finger "hung up" in an opponent's jersey or otherwise trying to grip something firmly with the object being forcibly pulled away
    - Pain over the volar distal finger

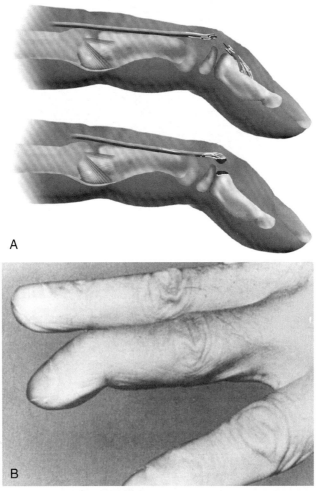

Figure 5E.9. Illustration (A) and clinical photograph (B) of a zone I terminal extensor tendon injury (mallet finger). This injury can be a tendinous rupture or bony avulsion fracture (A). Clinically, the resting posture of the affected digit will be altered with the DIP joint held in approximately 45° of flexion (B). There will absent active DIP extension. ((A) From Brinker MR. *Review of Orthopaedic Trauma*. 2nd ed. Philadelphia, PA: Wolters Kluwer and Lippincott Williams & Wilkins; 2013 and (B) Salter RB. *Textbook of Disorders and Injuries of the Musculoskeletal System: An Introduction to Orthopaedics, Fractures, and Joint Injuries, Rheumatology, Metabolic Bone Disease, and Rehabilitation*. 3rd ed. Baltimore: Williams & Wilkins; 1999.)

- In the resting position, the DIP joint of the affected digit will be held in more extension relative to the other digits
- Passive wrist extension will not result in DIP flexion due to the disrupted tenodesis effect
- May have a palpable nodule more proximally in the digit or palm
  • Represents the retracted tendon
• Zones II to V are typically open laceration injuries
  - Must examine each FDS and FDP tendon in isolation as described earlier
  - The resting posture and tenodesis effect (both described earlier) are useful examination tools for these injuries
  - Careful neurovascular examination is critical
    • Neurovascular injury portends worse prognosis for zones II to V injuries

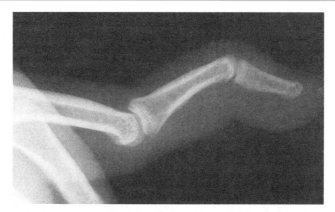

Figure 5E.10. Radiograph a classic swan neck deformity secondary to a chronic untreated terminal extensor tendon injury. There is persistent DIP flexion and associated compensatory PIP hyperextension, the latter of which occurs as the volar plate of the PIP attenuates and the lateral bands migrate dorsally. (From Bucholz RW, Heckman JD. *Rockwood & Green's Fractures in Adults*. 5th ed. Lippincott: Williams & Wilkins; 2001.)

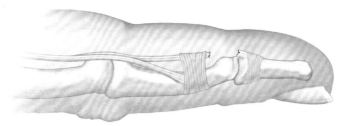

Figure 5E.11. Illustration of a zone I flexor tendon rupture, which by definition involves only the FDP (flexor digitorum profundus) tendon. This can be a purely tendinous injury as depicted above or can be associated with a bony avulsion fracture. (From Miller MD, ed. *Sports Medicine Conditions: Return to Play: Recognition, Treatment, Planning*. Philadelphia, PA: Lippincott Williams & Wilkins; 2014.)

- Other zone-specific examination considerations:
  - Zone II
    - Typically has concurrent FDP and FDS injury due to the close proximity within the fibro-osseous sheath
  - Zone III
    - Highest association with neurovascular injury due to the close proximity to the common digital nerves and arteries as well as the superficial palmar arch
  - Zone IV
    - Relatively small-sized laceration can lead to injury in multiple digits due to tight association of all flexor tendons within the carpal tunnel
      - Must evaluate all tendons to all fingers in isolation
  - Zone V
    - Also in high association with neurovascular injury
  - Flexor tendon pulley rupture
    - Most common in rock climbers
    - Typically presents as pain +/− ecchymosis along the volar surface of the proximal phalanx after feeling a "pop" in the finger during forceful gripping activity
    - Examination will reveal bowstringing of the flexor tendons during active flexion of the digit
    - Typically involves the A2 and A3 pulleys
      - Can involve A4 as well

IMAGING

- Plain radiographs are standard in the workup for most of these injuries
  - Evaluate for bony avulsions and associated dislocations in closed injuries and assess for retained foreign bodies in open injuries
- Ultrasonography and/or MRI can be useful for assessing tendon retraction, evaluating for other concurrent soft tissue injuries, or in equivocal cases
  - Dynamic ultrasonography can be a useful adjunct in certain cases

REFERENCES

1. Townley WA, Swan MC, Dunn RLR. Congenital absence of flexor digitorum superficialis: implications for assessment of little finger lacerations. *J Hand Surg.* 2017;35(5):417-418.
2. Colzani G, Tos P, Battiston B, Merolla G, Porcellini G, Artiaco S. Traumatic extensor tendon injuries to the hand: clinical anatomy, biomechanics, and surgical procedure review. *J Hand Microsurg.* 2016;8(1):2-12. doi:10.1055/s-0036-1572534.
3. Elson RA. Rupture of the central slip of the extensor hood of the finger: a test for early diagnosis. *J Bone Joint Surg Br.* 1986;68:229-231.
4. Bachoura A, Ferikes AJ, Lubahn JD. A review of mallet finger and Jersey finger injuries in the athlete. *Curr Rev Musculoskelet Med.* 2017;10(1) 1-9.
5. Strauch RJ. Extensor tendon injury. In: Wolfe SW, Pederson WC, Hotchkiss RN, Kozin SH, eds. *Green's Operative Hand Surgery.* 6th ed. Philadelphia, PA: Elsevier Churchill Livingstone; 2011:159-188.
6. Seiler III JG. Flexor tendon injury. In: Wolfe SW, Pederson WC, Hotchkiss RN, Kozin SH, eds. *Green's Operative Hand Surgery.* 6th ed. Philadelphia, PA: Elsevier Churchill Livingstone; 2011:189-238.

SECTION F
Ligamentous Injury to the Thumb

Daniel E. Hess

HISTORY

- Ligamentous injuries to the thumb are a common problem seen in a clinic and can be from various etiologies. The following items in a patient's clinical history are common for ligamentous injuries to the thumb:
  - Patients may report acute or chronic symptoms. Acute symptoms are typically the result of specific injury, whereas chronic symptoms may be the resulting attritional damage over time, potentially from the patients' occupation or hobbies
    - A forced radial deviation/hyperabduction mechanism should raise suspicion for an ulnar collateral ligament injury, which is much more common than a radial collateral ligament. Radial collateral ligament injuries typically occur with forced adduction or torsion of the flexed thumb
    - An axial force to a flexed thumb should raise suspicion for a thumb CMC dislocation. Less commonly, a dorsally directed force in the first web space can result in the same injury
    - Hyperextension injuries can cause thumb MCP dislocations, often resulting in simultaneous volar plate, capsule, and collateral ligament injuries
  - Sports or occupations requiring repetitive and forced gripping or high-contact activities have a higher rate of injuries to the thumb[4]

PHYSICAL EXAMINATION

General Inspection

- Associated deformity
  - Acute deformities are seen with MCP and CMC dislocations. Partial injuries are common and can result in varying degrees. MCP dislocations are most commonly volar, whereas CMC dislocations are most commonly dorsal
  - Hyperextension deformity of the MCP joint and dorsal subluxation of the CMC joint are commonly seen with chronic CMC arthritis
  - A palpable mass over the ulnar aspect of the MCP joint can represent a torn UCL with interposed adductor aponeurosis (Stener lesion)
    - First described in 1962 by Dr Bertil Stener[6]; the presence of this lesion means that the distal UCL cannot reapproximate to its insertion on the proximal phalanx and requires surgical intervention. It represents a tear of both the proper and accessory bands of the ulnar collateral ligament

- **Valgus Stress Test** 🔊 (Figure 5F.1)
  - Dr. CS Campbell, who coined the term "gamekeeper's thumb" after seeing the injury commonly in English rabbit poachers, also described the valgus stress test in 1955.[2]
  - Helps to determine the presence/amount of ulnar-sided instability of the thumb at the MCP joint
  - **Maneuver:**
    - Stress the thumb joint with radial deviation
    - Test the thumb with thumb in 30° of flexion and neutral/extension
    - Compare with the contralateral (uninjured) side
    - Instability (greater that 30° total or more than 15° when compared with the contralateral side or lack of a firm endpoint) in flexion is indicative of a tear of the more dorsal proper ulnar collateral ligament. Instability in extension suggests a tear of the more volar accessory ulnar collateral ligament and volar plate as well. Instability in both flexion and extension represents a complete rupture and warrants surgical attention[3,5]
    - Note: Varus stress examinations can help determine an injury to the radial collateral ligament. There is no radial sided equivalent to a Stener lesion, as the RCL is broad and the abductor aponeurosis does not commonly interpose beneath the torn ligament
  - **Limitations of Maneuver:**
    - Can be limited by pain in acute injuries. Consider local infiltration of 1% lidocaine before the maneuver
    - Chronic UCL injuries from occupations/hobbies can occur bilaterally, leaving no control side for comparison
    - May be difficult to objectively quantify or to distinguish a partial from a complete injury. Can measure the amount of ulnar-sided gapping or radial translation if examination is performed under fluoroscopy

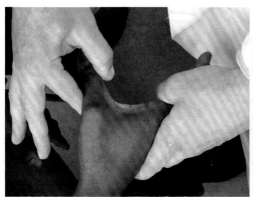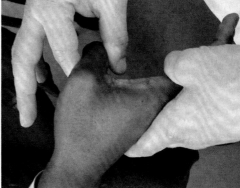

Figure 5F.1. A, Valgus stress test with the thumb in the neutral position. B, Valgus stress test with the thumb in 30° of flexion.

IMAGING

Plain Radiographs

- Standard PA, true lateral
- "Roberts view"—fully pronate the forearm with the dorsum of the thumb on the cassette with the X-ray at a 15° angle distally facing proximal. Best assesses the thumb CMC joint
- Stress radiographs of the CMC joint to evaluate for subtle subluxation. Make sure plain films are obtained first to avoid displacing a nondisplaced fracture with a stress film

Computed Tomography

- Not typically obtained

Magnetic Resonance Imaging

- In general: static imaging, typically highly sensitive for pathology but may have incidental findings, and important to correlate clinically
- MRI has proven useful in suspected collateral injuries, although it is not needed if the clinical examination is obvious for a complete tear. It can, however, be used to distinguish between partial and complete tears, which has prognostic implications
- Preferable to have a musculoskeletal trained radiologist to read the MRI, as findings can be subtle

Ultrasonography

- In general: cost-effective, easily accessible, and can be performed dynamically and compared with the contralateral side. It is, however, highly operator-dependent
- Studies have shown that it has a 76% sensitivity and 81% specificity in diagnosis of UCL tears[1]

Classic Surgical Findings

- The classic surgical finding for a UCL repair with a Stener lesion is the interposition underlying the ruptured UCL, preventing it from reapposing with its metacarpal insertion site. This needs to be freed before the UCL can be repaired

REFERENCES

1. Höglund M, Tordai P, Muren C. Diagnosis by ultrasound of dislocated ulnar collateral ligament of the thumb. *Acta Radiol*. 1995;36(6):620-625.
2. Campbell CS. Gamekeeper's thumb. *J Bone Joint Surg Br*. 1955;37-B(1):148-149.
3. Heyman P, Gelberman RH, Duncan K, Hipp JA. Injuries of the ulnar collateral ligament of the thumb metacarpophalangeal joint. Biomechanical and prospective clinical studies on the usefulness of valgus stress testing. *Clin Orthop Relat Res*. 1993;292:165-171.
4. Owings FP, Calandruccio JH, Mauck BM. Thumb ligament injuries in the athlete. *Orthop Clin North Am*. 2016;47(4):799-807. doi:10.1016/j.ocl.2016.06.001.
5. McKeon KE, Gelberman RH, Calfee RP. Ulnar collateral ligament injuries of the thumb: phalangeal translation during valgus stress in human cadavera. *J Bone Joint Surg Am*. 2013;95(10):881-887. doi:10.2106/JBJS.L.00204.
6. Stener B. Skeletal injuries associated with rupture of the ulnar collateral ligament of the metacarpophalangeal joint of the thumb. A clinical and anatomical study. *Acta Chir Scand*. 1963;125:583-586.

SECTION G
Dupuytren Disease

Kevin L. Laroche

HISTORY

- Commonly seen in Caucasian males of northern European ancestry[3]
- Positive family history
  - Autosomal dominant disease
- Complaints of skin tightness, nodules in palmar fascia, cords with contractures (Figure 5G.1), flexion contractures involving the MCP and/or PIP joint that affect simple activities
- Commonly affects small and ring fingers
- Associated with DM, tobacco use, HIV, and antiseizure medications[2]
- Radial-sided involvement or bilateralism is indicative of more aggressive disease
- Palmar nodularity alone does not confirm Dupuytren disease
  - Differential includes palmar fibromatosis and inclusion cyst
- Ask about ectopic cord locations[4]
  - Sole of the foot (Ledderhose disease) (Figure 5G.2)
  - Penis (Peyronie disease) (Figure 5G.3)
  - Common in Dupuytren diathesis

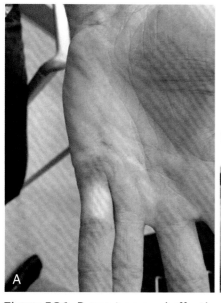
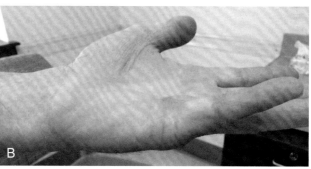

Figure 5G.1. Dupuytren cord affecting the small finger.

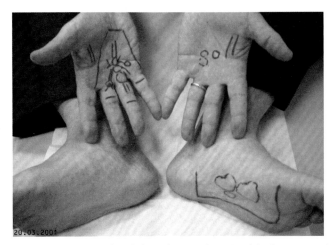

Figure 5G.2. Morbus Dupuytren on both hands. Morbus Ledderhose on the left foot. (From Halperin EC, Perez CA, Wazer DE, Brady LW, eds. *Perez and Brady's Principles and Practice of Radiation Oncology*. 6th ed. Philadelphia: Wolters Kluwer/Lippincott Williams & Wilkins; 2013.)

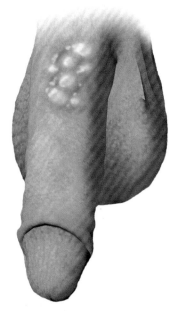

Figure 5G.3. In Peyronie disease, there are palpable nontender hard plaques just beneath the skin, usually along the dorsum of the penis. The patient complains of crooked, painful erections.

PHYSICAL EXAMINATION

Observation

- Flexion contractures that impair simple activities[5]
  - Examples: wearing gloves, hands in pockets
- Look for knuckle pads (Figure 5G.4)

Palpation

- Nodules in the pretendinous bands
- Skin adhesion and dimpling
- Pathologic cords (Figures 5G.5)
  - The key to cord palpation is to feel for a change from soft to firm, as the finger is passively ranged from flexion to extension
  - Pretendinous cords are midline
  - Spiral cords run lateral along the proximal phalanx
  - Retrovascular cords cause DIP contracture

Range of Motion

- Passive extension deficit due to a contracted cord[6]
  - Most often affecting the MCP and PIP joints of the fingers
  - Location of cord dictates which joint is involved
- Range-of-motion measurement of individual joints using a goniometer

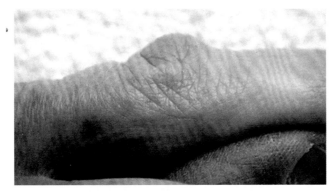

Figure 5G.4. Garrod node over the dorsum of the proximal interphalangeal joint. (From Wiesel SW, ed. *Operative Techniques in Orthopaedic Surgery*. Vol 4. Wolters Kluwer; 2010.)

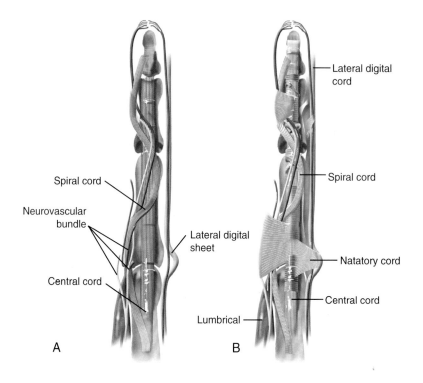

Spiral cord

Neurovascular
bundle

Central cord

Lateral digital
sheet

A

Lateral digital
cord

Spiral cord

Natatory cord

Central cord

Lumbrical

B

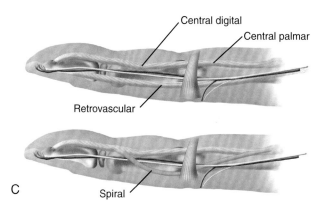

Central digital

Central palmar

Retrovascular

C

Spiral

Figure 5G.5. A, The formation of a spiral cord showing displacement of the neurovascular bundle. B, Pathologic anatomy of Dupuytren disease in the fingers. C, Spiral and retrovascular cords.

KEY EXAMINATION MANEUVERS

- Ensure full active and passive flexion

- **Hueston Tabletop Test** 🖥 (Figure 5G.6)
  - First described by Dr J Hueston[7] in 1982
  - **Maneuver:**
    - Ask the patient to place the palm flat on the table
    - The examiner looks for MCP or PIP contracture
    - The test is positive if the patient is unable to place fingers flat on the table
  - **Limitations of Maneuver:**
    - May be positive for other reasons such as previous injury to MCP or PIP joints causing a contracture or arthritis changes

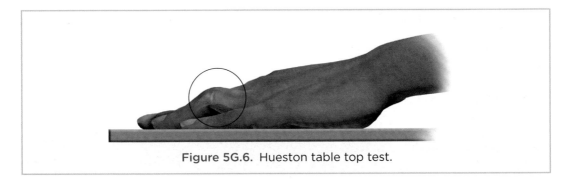

Figure 5G.6. Hueston table top test.

IMAGING

Plain Radiographs

- Limited usage
- PA, lateral, and oblique imaging
  - Visualize the extent of degenerative joint changes or heterotopic ossification of cords[1]

Ultrasonography

- Seen as hypoechoic nodules in the subcutaneous tissues superficial to flexor tendons (Figure 5G.7)
- Identify neurovascular displacement from a spiral cord
  - With progressive flexion, the bundle moves volar and midline

Magnetic Resonance Imaging

- Evaluate the cellularity of the disease (Figures 5G.8 and 5G.9)
- Rule out inclusion cyst or malignancy

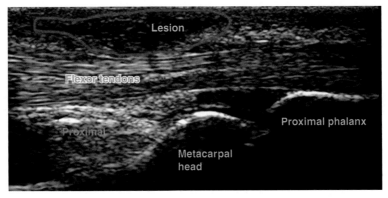

Figure 5G.7. Stage 1—Dupuytren contracture (palmar fibromatosis). Rounded hypoechoic solid fibroma on the palmar aspect of the flexor tendon is the earliest sign of Dupuytren contracture of the hand. (From Waldman SD. *Comprehensive Atlas of Ultrasound-Guided Pain Management Injection Techniques*. Philadelphia: Wolters Kluwer Health/Lippincott Williams & Wilkins; 2014.)

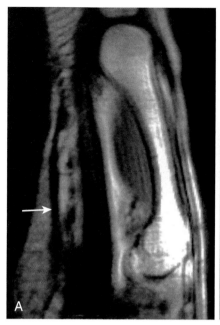
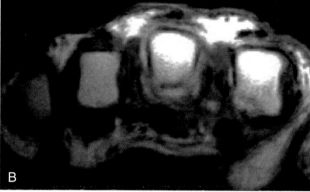

Figure 5G.8. Magnetic resonance imaging of Dupuytren contracture. A, Sagittal T1-weighted image of the fifth metacarpal showing low-intensity cord (arrow). B, Axial T1-weighted image showing a classic subcutaneous nodule. (From Berquist TH, ed. *MRI of the Musculoskeletal System*. 6th ed. Philadelphia, PA: Lippincott Williams & Wilkins; 2013:870-995.)

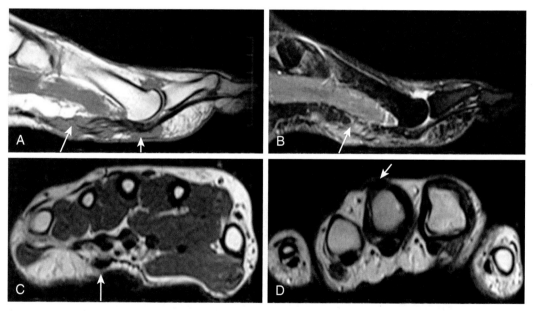

Figure 5G.9. Magnetic resonance imaging of palmar (Dupuytren contracture) and plantar (Ledderhose disease) fibromatosis. A, Sagittal T1-weighted image of the right foot demonstrating nodular soft tissue masses in the distal plantar fascia, which are isointense to muscle (arrows). B, Sagittal T2-weighted image of the same foot showing plantar nodules that are of heterogeneously high signal intensity (arrow). C, MRI of the left hand at the level of the palmar aponeurosis. Short-axis T2 fast spin echo shows focal nodular low signal intensity on the ulnar aspect of the palmar aponeurosis (arrow). D, Short-axis T2 fast spin-echo sequence of the hand at the level of the PIP joints shows focal subcutaneous thickening of the dorsal pads. (From English C, Coughlan R, Carey J, et al. Plantar and palmar fibromatosis: characteristic imaging features and role of MRI in clinical management. *Rhuematology*. 2012;51(6):1134-1136.)

REFERENCES

1. Sadideen H, Athanasou N, Ashmore A, et al. Heterotopic ossification in Dupuytren's disease: clinical and histological significance. *J Bone Joint Surg Br.* 2011;93:1676-1678.
2. Burge P, Hoy G, Regan P, et al. Smoking, alcohol and the risk of Dupuytren's contracture. *J Bone Joint Surg Br.* 1997;79:206-210.
3. Dibenedetti DB, Nguyen D, Zografos L, et al. Prevalence, incidence, and treatments of Dupuytren's disease in the United States: results from a population-based study. *Hand.* 2011;6:149-158.
4. Geoghegan JM, Forbes J, Clark DI, et al. Dupuytren's disease risk factors. *J Hand Surg Br.* 2004;29:423-426.
5. Rayan G. Dupuytren disease: anatomy, pathology, presentation and treatment. *J Bone Joint Surg Am.* 2007;89A:190-198.
6. Hueston J. The control of recurrent Dupuytren's contracture by skin replacement. *Br J Plast Surg.* 1969;22:152-156.
7. Hueston JT. The table top test. *Hand.* 1982;14(1):100-103.

SECTION H
Ulnar Nerve Compression at the Hand

Daniel E. Hess

HISTORY

- Compression of the ulnar nerve in the hand is less common than compression at the elbow but is still an important diagnosis to keep in mind. Compression can occur in 1 or more of 3 anatomic zones and will cause a purely sensory, purely motor, or mixed picture depending on the level of the compression. The following items in a patient's clinical history are common for ulnar nerve compression at the hand:
  - Patients may describe weakness, numbness, or both
  - Patients should describe the activities they are involved in
    - Ulnar tunnel syndrome has been well described in cyclists because of prolonged grip pressures on handlebars[9]
    - Hook of the hamate fractures are often caused by a direct blow while swinging a baseball bat or a golf club
    - Heavy handheld impact or vibratory occupational tools, such as a jackhammer, has been linked to development of hypothenar hammer syndrome, which is a vascular injury to the ulnar artery with resultant ischemia and compression to the ulnar nerve in Guyon canal[1,3,7,8]
  - A history of trauma or injury to the hand/wrist is very important
    - Often the mechanism is a fall on an outstretched hand or, in the case of the hook of the hamate, a direct blow can cause a fracture
    - Fractures of the distal radius, hamate, pisiform, trapezium, and metacarpal base of the ring and small fingers have been reported to cause ulnar neuropathy
    - Typically, the neuropathy is a result of compression from surrounding swelling although direct damage to the nerve can happen, especially in hook of the hamate fractures

PHYSICAL EXAMINATION

General Examination

- Inspection
  - Look for signs of atrophy in the hypothenar eminence or interossei wasting
  - In severe cases the ring and small fingers will be held in flexion
  - Inspect/palpate for any deformity from trauma or masses
  - Wartenberg sign: slight abduction posturing of the small finger secondary to weak adducting intrinsics and unopposed ulnar pull of extensor digiti minimi
- Sensory testing in the hand
  - Altered 2-point discrimination or Semmes-Weinstein suggest more severe pathology
- Motor testing of the hand
  - Intrinsic weakness or inability to cross fingers
  - Comparison of grip and pinch to the contralateral side

- Vascular examination
  - Assessment of radial and ulnar pulses
  - Doppler examination can be helpful to find bruits or thrills over the ulnar artery suggestive of aneurysmal dilation, a potential cause of compression
- Full cervical spine examination
  - Spurling maneuver can be used to help distinguish radiculopathic pain/numbness, which can mimic ulnar tunnel syndrome
  - Reflexes

KEY EXAMINATION MANEUVERS

- **Tinel Sign** (Figure 5H.1) (Sensitivity 26%-79%, Specificity 40%-100%)
  - First described in the literature by Jules Tinel in 1915 who reported a "tingling sign" with percussion of peripheral nerves[10]
  - Helps to isolate median nerve compression at the wrist
  - **Maneuver**:
    - The examiner will sit across from the patient. By gently tapping on the hand over the pisiform, one may elicit an electrical shocklike sensation into the ulnar 2 digits, which is a positive response
  - **Limitations of Maneuver:**
    - Too much force during percussion can cause paresthesias without ulnar tunnel syndrome (false-positive results)
    - Injuries to the wrist can limit effectiveness of this examination maneuver

- **Allen Test** (Figure 5H.2)
  - First described in the literature in its original form in 1929 by Edgar Van Nuys Allen.[11] A modified version described by Irving S. Wright in 1966 is the more commonly used form of the test in contemporary times[12]
  - Helps to diagnose ulnar artery thrombosis, a cause of hypothenar hammer syndrome[4]
  - **Maneuver:**
    - The patient elevates hands and clenches first for 30 seconds. Pressure is then applied over the ulnar and radial arteries to provide occlusion. The hand is then opened and the examiner releases the ulnar pressure while keeping radial pressure. A positive test is if the color in the hand does not return within 5 to 15 seconds
  - **Limitations of Maneuver:**
    - A percentage of patients lack sufficient anastomosis for a dual blood supply
    - Unknown sensitivity and specificity for hypothenar hammer syndrome

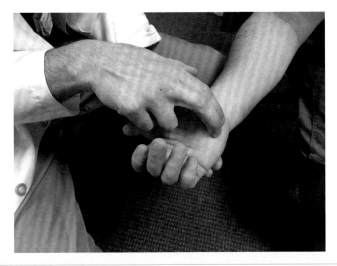

Figure 5H.1. Tinel sign at Guyon canal.

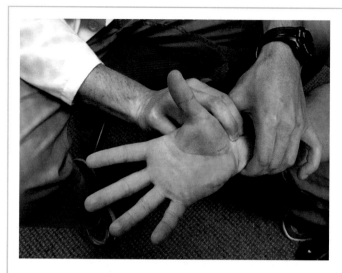

Figure 5H.2. Allen test. Clinical photograph is taken after release of the tourniquet/blood pressure cuff while maintaining occlusion of the radial artery; the hand reperfuses indicating a patent ulnar artery and full arterial arch.

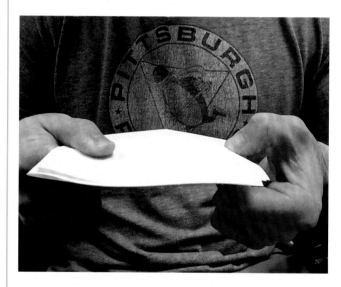

Figure 5H.3. Froment sign. Note that the right hand is the unaffected side and the left hand is recruiting the FPL (median nerve) to aid with pinch because of the weakness of the adductor pollicis (ulnar nerve).

- **Froment Sign** (Figure 5H.3)[13]
  - First described in the literature in 1915 by Jules Froment
  - Helps to distinguish motor involvement with ulnar nerve compression from purely sensory
  - **Maneuver**
    - The patient is asked to pinch a piece of paper between the pulp of the thumb and index finger. The examiner, sitting across from the patient, pulls the paper away from the patient and, if positive for ulnar motor neuropathy, the patient will flex the thumb IP joint to hold onto the paper. The adductor pollicis (innervated by the ulnar nerve) is weak and cannot hold onto the paper and requires the flexor pollicis longus (innervated by the median nerve) to fire and provide pinch
  - **Limitations of Maneuver:**
    - Not specific to ulnar nerve compression at the wrist
    - Would not be positive in zone III compression (pure sensory)

IMAGING

Plain Radiographs

- Standard hand and wrist radiographs should be obtained, especially in the setting of trauma or occupational/recreational stress/overuse
- A "carpal tunnel view" can be obtained to better evaluate the hook of the hamate if such a fracture is suspected

Computed Tomography

- Can be helpful to visualize a hook of the hamate fracture or monitor for appropriate union when following a hook of the hamate fracture

Magnetic Resonance Imaging

- In general: static imaging, typically highly sensitive for pathology but may have incidental findings, and important to correlate clinically
- Can be helpful in localizing ganglia, accessory or hypertrophic muscles, aneurysms, or other space-occupying lesions[2,5]

Ultrasonography

- In general: cost-effective, easily accessible, and can be performed dynamically and compared with the contralateral side. It is, however, highly operator-dependent[6]
- Can also detect space-occupying lesions such as anomalous muscles or ganglia
- Can also be used to aid in ganglion aspiration

Electromyography

- Can be helpful to localize the level of neuropathy. Should include conduction velocity across the elbow and wrist to evaluate for associated cubital tunnel and carpal tunnel

Classic Surgical Findings

- The classic surgical finding for ulnar tunnel syndrome is associated with a space-occupying lesion (eg, Ganglion, malunited hamate, pseudoaneurysm). It is important to decompress the more superficial sensory branch as well as the deeper motor branch, which is located just below the leading tendinous edge of the hypothenar muscle origin

REFERENCES

1. Murata K, Shih J-T, Tsai T-M. Causes of ulnar tunnel syndrome: a retrospective study of 31 subjects. *J Hand Surg Am*. 2003;28(4):647-651.
2. Maroukis BL, Ogawa T, Rehim SA, Chung KC. Guyon canal: the evolution of clinical anatomy. *J Hand Surg Am*. 2015;40(3):560-565. doi:10.1016/j.jhsa.2014.09.026.
3. Marie I, Hervé F, Primard E, Cailleux N, Levesque H. Long-term follow-up of hypothenar hammer syndrome: a series of 47 patients. *Medicine (Baltimore)*. 2007;86(6):334-343. doi:10.1097/MD.0b013e31815c95d3.
4. Hui-Chou HG, McClinton MA. Current options for treatment of hypothenar hammer syndrome. *Hand Clin*. 2015;31(1):53-62. doi:10.1016/j.hcl.2014.09.005.
5. Harvie P, Patel N, Ostlere SJ. Prevalence and epidemiological variation of anomalous muscles at guyon's canal. *J Hand Surg Br*. 2004;29(1):26-29.
6. Ginanneschi F, Filippou G, Reale F, Scarselli C, Galeazzi M, Rossi A. Ultrasonographic and functional changes of the ulnar nerve at Guyon's canal after carpal tunnel release. *Clin Neurophysiol*. 2010;121(2):208-213. doi:10.1016/j.clinph.2009.09.031.

7. Chen S-H, Tsai T-M. Ulnar tunnel syndrome. *J Hand Surg Am*. 2014;39(3):571-579. doi:10.1016/j.jhsa.2013.08.102.

8. Bachoura A, Jacoby SM. Ulnar tunnel syndrome. *Orthop Clin North Am*. 2012;43(4):467-474. doi:10.1016/j.ocl.2012.07.016.

9. Akuthota V, Plastaras C, Lindberg K, Tobey J, Press J, Garvan C. The effect of long-distance bicycling on ulnar and median nerves: an electrophysiologic evaluation of cyclist palsy. *Am J Sports Med*. 2005;33(8):1224-1230. doi:10.1177/0363546505275131.

10. Tinel J. "Tingling" signs with peripheral nerve injuries.1915. *J Hand Surg Br*. 2005;30(1):87-89. doi:10.1016/j.jhsb.2004.10.007.

11. Allen EV. Thromboangiitis obliterans: methods of diagnosis of chronic occlusive arterial lesions distal to the wrist with illustrative cases. *Am J Med Sci*. 1929;178:237-243.

12. Ejrup B, Fischer B, Wright IS. Clinical evaluation of blood flow to the hand. *Circulation*. 1966;33(5):778-780.

13. Froment J. La préhension dans les paralysies du nerf cubital et le signe du pouce. *Presse Med*. 1915;1:409.

SECTION I
Superficial Sensory Radial Nerve Compression (Wartenberg Syndrome)

Trenton Gause

HISTORY

- Described by Wartenberg[7] in 1932 case series involving a compression neuropathy of the superficial radial nerve (SRN), but actually first reported by Matzdorff in 1926[8]
- Originally coined *cheiralgia paresthetica*
- Thought to be due to superficial positioning of the sensory branch of the radial nerve with minimal soft tissue coverage[2]
  - Enters subcutaneous tissue approximately 8 to 9 cm proximal to the radial styloid **(Figure 5I.1)**
  - Traverses between the brachioradialis and the ECRL tendons to become subcutaneous
  - As the wrist pronates, the interval between the above tendons narrows
    - Creates a potential site of tethering of the SRN
- Patients present with typical compression neuropathy complaints with gradual onset, ie, paresthesia, ill-defined pain or numbness largely in the SRN distribution
  - No motor deficits, as the SRN is purely sensory
- The following have been implicated in the literature as precipitating factors[5]:
  - Wrist watches
  - Handcuffs
  - Bracelets
  - Splints or casts that are overly tight

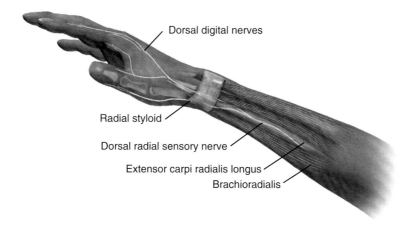

Figure 5I.1. Course of the superficial radial nerve through the forearm, note the potential entrapment area between the ECRL and BR proximally, ie, Wartenberg point and the target area for the Tinel sign. ECRL, extensor carpi radialis longus; BR, brachioradialis.

- Activities requiring repetitive wrist motion
  - Most commonly those involving excessive pronation/supination
- Trauma
- Iatrogenic
- de Quervain tenosynovitis
- Epidemiology:
  - M:F ratio is estimated to be 1:4
  - Typically occurs in middle to older age

Physical Examination

- Diagnosis usually revolves around reproduction of the symptoms upon pronation and wrist flexion with ulnar deviation

KEY EXAMINATION MANEUVERS

- **Tinel Sign**
  - Described in the literature by Braidwood et al[1] in 1975 and in Matzdorff's 1926 paper
  - There have been no recent modifications
  - **Maneuver:**
    - The examiner sits in front of or to the side of patient and may use one hand to support the patient's affected forearm
    - With the patient's arm in neutral pronosupination, the gently percusses, using 2 fingers on the free hand repeatedly over the radial aspect of the forearm
    - The examiner begins at the Wartenberg point and moves distally to approximate the course of the SRN
    - Reproduction of pain or paresthesia at any point is considered positive
    - The physician may ask the patient to hyperpronate the affected forearm if so desired to increase the tethering of the nerve
  - **Limitations of Maneuver:**
    - Requires skill of the physician in regard to anatomy
    - No published studies that define sensitivity and specificity

- **Pronation, Flexion, and Ulnar Deviation Test**
  - Described in Wartenberg's[7] original article in 1932 and also in Ehrlich et al's article in 1986[4]
  - No recent modifications
  - **Maneuver:**
    - Standing or sitting in front of the patient, the examiner may stabilize the patients forearm with one hand
    - The examiner then forcefully pronates, flexes, and ulnarly deviates the affect wrist
      - Physicians may also flex the patients thumb on the affected side to further increase tension on the nerve
      - The examiner may also request that the patient rapidly pronate and supinate the arm using an object such as a pen or screwdriver
    - Any neurologic symptoms or pain renders the examination positive
  - **Limitations of Maneuver:**
    - No clear standardized form exists in the literature
    - Much of the physical examinations were detailed as case series
    - As in the above examination, this maneuver is passive and requires knowledge

- **False-positive Finkelstein or Eichhoff Test**[6]
  - Originally detailed in Wartenberg's[7] original 1932 article and again in Eaton's[3] 1992 article
  - Care must be taken to differentiate paresthesia and neurologic symptoms from the pain of de Quervain
  - No recent modifications

- **Maneuver:**
  - See the corresponding section on de Quervain tenosynovitis for a complete description of the maneuver
  - Must differentiate from true positive for de Quervain and false positive for Wartenberg according to the following:
    - de Quervain will lack neurologic symptoms in the distribution of the SRN **(Figure 51.2)**
    - False-positive Finkelstein test will be independent of the thumb position
- **Limitations of Maneuver:**
  - Multiple disease entities are possible with a positive Finkelstein or Eichhoff test
  - Can be confused with diagnosis of de Quervain
  - Requires a clear description of pain by the patient to accurately interpret results

- A corticosteroid injection that leads to symptomatic relief at the Wartenberg point may differentiate between Wartenberg syndrome and neuritis of the lateral antebrachial cutaneous nerve, which may have a similar overlap in sensory distribution

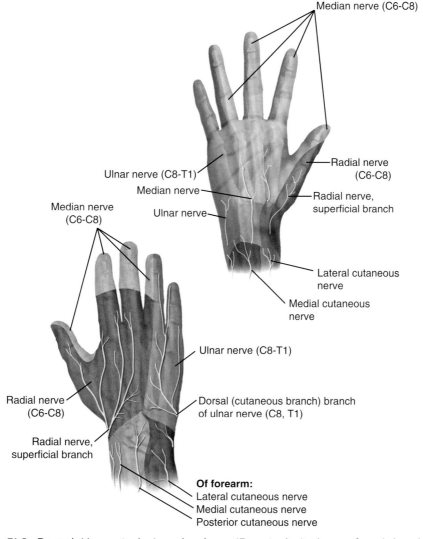

Figure 51.2. Dorsal (A, posterior) and palmar (B, anterior) views of peripheral nerve sensory distribution.

IMAGING

- There is no routine imaging indicated in the diagnosis of Wartenberg syndrome
- Imaging may be useful to rule out other disease entities that may present similarly, ie:
  - Cervical disk disease
  - Basilar arthritis of the thumb or wrist joint
- Electrodiagnostic studies are rarely indicated as well
- Clinical presentation, history, and examination still remain to be the major diagnostic tools

REFERENCES

1. Braidwood AS. Superficial radial neuropathy. *J Bone Joint J*. 1975;57(3):380-383.
2. Mackinnon SE, Novak CB. Compression neuropathies. In: Scott WF, et al, eds. *Green's Operative Hand Surgery*. Philadelphia, PA: Elsevier; 2017:921-959.
3. Eaton CJ, Lister GD. Radial nerve compression. *Hand Clin*. 1992;8(2):345-357.
4. Ehrlich W, Dellon AL, Mackinnon SE. Cheiralgia Paresthetica (entrapment of the radial sensory nerve). *J Hand Surg*. 1986;11(2):196-199.
5. Knutsen EJ, Calfee RP. Uncommon upper extremity compression neuropathies. *Hand Clin*. 2013;29(3):443-453.
6. Lanzetta M, Foucher G. Entrapment of the superficial branch of the radial nerve (Wartenberg's syndrome). *Int Orthop*. 1993;17(6):342-345.
7. Wartenberg R. Cheiralgia Paraesthetica. (Isolierte Neuritis Des Ramus Superficialis Nervi Radialis.). *Z gesamte Neurolo Psychiatr*. 1932;141(1):145-155.
8. Matzdorff P. Zwei Seltene Fälle von Peripherer Sensibler Lähmung (I. Sensible Armbanduhrlähmung, II. Isolierte Rheumatische Lähmung des 2. Astes des Nervus Trigeminus). *J Mol Med*. 1926;5(26):1187.

SECTION J
Carpal Tunnel Syndrome

Daniel E. Hess

HISTORY

- Compression of the median nerve within the carpal tunnel is the most common neuropathy of the upper extremity. The following items in a patient's clinical history are common for CTS[2,4-6,8]:
  - Symptoms often predominate at nighttime. Daytime symptoms are typically activity-related and wrist position–related. A classic story is the affected hand going numb while driving a vehicle with the wrist in a flexed position holding the steering wheel
  - Patients may report being involved in sports or occupations requiring repetitive/excessive use of the hands/digits, repeated impact to the palm, or operating vibratory tools
  - Typically insidious onset on numbness in the radial 3 fingers
  - Pain can accompany the numbness
  - Patients can report difficulty with fine sensory discrimination such as determining the type of coin in a pocket full of change
  - Occasionally report a history of recent injury or wrist surgery. Acute CTS can result from wrist trauma, wrist hemorrhage/edema, or high-pressure injection injury
  - Patients history of prior treatments and their response is very important. This includes noting the type of brace used, symptomatic position of hand, and type of injection used
  - A patient may report a complex medical history. Medical comorbidities such as those affecting fluid balance, inflammatory conditions, neuropathic conditions, and hemorrhagic conditions can have an association with CTS

PHYSICAL EXAMINATION
General Examination[4-6,8]

- Inspection
  - Look for signs of atrophy in the soft tissues (especially thenar atrophy)
  - Cold intolerance, dryness, and other signs of sympathetic dysfunction in the radial 3 digits
- Sensory testing in the hand
  - Altered 2-point discrimination or Semmes-Weinstein suggest more severe pathology
- Motor testing of the thenar musculature
  - Flexion and opposition
- Full cervical spine examination
  - Spurling maneuver can be used to help distinguish radiculopathic pain/numbness, which can mimic CTS
  - Reflexes

- **Tinel Sign** (Figure 5J.1) (Sensitivity 26%-79%, Specificity 40%-100%)
  - First described in the literature by Jules Tinel[7] in 1915 who reported a "tingling sign" with percussion of peripheral nerves
  - Helps to isolate median nerve compression at the wrist
  - **Maneuver:**
    - Have the patient rest the affected hand on a table or held by the physician with the volar wrist pointing toward the ceiling. The physician will then gently tap on the median nerve at the level of the carpal tunnel with his/her index and long fingers. A positive response is recorded if the tapping sends an electrical shocklike sensation into the radial 3 digits
  - **Limitations of Maneuver:**
    - Too much force during percussion can cause paresthesias without CTS (false-positive results)

- **Phalen wrist Flexion Test** (Figure 5J.2) (Sensitivity 10%-88%, Specificity 47%-100%)
  - First described in the literature in 1951 by Phalen[9]
  - Helps to isolate median nerve compression at the wrist

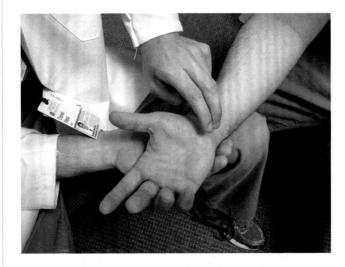

Figure 5J.1. Tinel sign at the carpal tunnel.

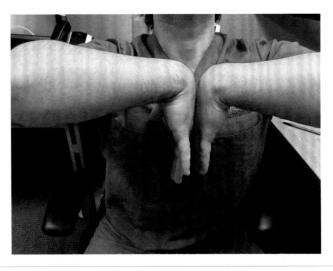

Figure 5J.2. Phalen wrist flexion sign.

- **Maneuver**:
  - Place patient's elbows on the examination table and allow wrists to terminally flex, and the dorsum of each hand presses against the other. This position is held for 60 seconds, and a positive finding is paresthesias in the median nerve distribution
- **Limitations of Maneuver:**
  - Patients with wrist stiffness (eg, from prior injury or prior surgery) often have a difficult time reaching significant enough wrist flexion
- **Durkan Compression Test** (Figure 5J.3) (Sensitivity 87%, Specificity 90%)
  - First described in the literature by Durkan in 1992.[1]
  - Helps to isolate median nerve compression at the wrist
  - **Maneuver:**
    - Direct compression of the median nerve at the carpal tunnel with the examiner's thumb for 30 seconds with the wrist in a neutral position. Paresthesias should resolve when the pressure is released. Sensitivity and specificity increase even higher with a calibrated compression device (13-14 psi)
  - **Limitations of Maneuver:**
    - If pressure is placed too proximal or distal, the findings will be falsely negative

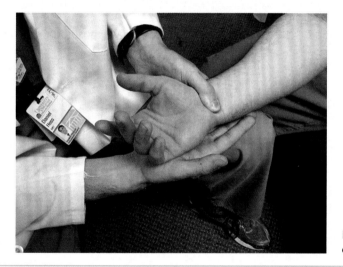

Figure 5J.3. Durkan wrist compression test.

IMAGING

Plain Radiographs

- Standard wrist films are typically obtained on the initial visit and can rule out any underlying bony pathology, although it has been reported to be very low yield

Computed Tomography

- Not typically obtained

Magnetic Resonance Imaging

- In general: static imaging, typically highly sensitive for pathology but may have incidental findings, and important to correlate clinically
- Can show intratunnel space-occupying lesions that can cause compression

- Can compare findings of the cross-sectional area of the median nerve and the space available for the nerve in the carpal tunnel and compare those values to established norms
- Not routinely needed

Ultrasonography

- In general: cost-effective, easily accessible, and can be performed dynamically and compared with the contralateral side. It is, however, highly operator-dependent
- Sensitivity of 89% and specificity of 90%
- Can show intratunnel space-occupying lesions that can cause compression although less accurate than MRI
- Can compare findings of the cross-sectional area of the median nerve and the space available for the nerve in the carpal tunnel and compare those values to established norms although less accurate than MRI
- Not routinely ordered currently but growing support in the literature

Electromyography

- Controversial in the literature whether it should be routinely performed. If physical examination and history suggest CTS, electrodiagnostic tests do not routinely change management[3]
- Sensitivity of 89% and specificity of 80%
- Distal motor latency >4.5 ms and distal sensory latency >3.5 ms are diagnostic for compression of the median nerve
- In severe and chronic cases, the EMG will show signs of denervation, such as fibrillation potentials, positive sharp waves, and fasciculations of the abductor pollicis brevis muscle

Classic Surgical Findings

- The classic surgical finding for CTS:
  - In idiopathic cases, edematous and hypertrophic fibrous tissue encase the transverse carpal ligament with minimal findings of inflammation

REFERENCES

1. Durkan JA. A new diagnostic test for carpal tunnel syndrome. *J Bone Joint Surg Am*. 1991;73(4): 535-538.
2. Cranford CS, Ho JY, Kalainov DM, Hartigan BJ. Carpal tunnel syndrome. *J Am Acad Orthop Surg*. 2007;15(9):537-548.
3. Graham B. The value added by electrodiagnostic testing in the diagnosis of carpal tunnel syndrome. *J Bone Joint Surg Am*. 2008;90(12):2587-2593. doi:10.2106/JBJS.G.01362.
4. Padua L, Coraci D, Erra C, et al. Carpal tunnel syndrome: clinical features, diagnosis, and management. *Lancet Neurol*. 2016;15(12):1273-1284. doi:10.1016/S1474-4422(16)30231-9.
5. Palumbo CF, Szabo RM. Examination of patients for carpal tunnel syndrome sensibility, provocative, and motor testing. *Hand Clin*. 2002;18(2):269-277, vi.
6. Stevens JC, Beard CM, O'Fallon WM, Kurland LT. Conditions associated with carpal tunnel syndrome. *Mayo Clin Proc*. 1992;67(6):541-548.
7. Tinel J. "Tingling" signs with peripheral nerve injuries. 1915. *J Hand Surg Br*. 2005;30(1):87-89. doi:10.1016/j.jhsb.2004.10.007.
8. Wipperman J, Goerl K. Carpal tunnel syndrome: diagnosis and management. *Am Fam Physician*. 2016;94(12):993-999.
9. Phalen GS. Spontaneous compression of the median nerve at the wrist. *J Am Med Assoc*. 1951;145(15):1128-1133.

SECTION K
Hand Infections

Jeffrey D. Boatright

HISTORY

- Wide range of conditions ranging from mild local superficial soft tissue involvement to potentially rapidly life-threatening systemic infection
- Presentation and physical examination varies widely depending on the anatomic region of hand, virulence of causative organism, and a variety of host factors
- Important to elucidate timing of onset, history of penetrating trauma, rapidity of progression, immunocompromised conditions, and tetanus and vaccination status
- Important to inquire about signs of systemic illness such as fever, lymphadenopathy, and constitutional symptoms
- Serologic laboratory findings should be used to augment diagnosis judiciously
  - WBC and CRP normal in up to 75% of cases; ESR normal in approximately 50%
- Most common causative organisms are *Staphylococcus aureus* (up to 60% of all hand infections) and β-hemolytic streptococcus
- Certain mechanisms and infections are associated with a particular microbe
  - Fight bite—α-hemolytic streptococcus (*Streptococcus viridans*), *S. aureus*, and *Eikenella corrodens* are common
  - Cat bite—often polymicrobial, 70% to 80% contain *Pasteurella* sp
  - Dog bite—often polymicrobial, 50% contain *Pasteurella* sp
  - Dental workers—herpetic whitlow (Figure 5K.1)
  - Diabetic infections—often polymicrobial and more aggressive, consider anaerobe involvement, chronic fungal infections
  - Intravenous drug users—often polymicrobial, consider anaerobe involvement
  - Necrotizing fasciitis—Group A streptococcus

PHYSICAL EXAMINATION

- Physical examination is highly variable depending on the anatomic location and type of infection
- Systematic inspection of the entire hand and wrist is imperative. Observe for classic signs of infection: swelling, erythema, areas of warmth, fluctuance, open wounds, signs of penetrating trauma, drainage, pain, decreased joint range of motion
  - Observe for proximal streaking or lymphangitis
  - Areas of fluctuance or erythema demarcation should be outlined with a marker to observe for interval progression and recession over time
- Hand cellulitis
  - Diffuse swelling, erythema, and warmth often along the dorsum of the hand and extensor tendons
  - Early cellulitis will have no discrete abscesses or regions of fluctuance
    - This can develop over time

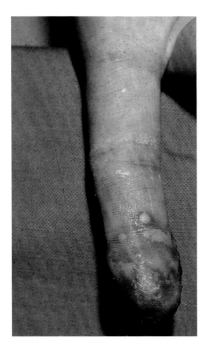

Figure 5K.1. Clinical appearance of herpetic whitlow. Note the clear vesicles some of which have begun to coalesce. (From Dr. Barankin Dermatology Collection.)

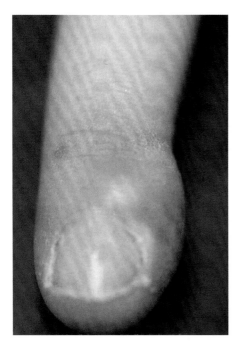

Figure 5K.2. Clinical appearance of an acute paronychial infection. (From Salimpour RR, Salimpour P, Salimpour P, Lippincott Williams & Wilkins. *Photographic Atlas of Pediatric Disorders and Diagnosis*. Philadelphia: Wolters Kluwer Health/Lippincott Williams & Wilkins; 2014.)

- Must be treated aggressively with antibiotics, especially in diabetics or immunocompromised
- Close observation required
- Paronychia (Figure 5K.2)
  - Swelling, erythema, warmth, fluctuance along nail fold
  - Common in nail-biters
  - Observe for extension under the nail plate in volar tracking into the pulp
  - Can typically be treated with warm soaks, +/− local bedside decompression and irrigation, and PO antibiotics

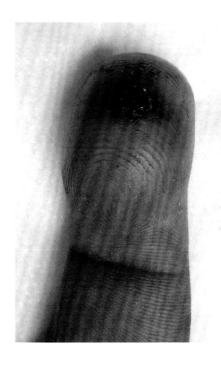

Figure 5K.3. Clinical appearance of an acute felon. (From Sherman SC. *Atlas of Clinical Emergency Medicine*. Wolters Kluwer Health; 2016.)

- Felon (Figure 5K.3)
  - Acute rapidly developing swelling, erythema, and often severe throbbing pain in the distal pulp of a digit
  - Typically will not cross the DIP flexion crease
  - Often associated with penetrating trauma
  - Can progress to tip necrosis, extension into the flexor tendon sheath or DIP joint septic arthritis, or osteomyelitis
- Clenched fist injury/fight bite infection (Figure 5K.4)
  - Open laceration over the dorsum of the MCP joint typically involving the long or ring fingers
    - Any laceration with signs of infection overlying the dorsum of the MCP joint should be considered a fight bite unless proven otherwise
  - Erythema, swelling, pain, frequently wound drainage, severe pain with active and passive MCP ROM
  - Must examine for extensor tendon injury, which is often retracted proximally relative to the laceration, given the change in position of the tendon in flexion (while making a fist) versus extension (while being examined) (Figure 5K.5)
- Acute pyogenic flexor tenosynovitis (FTS)
  - Presents with 4 classic Kanavel signs
    - Fusiform swelling of the digit, tenderness along the course of the flexor tendon sheath, severe pain with passive extension of the finger, and a semiflexed resting posture of the digit
    - No formal studies investigating the sensitivity of specificity or combined predicative probability of the 4 Kanavel signs
    - Pang et al investigated the presence of each Kanavel sign in 75 cases of known FTS
      - Fusiform swelling (97%), pain with passive extension (72%), semiflexed posture (69%), tenderness along the flexor sheath (64%)
  - Must examine proximally in the palm for potential development of a "horseshoe abscess," especially if the thumb or small finger is involved (Figure 5K.6)
    - Develops due to communication between the small finger flexor tendon sheath and the ulnar bursa, across the palm through a potential space between the pronator quadratus and FDP common sheath (space of Parona), to the radial bursa and into the thumb flexor tendon sheath

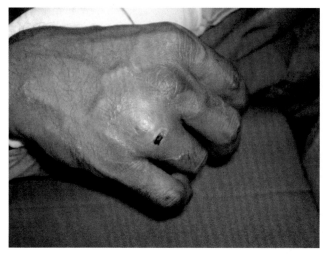

Figure 5K.4. Human bite injury after a fight with breach of the joint capsule (arrow). A. Pre-op appearance. (From Thorne C, Grabb WC, Beasley RW, et al. *Grabb and Smith's Plastic Surgery*. Wolters Kluwer; 2013.)

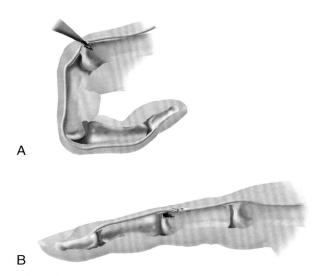

Figure 5K.5. Illustration demonstrating that the potential injury to the extensor tendon and metacarpal head does not align with the skin laceration during examination (finger extension) due to the relative changes in position of these structures compared with the moment of injury (finger flexion).

- Deep space hand infections
  - Presents after a history of penetrating trauma with severe focal palmar pain over the involved deep space with associated diffuse swelling, which is more pronounced dorsally (due to less adherent connective tissue dorsally)
  - Affected fingers may be held in an adducted position
- Septic arthritis
  - Usually in the setting of penetrating trauma
  - Painful passive and active range of motion of the affected joint
  - Fluctuance or fullness about the joint
  - Chronic PIP and DIP septic arthritis may cause boutonniere and mallet finger, respectively, due to the preferential destruction of the dorsal extensor structures

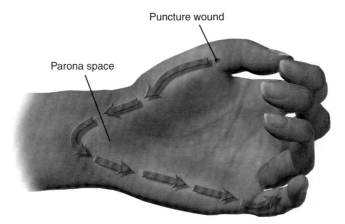

Figure 5K.6. Illustration demonstrating how a communication between the thumb flexor tendon sheath, radial bursa, Parona space, ulnar bursa, and small finger flexor tendon sheath can result in the development of a horseshoe abscess. (From Wiesel SW, ed. *Operative Techniques in Orthopaedic Surgery - 4 Volumes.* Wolters Kluwer Health/Lippincott Williams & Wilkins; 2011.)

- Osteomyelitis
  - Highly variable presentation and examination depending on chronicity, host factors, organism, and bone affected
  - Often can appear as a local skin and soft tissue infection, and failure for this to resolve with appropriate soft tissue infection treatment should raise suspicion for underlying osteomyelitis
- Necrotizing fasciitis
  - Rapidly progressive limb and life-threatening condition
  - Early infection may appear similar to cellulitis or other soft tissue infection
    - Often rapidly progressive (sometimes over a period of hours)
  - Subcutaneous crepitus, desquamation, formation of bullae, hypoesthetic skin, frank skin necrosis, dissection along fascial planes, venous or arterial thrombosis, and absence of frank purulence but rather thin gray watery exudate ("dishwater pus") are classic but variable findings
  - Pain to palpation or an orange peel appearance (peau d'orange) outside the region of cellulitic erythema should raise suspicion
  - Probing an open wound, if present, will typically reveal easy blunt dissection along fascial planes
  - Often have signs of systemic infection or sepsis, typically with markedly elevated WBC and inflammatory markers
    - Electrolyte derangements are common

IMAGING

- Not routinely indicated in the diagnosis of hand infections
- Ultrasonography may help elucidate the extent of a deep soft tissue infection
- Radiographs are needed if osteomyelitis is suspected (Figure 5K.7)
  - Also helpful in fight bite injuries and other penetrating trauma to rule out retained foreign body
- MRI is useful in distinguishing between severe cellulitis and deep space abscess
  - Surgical treatment should not be delayed for advanced imaging studies such as MRI if there is clinical suspicion for necrotizing fasciitis

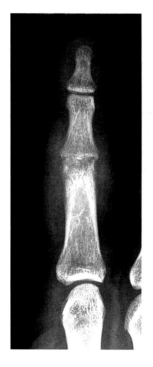

Figure 5K.7. This finger radiograph demonstrates PIP joint space narrowing, periarticular erosions, trabecular destruction, and soft tissue swelling consistent with proximal phalanx osteomyelitis likely secondary to a chronic PIP septic arthritis. (From Greenspan A, Gershwin ME. *Imaging in Rheumatology: A Clinical Approach*. Wolters Kluwer Health; 2018.)

REFERENCES

1. Stevanovic MV, Sharpe F. Acute infections. In: Wolfe SW, Pederson WC, Hotchkiss RN, Kozin SH, eds. *Green's Operative Hand Surgery*. 6th ed. Philadelphia, PA: Elsevier Churchill Livingstone; 2011:41-84.
2. Osterman M, Draeger R, Stern P. Acute hand infections. *J Hand Surg Am*. 2014;39:1628-1635.
3. Kanavel AB. The symptoms, signs, and diagnosis of tenosynovitis and fascial-space abscesses. In: *Infections of the Hand*. 1st ed. Philadelphia, PA: Lea & Febiger; 1912:201-226.
4. Pang HN, Teoh LC, Yam AK, Lee JY, Puhaindran ME, Tan AB. Factors affecting the prognosis of pyogenic flexor tenosynovitis. *J Bone Joint Surg Am*. 2007;89:1742-1748.

SECTION

The Foot and Ankle

Section Editor
M. Truitt Cooper

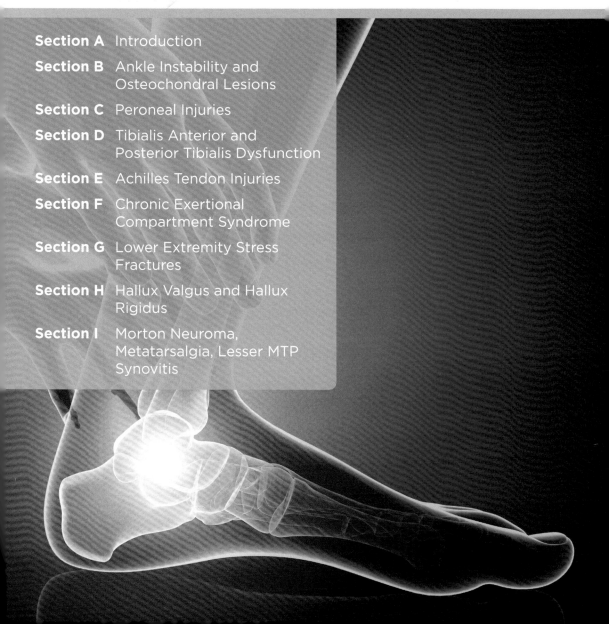

QUICK REFERENCE FLOW CHARTS

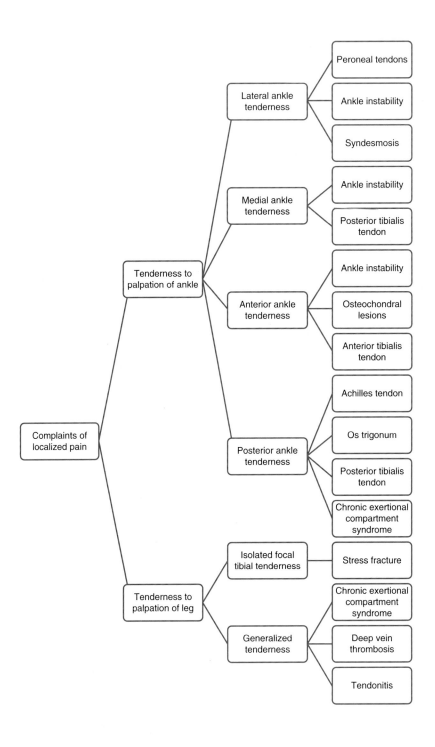

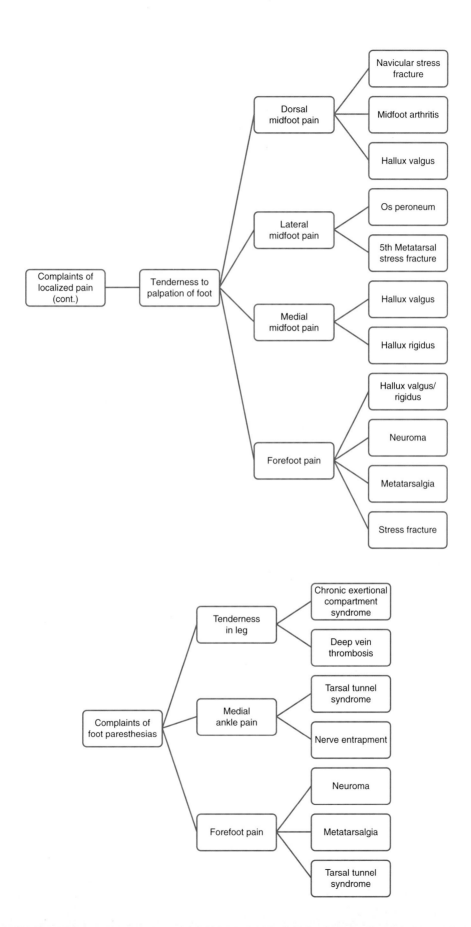

SECTION A
Introduction

Victor Anciano

HISTORY

It is important to consider the following parameters when a patient presents to the clinic with a foot or ankle complaint:

- Patient age
  - Younger patients are more likely to have an acute ligament tear
  - Older patients are more likely to have osteoarthritis and/or chronic tendinopathies
  - Younger patients commonly develop stress fractures of the lower extremities. In this age group, it is important to evaluate nutritional habits and, in female athletes, inquire about menstrual period. Special attention should be paid in sports where weight loss or weight goals are encouraged. Additionally, it is critical to evaluate changes in training patterns
  - Elderly or sedentary patients may develop stress fractures without significant activity
- Chronicity of symptoms
  - Acute injuries may involve ligament tears, fractures, and dislocations
  - Chronic injuries may represent untreated or unrecognized ligament injures (+/− recurrence), osteoarthritis, instability, or sequelae of deformity
  - Particularly in the ankle, degenerative joint disease is commonly associated with a history of trauma (up to 80%)
- Mechanism of injury (if any)
  - Noncontact injuries with immediate swelling may represent acute ligament rupture or fracture
  - Pivoting/twisting injuries of the ankle are commonly associated with high and low ankle sprains. History of sprains is a risk factor for chronic ankle instability
  - Rapid, sudden, or forced dorsiflexion of the foot is associated with Achilles tendon rupture or peroneal subluxation/dislocation. The position of the foot (inversion/eversion) at the time of the injury will cause strain on some tendons more than others
  - Ankle fractures caused by pronation and external rotation have been associated with high ankle sprains/syndesmosis injuries
  - History of trauma and or lacerations should raise suspicion for tendon tears
- Associated swelling (effusion)
  - The following conditions can be associated with acute or subacute swelling:
    – Lateral ankle instability
    – Osteochondral lesions
    – Achilles tendon rupture
    – Peroneal tendon tears/dislocations
    – Tibialis anterior tears
    – Chronic exertional compartment syndrome
- Mechanical symptoms (snapping)
  - Commonly associated with peroneal tendon subluxation/dislocation. Patient complain of feeling their tendons sliding anterior to the lateral malleolus
  - Patients with Achilles tendon rupture are likely to be disabled immediately after the injury. Patients will complain of inability to plantar flex the foot. Some will report a sensation as if they are falling forward

- History of ankle injury
  - One must be concerned about reinjury or instability from chronic tendinopathy
- History of ankle surgery
  - One must critically analyze the prior surgery to determine if there may have been any technical errors. Obtain prior operative reports, images; patient reports are often incomplete or inaccurate
- Prior treatment
- Current medications

PHYSICAL EXAMINATION

Observation

- Observe the patients' posture, how they get onto the examination table and how they describe their pain
- Observation of the patient's gait and foot position is important in evaluating risk factors and injuries. Always compare observations with the unaffected side
- Hip and knee alignment should be noted, as differences can lead to discovery of leg length discrepancies, genu varus/valgus that are risk factors for certain overuse injuries
- Evaluating the foot arches is an important aspect of the physical examination. Arches are evaluated both in weight-bearing and non–weight-bearing stances (Figure 6A.1)
  - The medial arch has usually about 1 cm of height but may be variable and thus comparison with the contralateral side is crucial
  - High arch (pes cavus) can be seen in congenital or neurologic cases
  - A low arch (pes planus) can be flexible or rigid. Flexible pes planus may appear as normal arches when non–weight-bearing, only to show collapse when weight-bearing
  - A convex arch (rocker bottom) can be seen in diabetic patients with Charcot neuropathic arthropathy
- Hindfoot alignment: The patient is examined from behind
  - The normal alignment of the hindfoot has 5° to 10° of valgus
  - Normally, 1 or 2 lateral toes are visible from the back. "Too many toes" sign can be seen in pes planus patients (Figure 6A.2)
  - Peek-a-boo sign may be seen in patients with cavovarus deformity (Figure 6A.3)
- Evaluation of gait pattern and standing attitude of the entire lower limb as it relates to the knee
  - Antalgic gait: Patients may walk with limp on the affected extremity. The stance (weight-bearing phase) is shorter on the affected extremity in antalgic gaits
  - Weak dorsiflexors gait: Patients who have weak dorsiflexors may have a "slap foot." Asking the patient to heel walk is a good evaluation of dorsiflexors strength
    - Slap gait: When the heel makes contact with the floor, the weak dorsiflexors cannot support the midfoot/forefoot. This leads to the foot slapping the floor as it contacts it
    - Steppage gait: Patients are unable to clear the floor during the swing phase due to inability to dorsiflex the foot. To compensate for this, patients will flex their hips and knees on the affected side. This is commonly seen in Charcot-Marie-Tooth patients
  - Toe-walking: This is a good test to evaluate the strength of the triceps surae complex
  - Lateral/medial foot walking: This is a good test for inversion and eversion strength, respectively. These tests may be difficult to perform by the patient and are not routinely performed
- Shoe wear: It is always important to evaluate the sole of the shoe when evaluating a patient for foot and ankle problems
  - Most runners wear down outer corner of the heel and the central region (Figure 6A.4)
  - Overpronators will show medial wearing vs oversupinators will show lateral wearing

Medial view   Posterior view

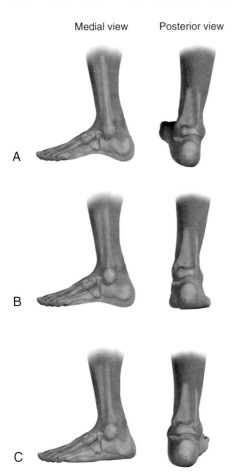

A

B

C

Figure 6A.1. A, Cavus foot, with elevation of the medial longitudinal arch and a slight hindfoot varus. B, Normal arch. C, Pes planus, with loss of the medial longitudinal arch and hindfoot valgus. From the posterior view, the "too many toes" sign can be noted.

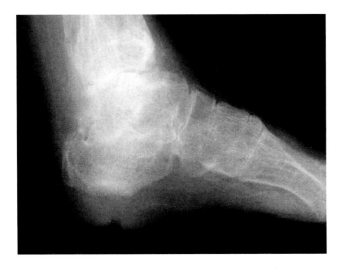

Figure 6A.2. Hindfoot valgus alignment as seen from the back. "Too many toes" signs can be seen laterally. (From Mosca VS. Calcaneal lengthening osteotomy for valgus deformity of the hindfoot. In: Tolo V, Skaggs D, eds. *Master Techniques in Orthopaedic Surgery: Pediatric Orthopaedics.* Philadelphia: Lippincott Williams & Wilkins; 2008.)

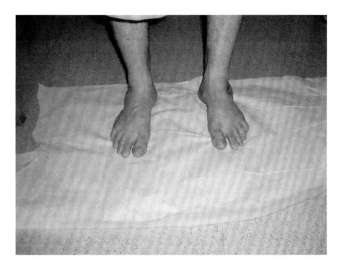

Figure 6A.3. Peek-a-boo sign indicating hindfoot varus: Notice the visibility of the medial aspect of the calcaneus, which is usually not visible. (From Fu F, ed. *Master Techniques in Orthopaedic Surgery: Sports Medicine*. Wolters Kluwer/Lippincott Williams & Wilkins; 2011.)

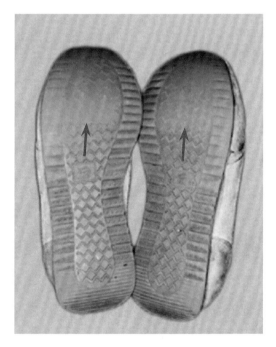

Figure 6A.4. Shoe wear on toes only. These shoes show typical wear patterns with loss of sole tread only on the toe regions (arrows). (From Staheli LT. *Fundamentals of Pediatric Orthopedics*. 5th ed. Philadelphia: Wolters Kluwer; 2016.)

Palpation

- Effusion
  - If an effusion is present, the patient will have difficulty with ankle dorsiflexion/plantar flexion
  - Check for swelling by comparing the contour of the lateral and medial malleolus to the contralateral ankle

- Tenderness
  - Medial tenderness may represent injury to medial-sided structures such as posterior tibial tendon, medial malleolus, deltoid ligament, and medial joint capsule
  - Lateral tenderness may represent injury to lateral structures such as peroneal tendons, lateral malleolus, lateral ankle ligaments, and lateral joint capsule
  - Focal tenderness over an area can be associated with both soft tissue and bony injury. Soft tissue injury tends to have a wider spread of tenderness vs bony injury, which can be more localized. For example, patients with tendinopathy may have tenderness along the length of the affected tendon. Patients with stress fractures have tenderness that is localized to the area of the fracture

KEY EXAMINATION MANEUVER

- **Homans Test** (Sensitivity: 10%-50%, Specificity: 40%-90%) (Figure 6A.5)
  - Commonly used as a screening examination for deep vein thrombosis. It is not discussed in any other section
  - Not considered a reliable test for deep vein thrombosis
  - First described by John Homans in 1944
  - **Maneuver:**
    - A positive Homan test is called **Homans sign**
    - The patient's knee should be flexed
    - The examiner then forcibly dorsiflexes the patient's ankle and observes for pain in the calf/popliteal region
  - **Limitations of Maneuver:**
    - Forceful dorsiflexion is needed, which can be uncomfortable in patients with other musculoskeletal injuries or recent surgery
    - Poor sensitivity and specificity

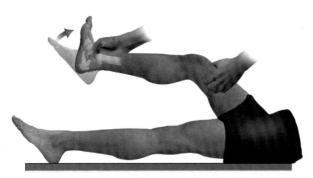

Figure 6A.5. Homans test. Eliciting pain with the knee flexed and forceful dorsiflexion is called a positive Homans sign.

Range of Motion (Figure 6A.6)

- Normal range of motion of the foot and ankle is typically in 3 planes
- Full dorsiflexion is close to 20°, whereas full plantar flexion has larger ROM (45°)

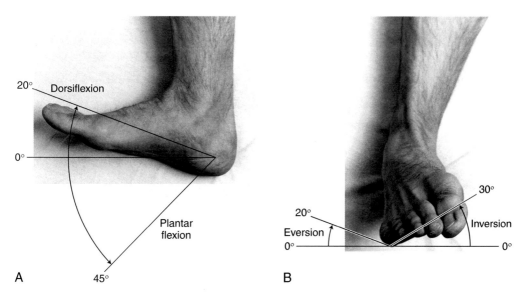

Figure 6A.6. Range of motion of the ankle and foot. A, Dorsiflexion and plantar flexion of the ankle. B, Eversion and inversion of the foot. (From Jones RM, Jones RM. *Patient Assessment in Pharmacy Practice*. Wolters Kluwer; 2016.)

KEY EXAMINATION MANEUVER

- **Silfverskiold Test** 🔵 (Sensitivity: n/a, Specificity: n/a) (Figure 6A.7)
  - First described in the literature by Nils Silfverskiold in 1924
  - This test allows the examiner to evaluate for Achilles tightness vs gastrocnemius tightness
  - A normal ankle has about 10° of dorsiflexion with the knee extended. Dorsiflexion should improve another 10° with the knee flexed
  - **Maneuver:**
    - The patient sits at the edge of the examination table allowing the knee to flex to 90°
    - The examiner then grabs the forefoot and dorsiflexes the ankle with the knee fully extended and with the knee flexed at 90°
    - The gastrocnemius muscle crosses the knee joint. Hence, with the knee in full extension (stretched gastrocnemius), the patient will have less ankle dorsiflexion than with the knee flexed (gastrocnemius relaxed)
    - Increased ankle dorsiflexion with the knee flexed is likely due to gastrocnemius tightness (gastrocnemius crosses both the ankle and knee joint; flexing the knee relaxes the gastrocnemius)
    - Equivalent ankle dorsiflexion with the knee extended and flexed is likely due to Achilles tightness but could also be due to an anterior osteophyte of the tibial plafond or another possible block to motion

- **Dorsiflexion-Eversion Test** (Sensitivity: n/a, Specificity: n/a) (Figure 6A.8)
  - First described in the literature by Kinoshita[3] in 2001
  - The test evaluates for tarsal tunnel syndrome
  - **Maneuver:**
    - The examiner passively maximally dorsiflexes and everts the ankle as well as passively maximally dorsiflexing the metatarsophalangeal (MTP) joints
    - The position is maintained between 10 to 30 seconds
    - The examination is positive if the patient complains of increasing pain, numbness, or aggravation of symptoms
    - It is helpful to compare with the unaffected side

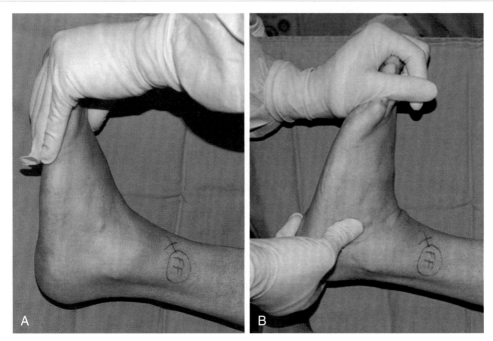

Figure 6A.7. Dorsiflexion in relation to knee flexion in Silfverskiold testing. A, Dorsiflexion to neutral with the knee extended. B, Dorsiflexion improves with the knee flexed. (From Wiesel SW, ed. *Operative Techniques in Orthopaedic Surgery - 4 Volumes*. Wolters Kluwer/Lippincott Williams & Wilkins; 2011.)

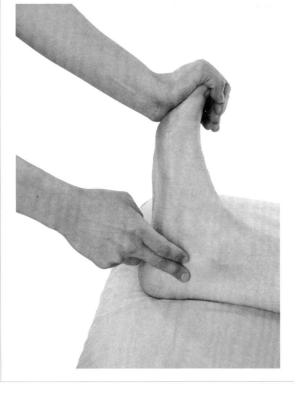

Figure   6A.8. Dorsiflexion-eversion test. Passively maximally dorsiflexing and everting the ankle while passively maximally dorsiflexing the MTP joints may aggravate symptoms in patients with tarsal tunnel syndrome. In this image, the examiner also demonstrates compression testing of the tarsal tunnel (Tinel sign). (From Bucci C. *Condition-Specific Massage Therapy*. Philadelphia: Wolters Kluwer Health/Lippincott Williams & Wilkins; 2012.)

- **Limitations of Maneuver:**
  - – Limited in patients with poor ankle or MTP ROM
  - – Limited in patients with MTP joint pathology

- Eversion and inversion of the foot is a more limited motion but ranges from 30° of inversion to 20° of eversion

- Abduction/adduction ranges from 20° of adduction to 10° of abduction

- Pronation and supination are common terms used in foot and ankle injuries to describe the position of the foot at the time of injury. Pronation is a combination of eversion, dorsiflexion, and abduction. Supination is a combination of inversion, plantar flexion, and adduction (Figure 6A.9)

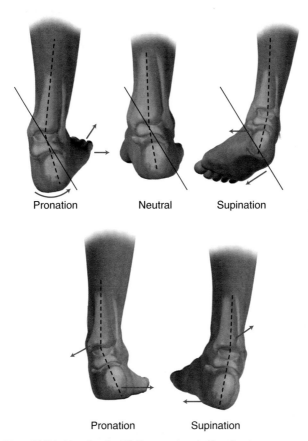

Pronation   Neutral   Supination

Pronation   Supination

Figure 6A.9. Top, With the foot off the ground, the foot moves on a fixed tibia, and the subtalar movement of pronation is produced by eversion, abduction, and dorsiflexion. Supination in the open chain is produced by inversion, adduction, and plantar flexion. Bottom, In a closed kinetic chain with the foot on the ground, much of the pronation and supination are produced by the weight of the body acting on the talus. In this weight-bearing position, the tibia moves on the talus to produce pronation and supination.

Muscular Strength

- Muscular strength is graded 1 to 5 as previously noted in other chapters
- Dorsiflexor weakness may represent an injury in the anterior compartment of the leg, ie, anterior tibialis tears
- Plantar flexor weakness may represent an injury to the posterior compartment of the leg, ie, Achilles tendon rupture and chronic exertional compartment syndrome
- Foot and toe loss of extension may represent a common peroneal nerve injury
- Bony injury may also cause muscular weakness secondary to pain
- Finally, it is important to always consider spine etiologies for muscular weakness when other signs and symptoms are present such as back pain and/or radicular pain

Sensation (Figure 6A.10)

- Can be viewed as dermatomes L2-S1 or as peripheral nerves listed below:
  - Saphenous
  - Sural
  - Superficial peroneal
  - Deep peroneal
  - Tibial

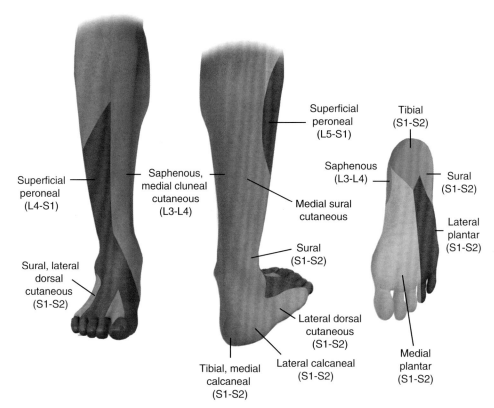

Figure 6A.10. Sensory distribution of the leg and foot.

KEY EXAMINATION MANEUVERS

Section A: Introduction

- Homans test
- Silfverskiold test
- Dorsiflexion-eversion test

Section B: Ankle Instability and Osteochondral Lesions

- Anterior drawer test
- Talar tilt test

Section C: Peroneal Injuries

- Peroneal subluxation test
- Peroneal compression test

Section D: Posterior Tibialis Dysfunction

- "Too many toes" sign
- Single limb heel rise
- First metatarsal rise test

Section E: Achilles Tendon Rupture

- Observation and palpation of achilles
- Thompson test
- Matles test
- Copeland test

Section F: Chronic Exertional Compartment Syndrome

- Compartment pressure monitoring

Section G: Lower Extremity Stress Fractures

- "N spot" sign

Section H: Hallux Valgus and Hallux Rigidus

- First TMT hypermobility
- Grind test

Section I: Morton Neuroma, Metatarsalgia, and Lesser MTP Synovitis

- Thumb-index finger squeeze
- Mulder click test
- Plantar percussion test
- Rocker concept
- Dorsal drawer test

IMAGING

Plain Radiographs (Figures 6A.11 and 6A.12)

- AP view of the foot and ankle
- Lateral view of the foot and ankle
- Mortise view of the ankle
- Medial/lateral oblique views of the foot
- Stress radiographs

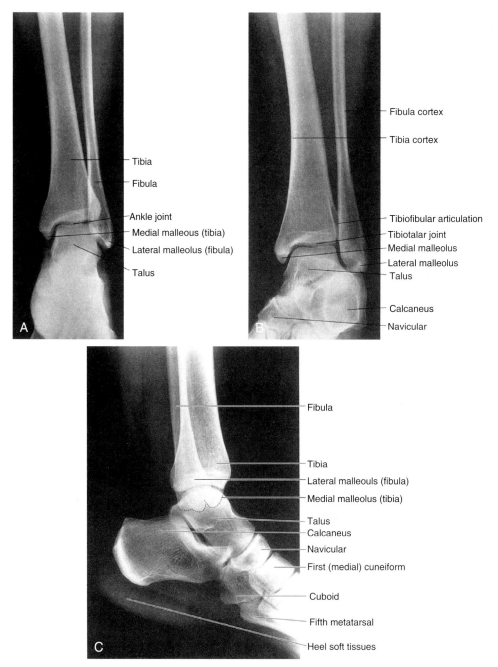

Figure 6A.11. Radiographic examination of the ankle. A, AP view. B, Mortise view. C, Lateral view. (From Erkonen WE, Smith WL. *Radiology 101: The Basics and Fundamentals of Imaging*. Philadelphia, PA: Wolters Kluwer/Lippincott Williams & Wilkins Health; 2010.)

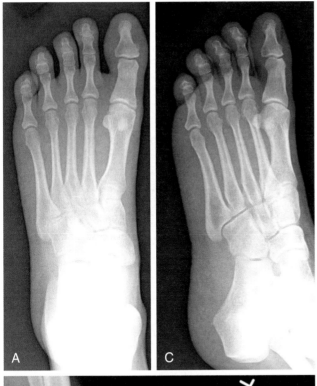

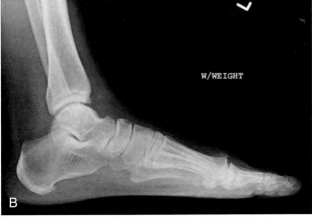

Figure 6A.12. Radiographic examination of the foot. A, DP view of the left foot. B, Lateral view of the left foot. C, Oblique view of the left foot.

Magnetic Resonance Imaging

Classic findings:

- Bone bruises, stress fractures, periosteal reactions
- Osteochondral lesions
- Tendon integrity
- Tendon sheath tears
- Ligament tears
- Neuromas

Computed Tomography

- Helpful in evaluating bony anatomy and ruling out subtle fractures

Ultrasonography

- Cost-effective imaging technique without radiation exposure
- Helpful in diagnosis of tendon tears, subluxations, and dislocations
- Can perform dynamic testing to evaluate tendon functionality

Ankle Arthroscopy (Figure 6A.13)

- Portals:
  - Anteromedial: a primary viewing portal to the anteromedial joint; tends to be established first during arthroscopy
    - Location is between tibialis anterior and medial malleolus
  - Anterolateral: a primary viewing portal to the anterolateral joint
    - Location is between peroneus tertius/superficial peroneal nerve (SPN) and lateral malleolus; important to trace SPN before incision to avoid injury
    - Risk: the portal with the highest risk of nerve injury to the intermediate dorsal cutaneous branch of the SPN
  - Anterocentral: used as an anterior viewing portal; not commonly used owing to the risk of injury to dorsalis pedis
    - Location is between extensor digitorum longus and extensor halluces longus
  - Posterolateral: used for access to os trigonum
    - Location is about 2 cm proximal to the tip of the lateral malleolus between the peroneal tendons and the Achilles tendon
  - Posteromedial: also used for access to os trigonum
    - Location is immediately medial to the Achilles tendon; avoid medializing the portal owing to the risk of injury to the posterior tibial artery and tibial nerve

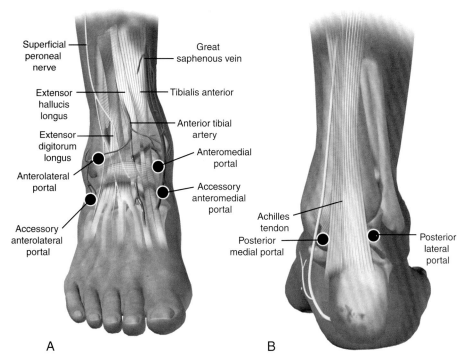

Figure 6A.13. A, Anterior anatomy pertinent to ankle arthroscopy. The anteromedial portal is placed immediately adjacent to the medial border of the tibialis anterior tendon at the level of the joint line. An accessory medial portal may be placed 1 cm or more from the anteromedial portal, as guided intraoperatively by the placement of a hypodermic needle. B, Posterior anatomy pertinent to ankle arthroscopy. The posterolateral portal is placed immediately adjacent to the lateral border of the Achilles tendon 1-2 cm distal to the level of the anterior portals.

REFERENCES

1. Barouk P, Barouk LS. Clinical diagnosis of gastrocnemius tightness. *Foot Ankle Clin.* 2014;19(4):659-667. doi:10.1016/j.fcl.2014.08.004.

2. Chao J. Deep vein thrombosis in foot and ankle surgery. *Orthop Clin North Am.* 2016;47(2):471-475. doi:10.1016/j.ocl.2015.10.001.

3. Kinoshita M, Okuda R, Morikawa J, Jotoku T, Abe M. The dorsiflexion-eversion test for diagnosis of tarsal tunnel syndrome. *J Bone Joint Surg Am.* 2001;83–A(12):1835-1839.

4. Maceira E, Monteagudo M. Subtalar anatomy and mechanics. *Foot Ankle Clin.* 2015;20(2):195-221. doi:10.1016/j.fcl.2015.02.001.

5. Bickley L. *Bates' Guide to Physical Examination and History-Taking.* 11th ed. Philadelphia: LWW; 2012.

6. Miller CM, Winter WG, Bucknell AL, Jonassen EA. Injuries to the midtarsal joint and lesser tarsal bones. *J Am Acad Orthop Surg.* 1998;6(4):249-258.

7. Mulligan ME. Ankle and foot trauma. *Semin Muscoskel Radiol.* 2000;4(2):241-253. doi:10.1055/s-2000-13015.

8. Pomeroy G, Wilton J, Anthony S. Entrapment neuropathy about the foot and ankle: an update. *J Am Acad Orthop Surg.* 2015;23(1):58-66. doi:10.5435/JAAOS-23-01-58.

9. Ray RG. Arthroscopic anatomy of the ankle joint. *Clin Podiatr Med Surg.* 2016;33(4):467-480. doi:10.1016/j.cpm.2016.06.001.

SECTION B
Ankle Instability and Osteochondral Lesions

Victor Anciano

HISTORY

- Patients with ankle instability tend to have a history of recurrent ankle sprains
- The anterior talofibular ligament (ATFL) is the weakest of all lateral ligaments and tends to be the most commonly injured in patients with ankle instability
- Lateral ankle instability is much more common than medial instability (85% of cases); it is associated with excessive inversion and internal rotation of the hindfoot when the leg is in external rotation
- Instability can be functional vs mechanical. Functional instability is associated with poor neuromuscular control and lack of proprioception. Mechanical instability can be identified on physical examination with true instability of the joint
- Osteochondral injuries to the talus and/or distal tibia can be associated with chronic instability. Often, patients with osteochondral lesions will report a sensation of instability, or that the ankle "gives out," even without mechanical instability

PHYSICAL EXAMINATION

OBSERVATION

- Evaluate for hindfoot varus misalignment and for midfoot cavus (high arch). These are risk factors for chronic ankle instability
- Mild swelling and some ecchymosis may be seen on the lateral aspect of the ankle

Palpation

- Chronic ankle instability may present with focal tenderness on the ATFL
- Additionally, they may demonstrate pain from synovitis, most commonly in the anterolateral ankle joint line
- Peroneal tendons should be palpated, and there is a high correlation with chronic ankle instability and peroneal pathology

Range of Motion

- Evaluate ROM of midtarsal and subtalar joints as well as ankle

Muscular Strength

- Evaluate strength of peroneal musculature with resisted eversion. Peroneal musculature has been found to be weak in cases of chronic ankle instability

Sensation

- Proprioception may be abnormal in chronic ankle instability. Some patients will have a positive Romberg maneuver

- **Anterior Drawer Test** 🎦 (Sensitivity: 0.71, Specificity: 0.33) (Figures 6B.1 and 6B.2)
  - First described by Landeros and colleagues
  - **Maneuver:**
    - The patient sits with the foot hanging and the hindfoot in a neutral position
    - The examiner stabilizes the distal leg with one hand and the hindfoot with the other hand
    - The patient's foot is placed in 10° to 15° of plantar flexion
    - The examiner then applies an anteriorly directed force to the rear of the foot assessing the amount of translation of the talus
    - New studies suggest that anterolateral drawer test may result in increased displacement
    - To perform the anterolateral drawer test, the patient is placed in the same position
    - The examiner places one hand on the distal tibia, making sure to palpate between lateral surface of talus and anterior aspect of fibula. The examiner uses the other hand to provide anterior force on the forefoot while internally rotating. More than 3 mm of displacement is considered positive

- **Talar Tilt Test** (Sensitivity: n/a, Specificity: n/a) (Figures 6B.2 and 6B.3)
  - No author is credited with discovery. It is not supported by literature as a diagnostic examination
  - **Maneuver:**
    - The examination is performed with the patient in a seated position with the knee bent and the foot in a neutral position
    - One hand is used to stabilize the distal tibia while the other hand applies an inversion force to the foot
    - The test is positive if the patient experiences pain or if the examiner senses laxity
    - It is very useful to perform this test under fluoroscopy to differentiate inversion through the subtalar joint versus true tibiotalar tilt

- **Limitations of Maneuver:**
  - Patients with acute lateral ankle sprains may have difficulty performing all physical examination maneuvers secondary to pain. Chronic ankle instability will likely demonstrate laxity with much more ease than an acute lateral ankle sprain

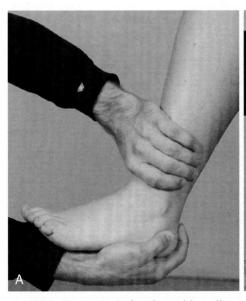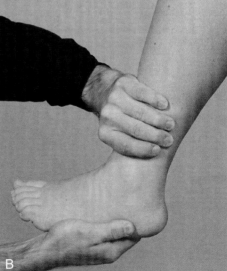

Figure 6B.1. Stress tests for the ankle collateral ligaments. A, Anterior drawer test. B, Talar tilt test. (From Anderson MK, Barnum M. *Foundations of Athletic Training: Prevention, Assessment, and Management.* Wolters Kluwer; 2017.)

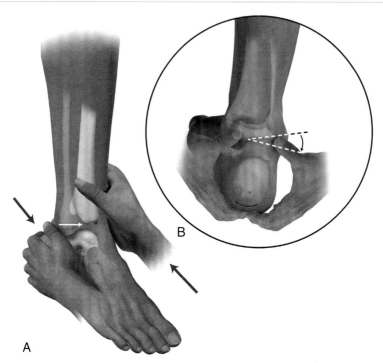

Figure 6B.2. Stress testing of the ankle. A, Positive anterior drawer sign (small arrow). The anterior drawer sign test is used to evaluate the intactness of the anterior talofibular ligament. B, Talar tilt test to evaluate the stability of the anterior talofibular and calcaneofibular ligaments. The ankle is unstable if the anterior talofibular and calcaneofibular ligaments are torn.

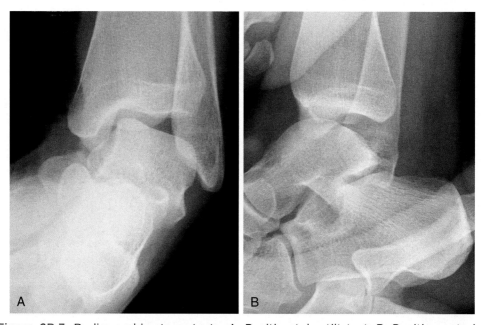

Figure 6B.3. Radiographic stress tests. A, Positive talar tilt test. B, Positive anterior drawer test. (From Easley ME, Wiesel SW. *Operative Techniques in Foot and Ankle Surgery*. Wolters Kluwer; 2017.)

IMAGING

Plain Radiographs

- Plain radiography of the ankle is helpful in ruling out other causes of ankle pain, such as acute fractures, stress fractures, osteochondral defects, or os subfibulare
  - It is important to look at the tibiotalar joint alignment as well
- AP and mortise views help in delineating the joint and evaluating for articular surface injury, syndesmosis pathology, or acute fractures
- Stress radiography:
  - Lateral radiographs may be used concomitantly with the anterior drawer maneuver to evaluate translation of the talus. 5 to 10 mm of translation or 3 mm difference compared with the contralateral ankle is considered abnormal (Figure 6B.3)
  - Talar tilt stress test can be done with weight-bearing films on an inversion stress platform. Alternatively, weights can be strapped to the ankle while the leg is on its lateral side on the table. Normal talar tilt is 5°. Abnormal values are considered >9° or twice the angle of the contralateral ankle

Computer Tomography

- CT has little role in evaluation of chronic instability. It is helpful in evaluating osteochondritis dissecans (OCD) lesions. However, MRI remains a better study for both OCD fragments and ligament evaluation. CT arthrogram can also be used for diagnosis of osteochondral lesions

Magnetic Resonance Imaging

- MRI is useful in ruling out other sources of ankle pain such as radiographically occult fractures, OCD lesions (Figure 6B.4), sinus tarsi injury, or tendon injuries
- Ligament injury may be visualized on MRI through ligament swelling, discontinuity, nonvisualization, or visualization of a wavy ligament

CLASSIC ARTHROSCOPIC FINDINGS

Chondral lesions may be seen during arthroscopy of the ankle that is performed for lateral ankle instability. Chondral lesions can be addressed at this time. Management of these lesions is beyond the scope of this textbook (Figure 6B.5).

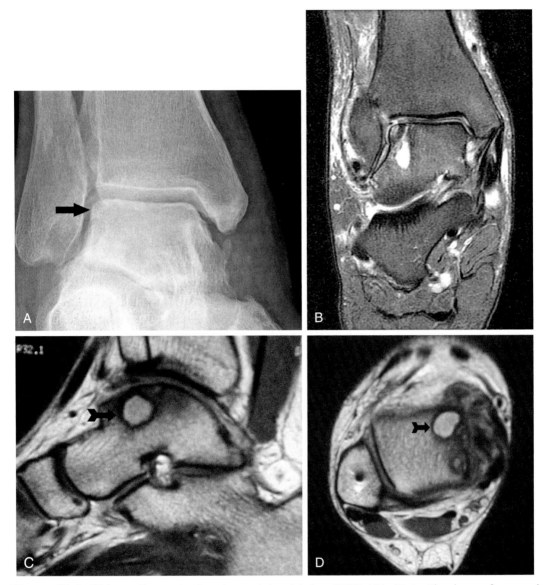

Figure 6B.4. Plain radiograph showing a lateral talus OCD (A). Note the loss of normal trabecular anatomy in the lateral talar dome with increased density in the adjacent subchondral bone (arrow). Corresponding T2-weighted MRI demonstrating the lesion with corresponding bone edema and cystic change (B). Sagittal (C) and axial (D) T1-weighted MRI of a large cystic lesion of the medial talar dome (arrow). (From Altchek D, DiGiovanni CW, Dines JS, Positano RG. *Foot and Ankle Sports Medicine.* 2013.)

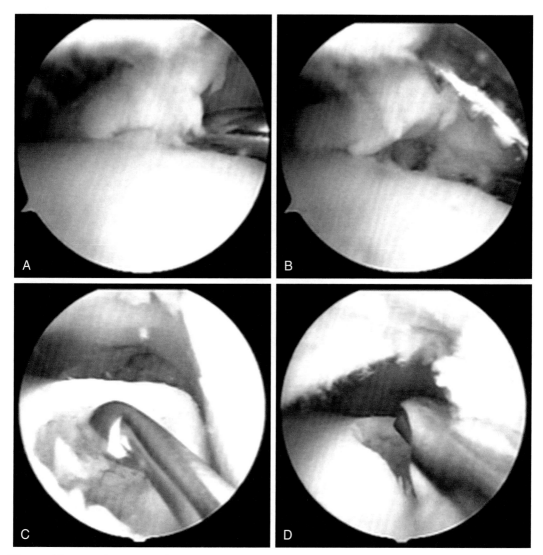

Figure 6B.5. Arthroscopic findings of an OCD lesion with a loose body. A and B, The loose body. C and D, Debridement of OCD lesion. (From Johnson D, Amendola NA, Barber F. *Operative Arthroscopy.* Philadelphia: Wolters Kluwer; 2015.)

REFERENCES

1. Al-Mohrej OA, Al-Kenani NS. Chronic ankle instability: current perspectives. *Avicenna J Med.* 2016;6(4):103-108. doi:10.4103/2231-0770.191446.
2. Croy T, Koppenhaver S, Saliba S, Hertel J. Anterior talocrural joint laxity: diagnostic accuracy of the anterior drawer test of the ankle. *J Orthop Sports Phys Ther.* 2013;43(12):911-919. doi:10.2519/jospt.2013.4679.
3. van Dijk CN, Lim LS, Bossuyt PM, Marti RK. Physical examination is sufficient for the diagnosis of sprained ankles. *J Bone Joint Surg Br.* 1996;78(6):958-962.
4. van Dijk CN, Mol BW, Lim LS, Marti RK, Bossuyt PM. Diagnosis of ligament rupture of the ankle joint. Physical examination, arthrography, stress radiography and sonography compared in 160 patients after inversion trauma. *Acta Orthop Scand.* 1996;67(6):566-570.
5. Ferran NA, Oliva F, Maffulli N. Ankle instability. *Sports Med Arthrosc Rev.* 2009;17(2):139-145. doi:10.1097/JSA.0b013e3181a3d790.
6. Maffulli N, Ferran NA. Management of acute and chronic ankle instability. *J Am Acad Orthop Surg.* 2008;16(10):608-615.

7. Miller AG, Myers SH, Parks BG, Guyton GP. Anterolateral drawer versus anterior drawer test for ankle instability: a biomechanical model. *Foot Ankle Int.* 2016;37(4):407-410. doi:10.1177/1071100715620854.

8. Phisitkul P, Chaichankul C, Sripongsai R, Prasitdamrong I, Tengtrakulcharoen P, Suarchawaratana S. Accuracy of anterolateral drawer test in lateral ankle instability: a cadaveric study. *Foot Ankle Int.* 2009;30(7):690-695. doi:10.3113/FAI.2009.0690.

9. Willems T, Witvrouw E, Verstuyft J, Vaes P, De Clercq D. Proprioception and muscle strength in subjects with a history of ankle sprains and chronic instability. *J Athl Train.* 2002;37(4):487-493.

SECTION C
Peroneal Injuries

Victor Anciano

HISTORY

- Both muscles of the lateral compartment are innervated by the SPN and receive their blood supply from the posterior peroneal artery
- There is a zone of hypovascularity in both tendons at the point where they wrap around the fibula. This is a common site for injury
- The superior peroneal retinaculum (SPR) maintains the tendons in the retrofibular groove
- Injury to the peroneal tendons is commonly found with lateral ankle instability
- Peroneal tendon tears can result from acute trauma or chronic overuse
- Damage to soft tissue or bony stabilizers can disrupt adequate function of the tendon. A grading system is in place to describe the etiology of the subluxation (Figure 6C.1)
- Peroneal subluxation/dislocation can occur from forced dorsiflexion with concomitant muscle firing
- Peroneal brevis tears may occur from repeated subluxation, as the tendon slides over the fibular ridge
- Peroneal longus tendon tears are less common but can occur at the distal fibula, at the peroneal tubercle or at an os peroneum. Os peroneum is an accessory bone on the lateral plantar aspect of the cuboid. It is actually a sesamoid bone within the peroneus longus tendon
- Painful Os peroneum syndrome (POPS) refers to acute or chronic injury of the os peroneum or the tendon around it
- Patients will usually present with lateral ankle pain and, usually, a history of trauma

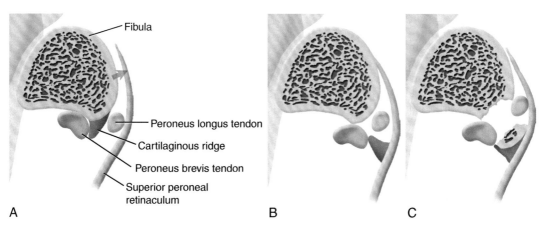

Figure 6C.1. Classification by Eckert and Davis of peroneal tendon subluxation/dislocation. A, Grade I: superior peroneal retinaculum (SPR) stripped off fibula; peroneus longus dislocated anteriorly. The arrow refers to the superior peroneal retinaculum being stripped off the fibula as described. B, Grade II: fibrous rim avulsed from posterolateral aspect of fibula along with SPR; peroneus longus dislocated anteriorly. C, Grade III: bony rim avulsion fracture attached to SPR with anterior dislocation of peroneus longus. (From Coughlin MJ, Mann RA, eds. *Surgery of the Foot and Ankle*. 7th ed. St. Louis, MO: Mosby; 1999:821; Modified from Eckert WR, Davis EAJ. Acute rupture of the peroneal retinaculum. *J Bone Joint Surg Am*. 1976;58A:670-672.)

PHYSICAL EXAMINATION

- **Inspection and Palpation with Active Firing of the Tendons**
  - Warmth, tenderness, and swelling may be palpated/elicited
  - In some instances, thickening of the tendon can be palpated
- **Strength Testing of the Peroneal Musculature** should be performed
  - **Maneuver:**
    - The patient should be seated with the leg hanging at the edge of the examination table
    - The patient is asked to perform 2 movements. (1) Ankle eversion and (2) plantar flexion of the first ray
    - The examiner provides gentle resistance to each movement
    - Pain with resistance may signal peroneal tendon injury
  - **Limitations of Maneuver:**
    - Isolating ankle movement may be difficult to the patient
    - Injury to surrounding structures may confuse the results from the examination
- **Peroneal Subluxation Test** (Sensitivity: n/a, Specificity: n/a)
  - Dynamic testing of peroneal function may result in subluxation
  - No author is credited with first description of examination
  - **Maneuver:**
    - The patient is asked to sit at the edge of the examination table with the knee flexed and leg hanging
    - The patient is then asked to actively plantar flex and dorsiflex the ankle with resisted eversion. The examiner may ask the patient to circumduct the ankle
    - A positive result will allow the examiner to feel or see the tendons sublux anterior to the lateral malleolus
    - Intrasheath subluxation may occur if the examiner can feel or see the tendons are noted to shift/translate relative to each other without subluxing anterior to the lateral malleolus
    - Examination may be performed with assistance of ultrasound imaging. The examiner uses one hand to provide resisted eversion while using an ultrasound probe directly over the tendons to visualize them (Figure 6C.2)
- **Peroneal Compression Test** (Sensitivity: n/a, Specificity: n/a)
  - First described by Sobel et al in 1994
  - The test can evaluate peroneus brevis tendonitis
  - **Maneuver:**
    - The patient is asked to allow the examiner to manipulate the foot passively
    - The patient sits with the affected foot hanging from chair or bed
    - The examiner uses one hand to evert and dorsiflex the patient's foot
    - The examiner uses the other hand to apply manual pressure against the fibular groove
    - The test is considered positive when the patient experiences pain

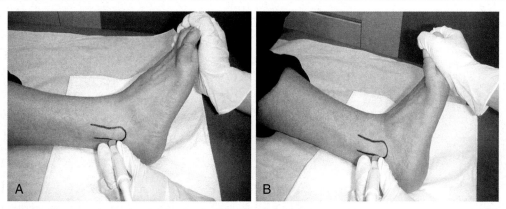

Figure 6C.2. Peroneal subluxation test. A, Neutral rest position: transducer placement for transverse view of peroneal tendons at the lateral malleolus (outlined in black) level. B, Stress maneuver: The transducer is held in the same position, and the ankle is dorsiflexed and everted. (From Sanders RC, Hall-Terracciano B. *Clinical Sonography: A Practical Guide*; Wolters Kluwer; 2016.)

IMAGING

Plain Radiographs

Weight-bearing radiographs should be obtained.

- Anteroposterior/internal rotation radiographs of the ankle:
  - A cortical avulsion fracture of the distal fibula may be observed, particularly in grade III SPR tears. This is referred to as the "fleck sign" or "rim fracture" (Figure 6C.3)
- Lateral radiographs of the foot:
  - These can show an avulsion fracture at the base of the fifth metatarsal (attachment of the plantar fascia) (Figure 6C.4)
- Oblique radiographs of the foot:
  - 20% of os peroneums are calcified and thus visible in plain radiographs. Acute fractures or diastasis of a bipartite os peroneum may be evaluated with this view (Figure 6C.5)
- Hindfoot alignment views: These are obtained with the patient standing on a platform. The beam is posterior to the patient and angled about 20° caudal
  - The midline of the calcaneal tuberosity is lateral to the middiaphyseal axis of the tibia in normal alignment. The normal alignment is 0° to 5° valgus on clinical examination (Figure 6C.6)
  - A varus hindfoot can predispose to peroneal tendonitis

Ultrasonography

It provides real-time assessment of peroneal function.

- It is a radiation-free and a very cost-effective tool for diagnosing peroneal subluxation; however, it is dependent on the experience of the operator (Figure 6C.2)
- Dynamic ultrasound studies offer accuracy of 94%, 100% sensitivity, 90% specificity, and a positive predictive value of 100% when diagnosing peroneal tendon subluxation

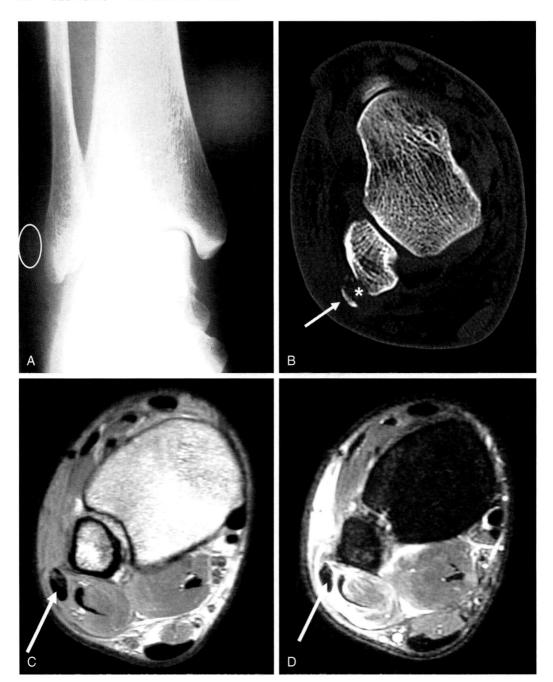

Figure 6C.3. A, AP radiograph of the ankle under a hot lamp shows a lateral rim fracture off the distal fibula (fleck sign, circle). B, Axial CT scan shows a grade III injury with an avulsion fracture of the lateral edge of the distal fibula (fleck sign, arrow) and dislocated peroneal tendon (asterisk). C and D, T1-and T2-weighted axial magnetic resonance images, respectively, show dislocated peroneal tendons (arrow) with abundant tenosynovitis. Note the shallow retrofibular groove and the torn SPR. (From Wiesel SW, ed. *Operative Techniques in Orthopaedic Surgery - 4 Volumes*. Wolters Kluwer; 2016.)

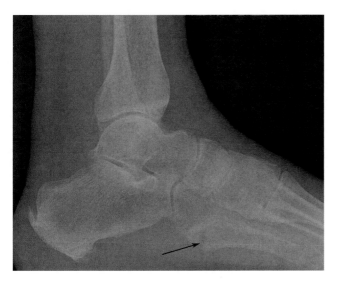

Figure 6C.4. Lateral radiograph of the ankle includes the base of the fifth metatarsal. There is an avulsion fracture at the fifth metatarsal base (arrow). (From Berquist TH, ed. *Imaging of the Foot and Ankle.* 3th ed. Philadelphia, PA: Wolters Kluwer/Lippincott Williams & Wilkins; 2011.)

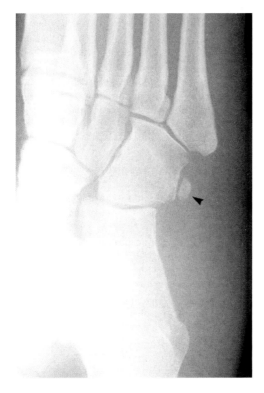

Figure 6C.5. Os peroneum (arrowhead): typical size and location adjacent to cuboid. (From Christman RA. *Foot and Ankle Radiology.* Wolters Kluwer; 2015.)

Computed Tomography

- Its role is very limited in peroneal tendon pathology
- It is helpful in evaluating bony injury and rule out other causes of lateral ankle pain
- It has been used to study the retromalleolar groove and its anatomic variants

Magnetic Resonance Imaging

- It provides the best imaging option to assess the integrity of the peroneal tendons
- It is helpful in evaluating key components of tendon stability such as the SPR and the tendon sheath (Figure 6C.3)
- It was shown to be 66% accurate with a 23% sensitivity and 100% specificity for peroneal tendon subluxation

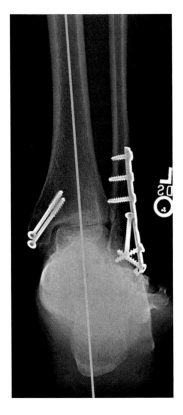

Figure 6C.6. Hindfoot alignment view of a 29-y-old patient after ORIF ankle fracture. A line is drawn from the center of the intramedullary canal through the center of the tibiotalar joint and extended distally. If there is no malalignment of the hindfoot, this line should pass through the most plantar portion of the calcaneus. This patient shows normal hindfoot alignment. (From Johnson D, Amendola NA, Barber F. *Operative Arthroscopy.* Philadelphia: Wolters Kluwer; 2015.)

REFERENCES

1. Bianchi S, Bortolotto C, Draghi F. Os peroneum imaging: normal appearance and pathological findings. *Insights Imaging.* 2017;8(1):59-68. doi:10.1007/s13244-016-0540-3.
2. Kumar Y, Alian A, Ahlawat S, Wukich DK, Chhabra A. Peroneal tendon pathology: pre- and post-operative high resolution US and MR imaging. *Eur J Radiol.* 2017;92:132-144. doi:10.1016/j.ejrad.2017.05.010.
3. Pesquer L, Guillo S, Poussange N, Pele E, Meyer P, Dallaudière B. Dynamic ultrasound of peroneal tendon instability. *Br J Radiol.* 2016;89(1063):20150958. doi:10.1259/bjr.20150958.
4. Roster B, Michelier P, Giza E. Peroneal tendon disorders. *Clin Sports Med.* 2015;34(4):625-641. doi:10.1016/j.csm.2015.06.003.
5. Sadamasu A, Yamaguchi S, Nakagawa R, et al. The recognition and incidence of peroneal tendon dislocation associated with a fracture of the talus. *Bone Joint J.* 2017;99–B(4):489-493. doi:10.1302/0301-620X.99B4.BJJ-2016-0641.R1.
6. Saragas NP, Ferrao PN, Mayet Z, Eshraghi H. Peroneal tendon dislocation/subluxation - case series and review of the literature. *Foot Ankle Surg.* 2016;22(2):125-130. doi:10.1016/j.fas.2015.06.002.

SECTION D
Tibialis Anterior and Posterior Tibialis Dysfunction

Michael M. Hadeed

RELEVANT ANATOMY

Tibialis Anterior

- Origin: lateral condyle of the tibia, proximal one-half to two-thirds of the tibial shaft, the anterior interosseous membrane
- Course: passes under the superior and inferior extensor retinacula; tendon can be palpated on the lateral aspect of the tibial crest proximal to the ankle joint
- Insertion: medial and plantar surfaces of the medial cuneiform and the base of the first metatarsal
- Innervation: deep peroneal nerve (L4, L5)
- Vascularity: supplied by the anterior tibial artery
- Action: it is the primary ankle dorsiflexor

Posterior Tibialis

- Origin: the posterior aspect of the tibia and fibula as well as the interosseous membrane
- Course: located in the deep posterior compartment of the leg, it is the most anterior tendon wrapping around the medial malleolus
- Insertion: broad insertion that includes 3 limbs with as many as 7 attachments
  - Anterior limb: inserts onto the navicular and medial cuneiform
  - Middle limb: inserts onto the middle and lateral cuneiforms, cuboid, and base of the second through the fourth metatarsal
  - Posterior limb: inserts on the sustentaculum tali anteriorly
- Innervation: tibial nerve (L4, L5)
- Vascularity: branches of the posterior tibial artery supply the tendon distally
  - There is a watershed area 2 to 6 cm proximal to the navicular insertion
- Action: the primary function is a dynamic stabilizer of the medial longitudinal arch
  - At heel strike, eccentric contraction slows the pronation of the foot
  - Concentric contraction inverts the hindfoot, which in turn allows locking of the transverse tarsal joints, creating a rigid lever arm for the toe-off phase of gait
  - Adducts and supinates the forefoot during stance phase of gait
  - Secondary plantar flexor of the ankle

HISTORY

Tibialis Anterior

- Can have acute or chronic rupture
  - Acute more common in young patients; presents with a "pop" due to strong eccentric contraction
    - Overall, these are extremely rare injuries
  - Chronic more common in those older than 65 years; attritional rupture; often presents with difficulty clearing the foot during the gait cycle
  - Often patients will describe prodromal pain that subsides after rupture

Posterior Tibialis

- Etiology of failure outside of traumatic mechanisms is unknown
- Early in the disease process, patients develop a loss of the medial longitudinal arch dynamic stabilization
- As the disease progresses, the loss of dynamic stabilization can lead to attritional failure of the static hindfoot stabilizers (spring ligaments, plantar fascia, plantar ligaments)
- Much of the foot deformity is caused by unopposed action of the peroneal tendons (particularly the peroneal brevis) (Figure 6D.1)

PHYSICAL EXAMINATION

Tibialis Anterior

Observation

- Can see swelling to the anterior ankle in acute cases
- Can see the toes extend during attempted dorsiflexion, as the patient tries to dorsiflex using the EHL and EDL muscles
- Gait would be altered to avoid hitting the toes
  - Steppage gait
    - Hip flexes more than normal
    - Foot slaps down after heel strike
  - Slap foot

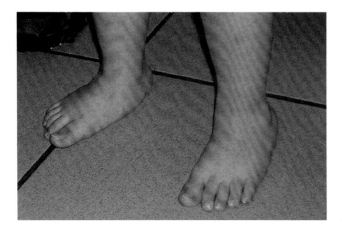

Figure 6D.1. Pes planus (flatfoot). (From Johnson D, Amendola NA, Barber F. *Operative Arthroscopy.* Philadelphia: Wolters Kluwer; 2015.)

Palpation

- May be able to palpate a mass as the anteromedial aspect of the ankle (tendon stump)
  - This is very commonly mistaken for a ganglion cyst or other soft tissue mass
- May lose the appropriate contour of the typical tibialis anterior tendon just proximal to the ankle
- May also feel crepitus in the area during ankle dorsiflexion and plantar flexion

Range of Motion

- May have limited active dorsiflexion of the ankle
- Should not impact passive motion

Strength

- Active dorsiflexion may be weak and demonstrate eversion
- Toe extensors (EHL and EDC) will be recruited to compensate

Posterior Tibialis

Observation

- Overall foot deformity
  - Pes planus–collapse of the medial longitudinal arch
  - Hindfoot valgus–flexible early in the disease process; may become rigid late or be rigid due to coalition (Figure 6D.2)
  - Forefoot varus/supination (Figure 6D.3)

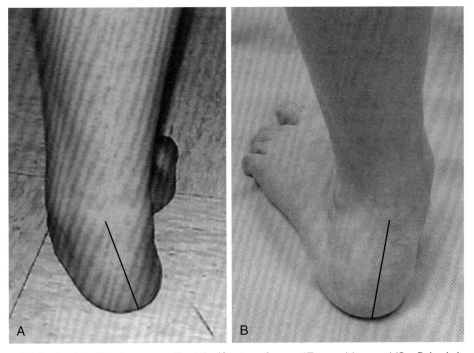

Figure 6D.2. A, Hindfoot varus. B, Hindfoot valgus. (From Mosca VS. *Principles and Management of Pediatric Foot and Ankle Deformities and Malformations.* Philadelphia: Wolters Kluwer; 2014.)

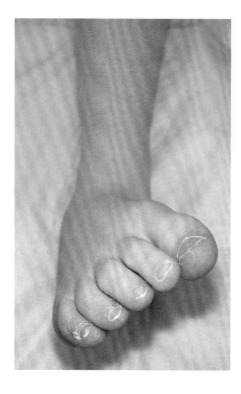

Figure 6D.3. Forefoot supination. (From Wiesel SW, ed. *Operative Techniques in Orthopaedic Surgery - 4 Volumes*. Wolters Kluwer; 2011.)

Range of Motion

● Important to determine if the foot deformities are correctable or if they are fixed (ie, hind-foot valgus)

Strength

● Place the foot in plantar flexion and inversion, apply an eversion force, and see if the patient can resist

KEY EXAMINATION MANEUVERS

● **"Too Many Toes" Sign** (Figure 6D.4)
  • First described by Kenneth A. Johnson in 1983
  • **Maneuver:**
    – Observe the patient's foot from behind the patient; there will be more toes than normally apparent on the lateral aspect of the foot

● **Single Limb Heel Rise** (Figure 6D.5A and 6D.5B)
  • First described by Kenneth A. Johnson in 1983
  • **Maneuver:**
    – The examiner asks the patient to stand on both feet
    – The examiner then asks the patient to stand alone on the affected foot and rise off on the toes and forefoot
    – "The test is positive if, during an attempt to rise onto the ball of the affected foot with the contralateral foot raised, the hindfoot does not assume a stable varus position and the heel is raised even slightly from the ground only with difficulty"
  • **Limitations of Maneuver**:
    – It is a complex maneuver that requires several other bone and muscle groups to be working appropriately
    – Unable to perform in more advanced stages of disease
    – Important to consider that this test is not specific, as there are many other reasons patients cannot perform (arthritis, general weakness, obesity)

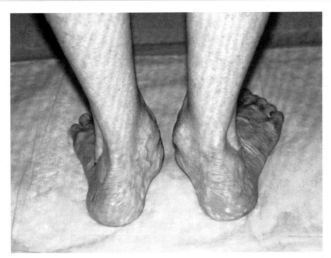

Figure 6D.4. Severe hindfoot valgus is observed in both feet. Abduction of the forefoot produces the "too many toes" sign. (From Kitaoka HB, ed. *The Foot and Ankle: Includes Fully Searchable Text and Image Bank Online*. 3rd ed. Philadelphia, PA: Wolters Kluwer Health/Lippincott Williams & Wilkins; 2013.)

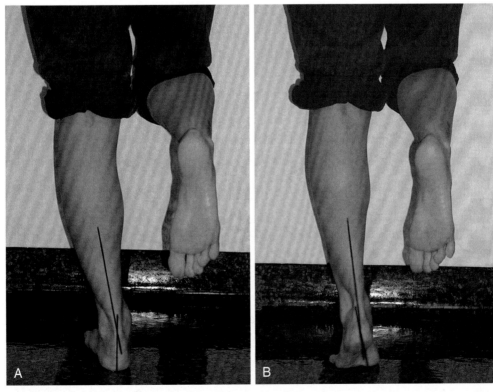

Figure 6D.5. A, Normal subject is being tested for strength of the posterior tibial tendon and muscle with a single heel rise test. The subject is standing with the left foot plantigrade, while the right foot is raised off the floor by flexing the knee. Notice the valgus position of the heel. B, The normal subject is easily able to raise the left heel off the floor. Notice the left heel position is in varus. (From Kitaoka HB, ed. *The Foot and Ankle: Includes Fully Searchable Text and Image Bank Online*. 3rd ed. Philadelphia, PA: Wolters Kluwer Health/Lippincott Williams & Wilkins; 2013.)

- **First Metatarsal Rise Test** (Sensitivity: 100%, Specificity: not reported)
  - First described by Beat Hintermann and Andre Gachter in 1996
  - **Maneuver:**
    - The examiner asks the patient to stand
    - The patient should be instructed to weight bear equally through both feet
    - The examiner should hold the heel and cause it to go into varus (toward the midline)
    - In patients with PT dysfunction, the first metatarsal will rise off the ground
    - In patients without PT dysfunction, the first metatarsal will stay on the ground
  - **Limitations of Maneuver:**
    - Questionable specificity, as many other foot and lower extremity conditions could potentially affect this test

IMAGING

Tibialis Anterior

Plain Radiographs

These confirm that there is no osseous injury.

Magnetic Resonance Imaging

It can help determine between a complete vs partial tear. It will often show degenerative changes within the tendon (Figure 6D.6).

Posterior Tibialis

Plain Radiographs

- AP foot
  - Increased talonavicular uncoverage (Figure 6D.7)
  - Increased talo-first metatarsal angle (Simmon angle)
- Lateral foot (weight-bearing) (Figure 6D.8)
  - Flattening of the plantar arch on a weight-bearing lateral view
    - Decreased medial cuneiform-floor height
    - Decreased calcaneal pitch (normal 17-32)
  - Increased talo-first MT angle (Meary angle) (Figure 6D.9)
  - Hindfoot or midfoot arthritis
- Mortise view
  - Talar tilt due to deltoid insufficiency in very advanced disease

Magnetic Resonance Imaging (Figure 6D.10)

- Normally the posterior tibial tendon is double the size of the adjacent FDL
- May see tenosynovitis with normal tendon
- Initially will get hypertrophy and rounding
- Slowly, the tendon will decrease in size to that of the FDL and smaller
- Eventually, the tendon will be absent altogether
- Will see injury to the spring ligament in more advanced stages
- Can see reactive edema in the navicular and retromalleolar groove of the distal tibia

Ultrasonography (Figure 6D.11)

- Heavily dependent on operators ability
- Low-grade injury is represented by hypertrophy
- More advanced injury is seen with atrophy and eventual lack of tendon
- You can also visualize the absence of the spring ligament in advanced disease

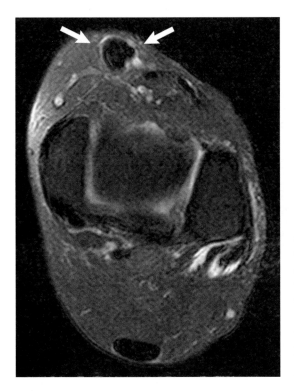

Figure 6D.6. MRI of tibialis anterior tenosynovitis. Axial proton density–weighted fat-suppressed MRI shows an additional fluid within the anterior tibialis tendon sheath (arrows) and tenosynovitis of the peroneus longus and brevis tendons. (From Kitaoka HB, ed. *The Foot and Ankle: Includes Fully Searchable Text and Image Bank Online*. 3rd ed. Philadelphia, PA: Wolters Kluwer Health/Lippincott Williams & Wilkins; 2013.)

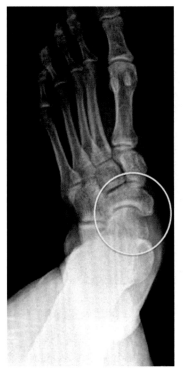

Figure 6D.7. AP X-ray of a foot in a patient with PTT dysfunction/AAFD. A key observation to be made on this X-ray is the abduction that is present through the talonavicular joint. In this instance, there is approximately 40% talar head uncoverage. (From Lotke PA, Abboud JA, Ende J, Ovid Technologies I. *Lippincott's Primary Care Orthopaedics*. Philadelphia: Wolters Kluwer/Lippincott Williams & Wilkins Health; 2008.)

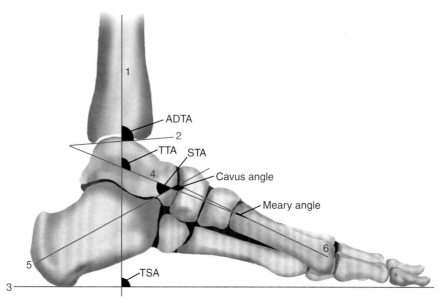

Figure 6D.8. Outline of the distal tibia and foot from a lateral radiograph for preoperative evaluation of ankle equinus demonstrating anatomic axis of the tibia (1), distal tibial ankle joint reference line (2), foot sole line (3), axis of the talus (4), axis of calcaneus (5), and axis of the first metatarsal (6). ADTA, anterior distal tibial angle; Cavus angle, calcaneal–first metatarsal angle; Meary angle, talar–first metatarsal angle; STA, sole–talar angle; TSA, tibial–sole angle; TTA, tibiotalar angle.

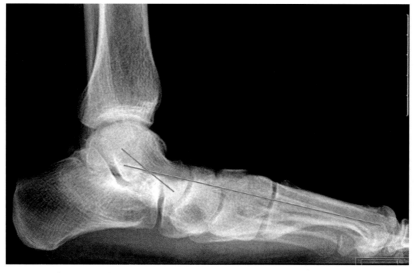

Figure 6D.9. Lateral X-ray of the foot showing an apex plantar Meary angle (the angle formed between a line down the center of the talar neck and the center of the first metatarsal). An apex plantar angle is typical of adult acquired flatfoot. Normal Meary angle ranges from 0° to 4°. (From Lotke PA, Abboud JA, Ende J, Ovid Technologies I. *Lippincott's Primary Care Orthopaedics*. Philadelphia: Wolters Kluwer/Lippincott Williams & Wilkins Health; 2008.)

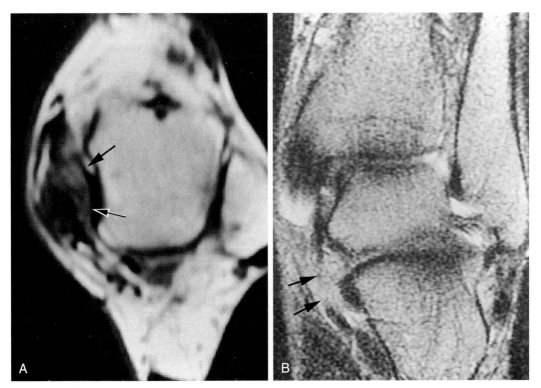

Figure 6D.10. A, T1-weighted MRI, axial ankle. Observe the intermediate signal intensity surrounding the posterior tibialis tendon (arrows), suggesting a tear. B, T2-weighted MRI, coronal ankle. Note the hyperintense signal within the partially disrupted posterior tibialis tendon (arrows). (From Terry R. Yochum, Lindsay JR. *Yochum and Rowe's Essentials of Skeletal Radiology*. 3rd ed. Philadelphia: Lippincott Williams & Wilkins; 2004.)

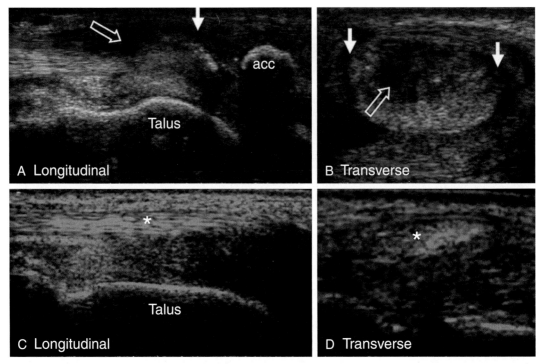

Figure 6D.11. Tibialis posterior tendinosis. A, Longitudinal ultrasound image of the distal tibialis posterior tendon with a degenerative tear (open arrow) just proximal to the accessory navicular (acc). Arrow, tenosynovial fluid. B, Transverse ultrasound image showing a markedly thickened tendon with hypoechoic cleft (open arrow) within the substance of the tendon, consistent with a partial longitudinal tear. A small amount of tenosynovial fluid is seen within the tendon sheath (arrows). C and D, Normal longitudinal and transverse ultrasound image of the distal tibialis posterior tendon (asterisk). (From Chew K, Stevens KJ, Wang TG, et al. Introduction to diagnostic musculoskeletal ultrasound: part 2: examination of the lower limb. *Am J Phys Med Rehab.* 2008;87(3):238-248.)

REFERENCES

1. Bong MR, Polatsch DB, Jazrawi LM, Rokito AS. Chronic exertional compartment syndrome: diagnosis and management. *Bull Hosp Jt Dis.* 2005;62(3-4):77-84. http://www.ncbi.nlm.nih.gov/pubmed/16022217.
2. Tzortziou V, Maffulli N, Padhiar N. Diagnosis and management of chronic exertional compartment syndrome (CECS) in the United Kingdom. *Clin J Sport Med.* 2006;16(3):209-213. http://www.ncbi.nlm.nih.gov/pubmed/16778540.
3. Coughlin MJ, Kaz A. Correlation of Harris mats, physical exam, pictures, and radiographic measurements in adult flatfoot deformity. *Foot Ankle Int.* 2009;30(7):604-612. doi:10.3113/FAI.2009.0604.
4. Churchill RS, Sferra JJ. Posterior tibial tendon insufficiency. Its diagnosis, management, and treatment. *Am J Orthop (Belle Mead NJ).* 1998;27(5):339-347. http://www.ncbi.nlm.nih.gov/pubmed/9604105.
5. Beals TC, Pomeroy GC, Manoli A. Posterior tibial tendon insufficiency: diagnosis and treatment. *J Am Acad Orthop Surg.* 1999;7(2):112-118. http://www.ncbi.nlm.nih.gov/pubmed/10336306.

SECTION E
Achilles Tendon Injuries

Victor Anciano

HISTORY

- Classically a noncontact mechanism of injury; common in the so-called weekend warriors, ie, jumping or sprinting injuries
- Many patients hear an audible "snap" during the injury
- It is commonly described by patients as been kicked or shot in the leg
- Immediate swelling and inability to bear weight on the affected leg
- The common mechanism of injury is sudden forced plantar flexion
- Risk factors include poor conditioning, steroid use, and use of quinolone antibiotics
- Patients may report inability to stand on toes

PHYSICAL EXAMINATION

KEY EXAMINATION MANEUVERS

- **Observation and Palpation** (Sensitivity: 0.73, Specificity: 0.89) (Figure 6E.1)
  - May demonstrate discontinuity of the tendon as well as bruising of the posterior ankle
  - Patients will have inability to dorsiflex or weak dorsiflexion
  - **Maneuver:**
    - With the patient lying prone, both legs should be placed side to side
    - The examiner then palpates along the border of the tendon on both legs
    - The test is positive if the examiner feels a gap along the tendon
  - **Limitations of Maneuver:**
    - Swelling may hinder proper evaluation of the tendon

- **Thompson Test** 🎥 (Sensitivity: 0.96, Specificity: 0.93) (Figure 6E.2)
  - First described by Thompson in 1955, then by Simmonds in 1957. Some people will refer to this as the Simmonds-Thompson test
  - Thompson did not publish his results until 1962
  - A reliable and easy test to perform
  - Does not cause significant discomfort to the patient
  - **Maneuver:**
    - The patient is placed in the prone position with the feet hanging off the table. Alternatively, the patient can kneel on a chair and have the foot hanging off the edge of the chair
    - The examiner then squeezes the patient's calf while looking at the foot
    - The test is considered positive if the foot stays in a neutral position or if minimal plantar flexion is noted
    - The test should be performed on both sides to have a "baseline" on the amount of plantar flexion expected

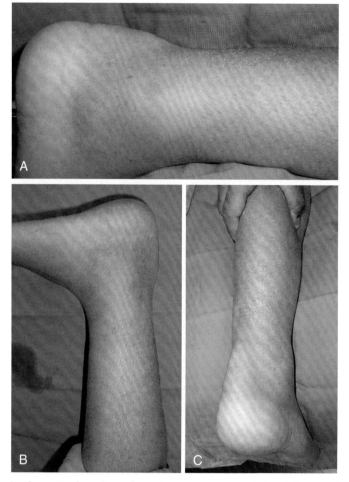

Figure 6E.1. A, Gap at the site of rupture, approximately 4-5 cm above Achilles insertion on calcaneus. B, Lack of physiologic resting tension demonstrated, also known as Matles test. C, Positive Thompson test: no ankle plantar flexion with calf squeeze. (From Easley ME, Wiesel SW. *Operative Techniques in Foot and Ankle Surgery*. Wolters Kluwer Health; 2017.)

- **Limitations of Maneuver:**
  - Minimal plantar flexion can confuse the examiner and may result in false negatives
  - Chronic injuries may have formed a hematoma providing a healing scaffolding, which can result in more plantar flexion than expected, thus resulting in a false negative
  - Some patients may be unable to get in a prone position, but kneeling is a viable option

- **Matles Test** (Sensitivity: 0.88, Specificity: 0.86) (Figure 6E.1)
  - First described by Matles in 1975
  - The test is helpful in that it can diagnose chronic as well as acute tears
  - **Maneuver:**
    - The patient is placed in the prone position
    - The examiner will then ask the patient to actively flex the knee through a range of motion of 0° to 90°
    - The examiner should pay close attention to the ankle as the knee flexes

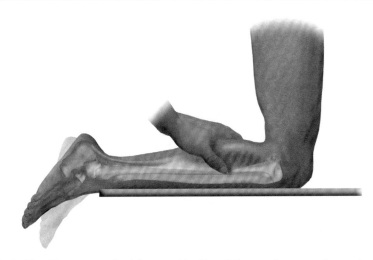

Figure 6E.2. The Thompson test for continuity of the gastrocnemius-soleus complex. Without rupture of the Achilles tendon, squeezing the calf causes active plantar flexion of the foot. With rupture, squeezing the superficial posterior compartment of the leg does not induce plantar flexion of the foot.

- In an intact Achilles tendon, the ankle will plantar flex as the knee gets closer to 90°
- The test is considered positive when the ankle remains in a neutral position or dorsiflexion is noted
- As with the Thompson test, the examiner should evaluate both extremities
- **Limitations of Maneuver:**
  - Unlike the Thompson test, Matles test requires the patient to be in a prone position
  - Results sometimes depend on the examiner noticing subtle differences in ankle plantar flexion vs dorsiflexion

- **Copeland Test** (Sensitivity: 0.78) (Figure 6E.3)
  - First described by Copeland in 1990
  - It applies the same principles as the Thompson and Matles test with the use of a blood pressure cuff
  - **Maneuver:**
    - The patient is placed in the prone position
    - The knee is flexed to 90°
    - A sphygmomanometer cuff is placed at the thickest aspect of the calf
    - With the ankle plantar flexed, the examiner then inflates the cuff to approximately 100 mm Hg
    - The ankle is then passively dorsiflexed by applying pressure on the sole of the foot
    - The test is considered positive if there is 0 to minimal change in the mercury column
    - An intact tendon will cause the pressure to rise to approximately 140 mm Hg
    - As with previous maneuvers, the test should be performed in both legs to obtain a baseline
  - **Limitations of Maneuver:**
    - Patients who cannot tolerate prone position may not tolerate the maneuver
    - The test requires additional tools including blood pressure cuffs and a sphygmomanometer

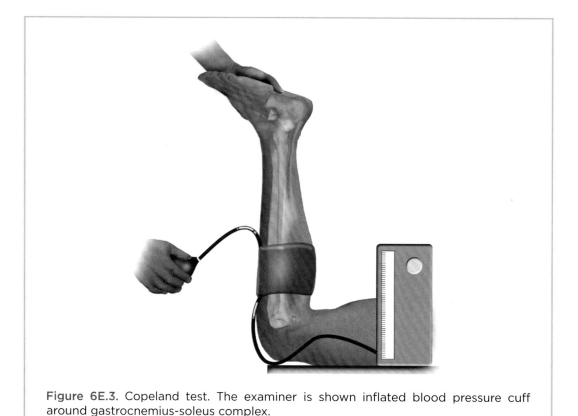

Figure 6E.3. Copeland test. The examiner is shown inflated blood pressure cuff around gastrocnemius-soleus complex.

IMAGING

Plain Radiographs

- The main role of radiography in Achilles tendon rupture is to rule out other causes of ankle pain. Radiographs should be obtained routinely to rule out fractures. Disruption of the soft tissue shadow of the Achilles tendon may be seen on radiography. Chronic tears may show ossification of the retracted tendon (Figure 6E.4)
- Lateral radiographs may show calcific tendinosis of the Achilles tendon, which is a risk factor for rupture

Ultrasonography

- A cost-effective tool for evaluating Achilles tendon injuries (Figure 6E.5)
- There is a high correlation between the size of rupture noted in ultrasonography and that seen by surgeons intraoperatively
- It is not much effective in diagnosing partial tears of the Achilles tendon

Magnetic Resonance Imaging

- The AAOS clinical guidelines in the treatment of Achilles tendon ruptures was unable to recommend against or for the use of MRI, ultrasonography, or radiography
- It has been shown to delay initial evaluation by a surgeon
- May play a role in patients with an inconclusive diagnosis (Figure 6E.4)

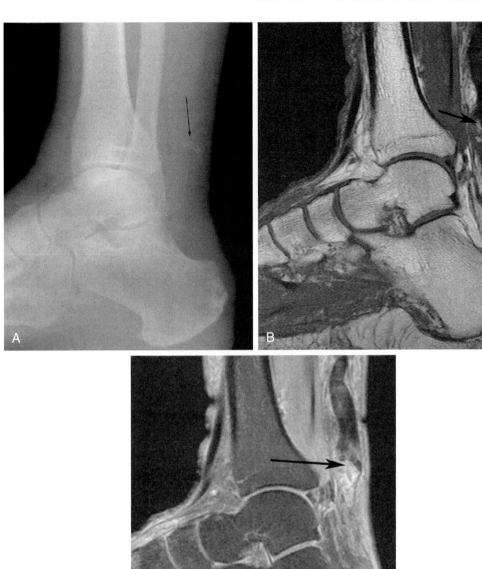

Figure 6E.4. Chronic complete tear of the Achilles tendon with retraction. A, Lateral radiograph demonstrating ossification in the retracted end of the torn tendon (arrow). Sagittal T1-weighted (B) and fast spin-echo fat-suppressed T2-weighted (C) images demonstrate a complete tear with retraction of the Achilles tendon. All arrows point to ossification of the tendon as described in the caption. (From Berquist TH, ed. *MRI of the Musculoskeletal System*. 6th ed. Philadelphia, PA: Wolters Kluwer; 2013.)

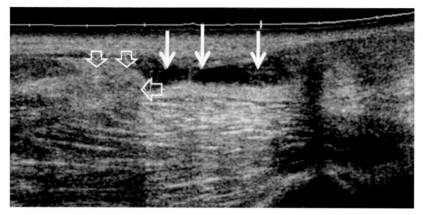

Figure 6E.5. Complete Achilles tendon tear. Longitudinal extended field-of-view scan demonstrates a complete gap (arrows) in the normal continuous echogenicity of the Achilles tendon. The fibrillar appearance of the Achilles tendon is lost as a result of retraction and shortening of the tendon. The retracted proximal tendon (open arrows) end appears nodular. (From Siegel MJ. *Pediatric Sonography*. Philadelphia: Wolters Kluwer/Lippincott Williams & Wilkins; 2011.)

REFERENCES

1. Dams OC, Reininga IHF, Gielen JL, van den Akker-Scheek I, Zwerver J. Imaging modalities in the diagnosis and monitoring of Achilles tendon ruptures: a systematic review. *Injury*. 2017. doi:10.1016/j.injury.2017.09.013.
2. Egger AC, Berkowitz MJ. Achilles tendon injuries. *Curr Rev Musculoskelet Med*. 2017;10(1):72-80. doi:10.1007/s12178-017-9386-7.
3. Gross CE, Nunley JA. Acute achilles tendon ruptures. *Foot Ankle Int*. 2016;37(no. 2):233-239. doi:10.1177/1071100715619606.
4. Kadakia AR, Dekker RG, Ho BS. Acute achilles tendon ruptures: an update on treatment. *J Am Acad Orthop Surg*. 2017;25(1):23-31. doi:10.5435/JAAOS-D-15-00187.
5. Longo UG, Petrillo S, Maffulli N, Denaro V. Acute achilles tendon rupture in athletes. *Foot Ankle Clin*. 2013;18(2):319-338. doi:10.1016/j.fcl.2013.02.009.
6. Singh D. Acute achilles tendon rupture. *Br Med J*. 2015;351:h4722.
7. Weinfeld SB. Achilles tendon disorders. *Med Clin North Am*. 2014;98(2):331-338. doi:10.1016/j.mcna.2013.11.005.

SECTION F
Chronic Exertional Compartment Syndrome

Michael M. Hadeed

HISTORY

- Often seen in runners or those who run a lot for their sport
- Anterior compartment most commonly affected (>70%)
- Unknown pathoanatomy, but may be associated with fascial hernias (most commonly near the intramuscular septum of the anterior and lateral compartments)
- Reproducible pain with exercise with predictable relief of pain after arresting the offending activity (not pathognomonic, as there are other syndromes with this presenting history, including popliteal outlet syndrome)

PHYSICAL EXAMINATION

Palpation

Compartments may feel firm, especially immediately after exercise.

Range of Motion

Passive stretch of the muscles in the affected compartment typically exacerbates the pain.

- Anterior
  - Tibialis anterior: ankle plantar flexion
  - Extensor hallucis longus: great toe flexion
  - Extensor digitorum longus: second to fifth toe flexion
- Lateral
  - Peroneal longus: ankle inversion
  - Peroneal brevis: ankle inversion
- Deep posterior
  - Posterior tibialis: ankle dorsiflexion
  - Flexor hallucis longus: great toe extension
  - Flexor digitorum longus: second to fifth toe extension
- Superficial posterior
  - Medial and lateral gastrocnemius, soleus-ankle dorsiflexion

Sensation

Patients may get paresthesias or numbness in the distribution of nerves from the affected compartment.

- Anterior
  - Deep peroneal nerve, first web space
- Lateral
  - SPN, dorsum of the foot

- Deep posterior
  - Tibial nerve, plantar surface of the foot
- Superficial posterior
  - Sural nerve, lateral aspect of the foot

KEY EXAMINATION MANEUVERS

- **Compartment Pressure Monitoring** (Sensitivity: 63%, Specificity: 95%) (Figure 6F.1)
  - Required to establish the diagnosis
  - First described by French and Price in 1962
  - Pressure must be measured at 3 timepoints (Figure 6F.2):
    - Resting
    - Immediate postexercise
    - Continuous postexercise for at least 30 minutes

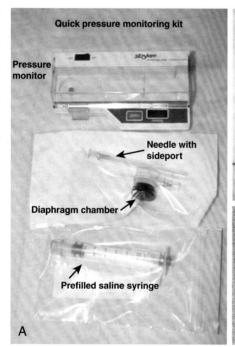
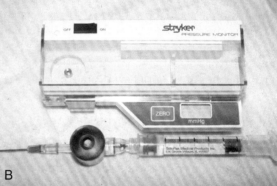
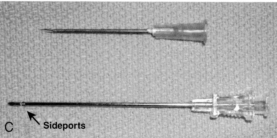

Figure 6F.1. Stryker intracompartmental pressure monitor. A, Quick pressure monitoring kit containing the intracompartmental pressure monitor, a prefilled saline syringe, a diaphragm chamber (transducer), and a needle. B, The assembled pressure monitor. To assemble the monitor kit, the needle is attached to the tapered end of the tapered chamber stem (transducer). The blue cap from the prefilled syringe is removed, and the syringe is screwed into the remaining end of the transducer, which is a Luer lock connection. The cover of the monitor is opened. The transducer is placed inside the well (black surface down). The snap cover is closed. Next, the clear end cap is pulled off the syringe end, and the monitor is ready to use. To prime the monitor, the needle is held 45° up from the horizontal and the syringe plunger is pushed slowly to purge air from the syringe. The monitor is then turned on. The assembled monitor is tilted at the approximate intended angle of insertion of the needle into the skin. The zero button is pressed to set the display at zero. The needle is then inserted into the appropriate location in the compartment. C, The intracompartmental pressure monitor needle has side ports to prevent soft tissue from collapsing around the needle opening. This is different from a regular needle that has only 1 opening at the end. (From Tornetta P, Wiesel SW. *Operative Techniques in Orthopaedic Trauma Surgery*. Wolters Kluwer; 2016.)

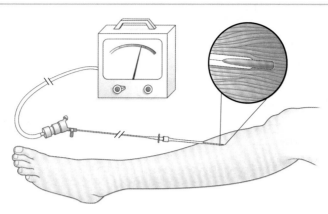

Figure 6F.2. The wick catheter is inserted into a muscle compartment and continuously monitors compartment pressure. (From Chapman MW, Szabo RM, Marder RA. *Chapman's Orthopaedic Surgery*. 3rd ed. Philadelphia, PA: Lippincott Williams & Wilkins; 2000:401.)

- Diagnostic criteria
  - Resting >15 mm Hg
  - Immediate postexercise >30 mm Hg *or* postexercise >20 mm Hg at 5 minutes, >15 mm Hg at 15 minutes

IMAGING

Near-infrared spectroscopy can show deoxygenation of muscle.

- Return to normal within 25 minutes of exercise cessation

REFERENCES

1. Markarian GG, Kelikian AS, Brage M, Trainor T, Dias L. Anterior tibialis tendon ruptures: an outcome analysis of operative versus nonoperative treatment. *Foot Ankle Int.* 1998;19(12):792-802. doi:10.1177/107110079801901202.
2. Sammarco VJ, Sammarco GJ, Henning C, Chaim S. Surgical repair of acute and chronic tibialis anterior tendon ruptures. *J Bone Joint Surg Am.* 2009;91(2):325-332. doi:10.2106/JBJS.G.01386.

SECTION G
Lower Extremity Stress Fractures

Timothy Maxwell Hoggard

HISTORY

- Classic "overuse" injuries seen in military personnel and competitive athletes, particularly common in distance runners, dancers, and basketball players
- Gradual onset of pain over a period of many days to weeks, typically exacerbated by activity and improved with rest
- Patients often endorse a recent, marked increase in the intensity, duration, and/or frequency of physical activity or a change in training-related equipment (eg, change in shoe wear, orthotics, and running surface)
- Commonly involves posteromedial tibia, calcaneus, distal fibula, and diaphysis of the second/third metatarsals but can also occur in high-risk locations such as the navicular, talus, fifth metatarsal, and hallux sesamoids (medial > lateral)
- A thorough medical history, specifically including diet, medications, and menstrual history in females, is important in identifying secondary causes of stress fractures (eg, female athlete triad)

PHYSICAL EXAMINATION

Observation

- Evaluation of limb biomechanics and any deformities may also prove beneficial in identifying precipitating factors, such as limb length discrepancy or soft tissue imbalance
- Patients with cavus feet have been shown to be at increased risk of fifth metatarsal stress fractures. Inversion of the foot may aggravate symptoms on examination

Palpation

- Focal bony tenderness with palpation is the most obvious examination finding
- Most sites of stress fractures are adequately superficial to elicit pain upon palpation or to identify overlying periosteal thickening and soft tissue swelling if present
- Location of pain in suspected tibial stress fractures is important to note, as anterior tibial stress fractures are at increased risk for progression to complete fracture and nonunion

Range of Motion

- Patients with hallux sesamoid stress fractures will endorse significant pain with passive dorsiflexion of the great toe

- **"N Spot" Sign** (Figure 6G.1)
  - First described by Kahn[4] in 1994
  - **Maneuver:**
    - Patients with navicular stress fractures may have point tenderness of the dorsal navicular between extensor hallucis longus and tibialis anterior
    - This spot coincides with the central third of the navicular, which has poor blood supply and experiences highest shear stresses during foot-strike phase of running
    - Percussion tenderness or tuning fork testing of the bone away from the fracture site may also elicit pain
    - A 1-legged hop test commonly reproduces pain in patients with navicular stress fractures (recreates axial load experienced during inciting activity)

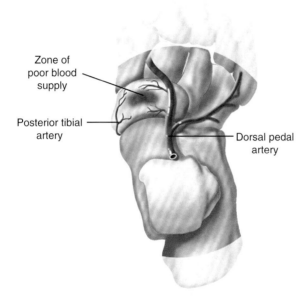

Zone of poor blood supply

Posterior tibial artery

Dorsal pedal artery

Figure 6G.1. Schematic of the blood supply of the navicular with watershed area in the central third.

IMAGING

Plain Radiographs

- Most appropriate imaging modality in the initial workup, as it is relatively inexpensive, commonly available, and can rule out more serious lesions
- Sensitivity ranges from 12% to 56%, specificity from 88% to 96%
- High false-negative rates suggest that these injuries are often missed, as radiographic findings may lag behind symptoms by weeks or may never appear at all
  - "Gray cortex sign": subtle intracortical striations initially seen in stress fractures involving cortical bone (eg, tibia and metatarsal diaphysis). A distinct radiolucent line with associated sclerosis/periosteal reaction may develop with continued damage (Figure 6G.2)
  - "Dreaded black line": linear lucency through the anterior diaphyseal cortex of the tibia, best seen on the lateral view (Figure 6G.3)

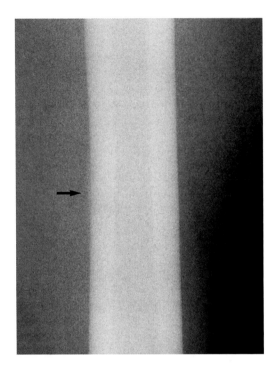

Figure 6G.2. The earliest radiographic changes of a stress fracture include "gray cortex" sign consisting of a subtle ill-defined cortical margin (arrow). (From Greenspan A, Beltran J, Ovid Technologies I. *Orthopedic Imaging: A Practical Approach*. Philadelphia: Wolters Kluwer Health/Lippincott Williams & Wilkins; 2015.)

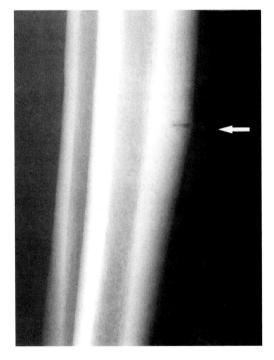

Figure 6G.3. Lateral radiograph demonstrates a stress fracture of the tibia (arrow). Note the perpendicular direction of the radiolucency to the long axis of the tibial cortex. (From Greenspan A, Beltran J. *Orthopedic Imaging: A Practical Approach*. Philadelphia: Wolters Kluwer Health/Lippincott Williams & Wilkins; 2015.)

- Navicular stress fractures are difficult to appreciate on plain radiographs, as they typically occur in the sagittal plane and are commonly incomplete, not involving the plantar surface. Further imaging should be obtained if there is clinical suspicion in setting of negative radiographs (Figure 6G.4)
- Fractures are especially difficult to identify in cancellous bone (eg, calcaneus) and typically appear as a faint band of sclerosis perpendicular to trabecular markings (Figure 6G.5)
- It is crucial to distinguish between the bipartite sesamoid and a stress fracture

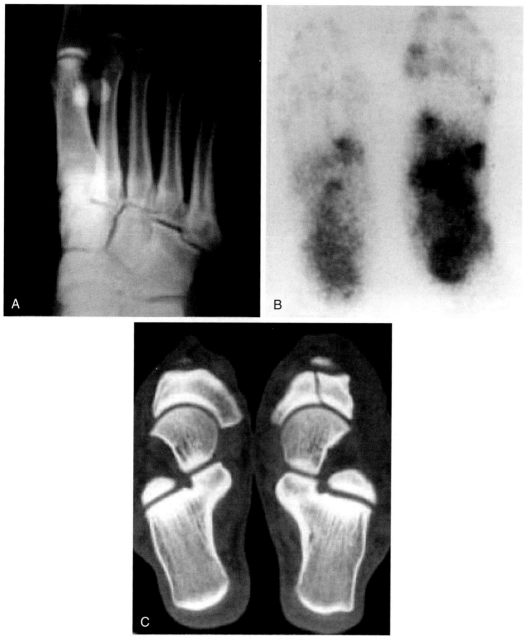

Figure 6G.4. A, Standard AP radiograph of a patient with midfoot pain does not reveal a stress fracture. B, Bone scan reveals increased uptake in the navicular bone. C, CT scan demonstrates a complete navicular stress fracture. (Reprinted from Boden BP, Osbahr DC. High-risk stress fractures. *J Am Acad Orthop Surg.* 2000;8:344-353, with permission.)

Magnetic Resonance Imaging

- Shown to be 68% to 99% sensitive and up to 97% specific
- Findings are typically presented weeks before radiographs
- Fracture appears as line of low signal on both T1 and T2/STIR sequences (Figure 6G.6)
- STIR sequences demonstrate periosteal and bone edema surrounding the fracture (Figure 6G.6)
- Noninvasive, no radiation exposure allows for soft tissue evaluation
- The major limitation is high cost, although part of this financial burden may be eliminated by no longer needing further diagnostic testing due to a low false-negative rate

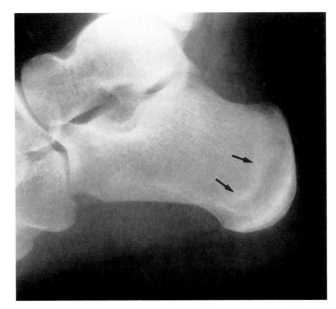

Figure 6G.5. A linear band of sclerosis is seen in the posterior calcaneus (arrows), which is diagnostic for a stress fracture of the calcaneus. (From Brant WE, Helms CA. *Brant and Helms Solution*. Wolters Kluwer Health/Lippincott Williams & Wilkins; 2007.)

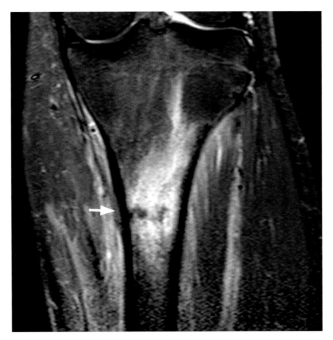

Figure 6G.6. Coronal T2-weighted MRI with fat suppression shows a focus of marrow edema traversed by a dark fracture line (arrow). Surrounding soft tissue edema is also present. (From Chew FS. *Skeletal Radiology the Bare Bones*. Philadelphia: Wolters Kluwer/Lippincott Williams & Wilkins Health; 2010.)

Computed Tomography

- Sensitivity ranges from 32% to 38% and specificity from 88% to 98%
- Primary advantage is delineation of suspected fractures not well depicted on plain radiographs, particularly those involving the navicular and cuneiforms
- Comparable false-negative rate with plain radiographs and increased radiation exposure

Nuclear Scintigraphy

- Sensitivity ranges from 50% to 97% and specificity from 33% to 98%
- Invasive, significantly higher radiation dose compared with other modalities
- Does not delineate chronicity of stress fracture or between other causes of increased bone uptake (eg, infection, tumor, arthritis)
- Valuable primarily for initial staging, as increased uptake may be seen up to 6 months after injury

REFERENCES

1. Boden BP, Osbahr DC. High-risk stress fractures: evaluation and treatment. *J Am Acad Orthop Surg.* 2000;8(6):344-353.
2. Caesar BC, McCollum GA, Elliot R, Williams A, Calder JDF. Stress fractures of the tibia and medial malleolus. *Foot Ankle Clin.* 2013;18(2):339-355.
3. Hossain M, Clutton J, Ridgewell M, Lyons K, Perera A. Stress fractures of the foot. *Clin Sports Med.* 2015;34(4):769-790.
4. Khan KM, Brukner PD, Kearney C, et al. Tarsal navicular stress fractures in athletes. *Sports Med.* 1994;17(1):65-76.
5. Mandell JC, Khurana B, Smith SE. Stress fractures of the foot and ankle, part 2: site-specific etiology, imaging, and treatment, and differential diagnosis. *Skeletal Radiol.* 2017:1-22.
6. Mann JA, Pedowitz DI. Evaluation and treatment of navicular stress fractures, including nonunions, revision surgery, and persistent pain after treatment. *Foot Ankle Clin.* 2009;14(2):187-204.
7. Muthukumar T, Butt SH, Cassar-Pullicino VN. Stress fractures and related disorders in foot and ankle: plain films, scintigraphy, CT, and MR imaging. *Semin Musculoskelet Radiol.* 2005;9(3):210-226.
8. Shindle MK, Endo Y, Warren RF, et al. Stress fractures about the tibia, foot, and ankle. *J Am Acad Orthop Surg.* 2012;20(3):167-176.
9. Smoliga JM, Wright AA, Hegedus EJ. Diagnostic accuracy of various imaging modalities for suspected lower extremity stress fractures: response. *Am J Sports Med.* 2016;44(7):NP33-NP34.

SECTION H
Hallux Valgus and Hallux Rigidus

Timothy Maxwell Hoggard

HISTORY

- **Hallux valgus**: defined as lateral deviation of the great toe (valgus) in conjunction with medial deviation of the first metatarsal (varus)
  - Most common disorder of the great toe
  - Patients may complain of cosmetic deformity more than pain
  - Upon presentation, patients primarily endorse pain over the medial eminence, classically worse with shoe wear
  - Etiology is likely multifactorial; intrinsic factors may include genetic predisposition, ligamentous laxity, and female sex, and extrinsic factors primarily include certain types of shoe wear (high heels, shoes with narrow toe box)
  - Pathoanatomy (Figure 6H.1)
    - Failure of medial support structures (capsule, collateral ligament, medial sesamoid ligament) allows the metatarsal head to migrate medially off of the sesamoid apparatus and leads to progressive medial capsular attenuation
    - Abductor hallucis is now more plantar and lateral relative to the metatarsal head, leading to pronation of the first metatarsal
    - Additionally, instability at the first tarsometatarsal has been suggested to contribute
    - Lateral migration of sesamoids and flexor hallucis longus contributes to valgus deformity of proximal phalanx, combined with unopposed adductor function, lateral shift of flexor hallucis longus and lateral capsular contraction
- **Hallux rigidus**: characterized by limited range of motion about the first MTP joint due to degenerative changes
  - Patients often initially endorse progressive pain over the dorsal aspect of the first MTP joint exacerbated with walking, particularly with toe off/heel rise
  - May be posttraumatic, inflammatory, or idiopathic
  - Patients may also complain of a dorsal prominence that becomes irritated with shoe wear
  - Barefoot activities are usually not well tolerated
  - Occasionally, some patients have burning or paresthesias related to pressure on the dorsomedial cutaneous nerve traversing over the dorsal osseous prominence

PHYSICAL EXAMINATION

Hallux Valgus

- **Inspection**
  - Valgus deformity with prominent medial eminence +/– bursal inflammation and skin irritation or breakdown (Figure 6H.2)
  - The great toe is often pronated and may be overlapping the second toe
  - Deformity exaggerated with weight-bearing
  - Patients may often demonstrate pes planus deformity

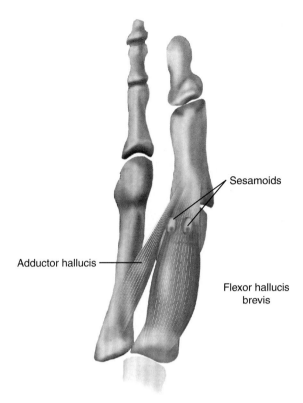

Figure 6H.1. Dorsal view of hallux valgus pathology with lateral subluxation of the sesamoids.

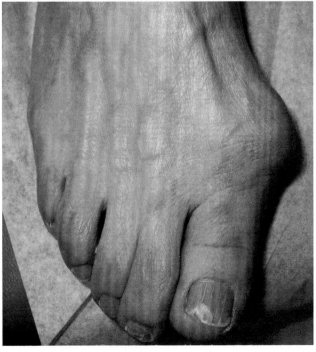

Figure 6H.2. Hallux valgus deformity. (Image provided by Stedman's Medical Dictionary, 2013.)

- **Palpation**
  - Patients endorse focal tenderness over the medial eminence, due to irritation of the dorsal cutaneous nerve of the great toe or an inflamed bursa overlying the medial metatarsal head
  - May be tender at the second MTP joint due to overload with incompetent first ray
  - May have positive Tinel sign or even numbness in region of dorsomedial cutaneous nerve
- **Range of motion**
  - Evaluation of MTP motion and the presence of crepitus are important to assess for contaminant degenerative changes in the first MTP joint

---

KEY EXAMINATION MANEUVERS

- **First TMT Hypermobility** 🔵 (Figure 6H.3)
  - First described by Root in 1971
  - **Maneuver:**
    - The examiner stabilizes the lesser metatarsals with one hand and brings the first metatarsal into full dorsiflexion and plantar flexion with the other hand
    - The amount of sagittal plane mobility is measured by comparing relative position of the examiner's fingers dorsally and thumbs plantarly
  - **Limitations of Maneuver**
    - Often present although difficult to assess on physical examination
    - Poor interrater reliability

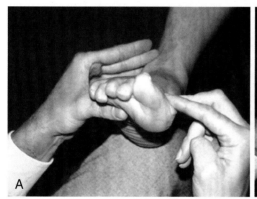 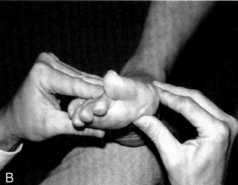

Figure 6H.3. First TMT hypermobility. The lesser metatarsals are stabilized in one hand while the examiner applies direct plantar (A) and dorsal (B) pressure to the first metatarsal. (From Easley ME, Wiesel SW. *Operative Techniques in Foot and Ankle Surgery*. Wolters Kluwer Health; 2017.)

Hallux Rigidus

- **Inspection**
  - Prominent dorsal prominence with overlying skin erythema (Figure 6H.4A)
- **Palpation**
  - Usually tender to palpation at the dorsal MTP joint line
  - The dorsal osteophyte is often palpable
  - If there is involvement of the dorsal digital nerve, there may be a positive Tinel sign
- **Range of motion**
  - Range of motion is diminished globally, dorsiflexion most significantly (Figure 6H.4B)

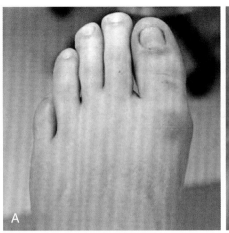
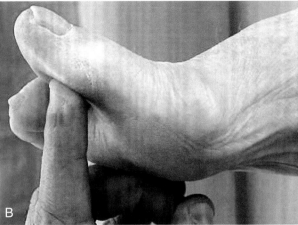

Figure 6H.4. A, Dorsal view of foot in hallux rigidus. Shoe wear may cause irritation over the dorsal bony prominence. B, Limited dorsiflexion is noted on the clinical examination. (From Easley ME, Wiesel SW. *Operative Techniques in Foot and Ankle Surgery*. Wolters Kluwer Health; 2017.)

KEY EXAMINATION MANEUVERS

- **Grind Test**
  - **Maneuver:**
    - The examiner grasps the proximal phalanx of the great near the MTP joint in neutral dorsiflexion
    - An axial load is applied with internal and external rotation
    - The test is considered positive if it elicits pain

- **Gait**
  - Patients often characteristically shift their weight laterally to off-load the first MTP and frequently exhibit signs of transfer metatarsalgia
  - To avoid dorsiflexion during the toe-off phase, patients may externally rotate the affected extremity to allow foot clearance during swing phase

IMAGING

Hallux Valgus

Plain Radiographs: Weight-Bearing AP and Lateral

- Hallux valgus angle (HVA): the angle formed by a line through the long axis of the first metatarsal and a line through the long axis of the proximal phalanx (Figure 6H.5)
  - Normal <15°
- Intermetatarsal angle (IMA): the angle formed between diaphysis of the first and second metatarsals (Figure 6H.5)
  - Normal <9°
- Distal metatarsal articular angle (DMAA): the angle formed between the long axis of the first metatarsal and a line perpendicular to the articular surface (Figure 6H.5)
  - Normal <10°

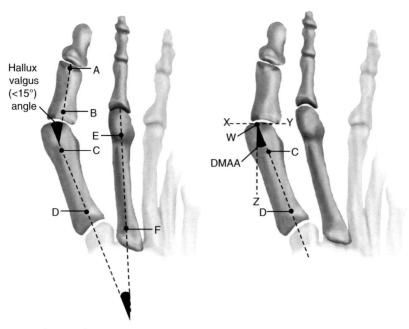

Figure 6H.5. Hallux valgus, intermetatarsal angle and distal metatarsal articular angle (DMAA): (A, B) axis of the proximal phalanx; (C, D) axis of the first metatarsal; (E, F) axis of the second metatarsal; (W) line perpendicular to the long axis of the first MT; (X, Y) the line along articular surface of the first metatarsal; (Z) the line perpendicular to the articular surface.

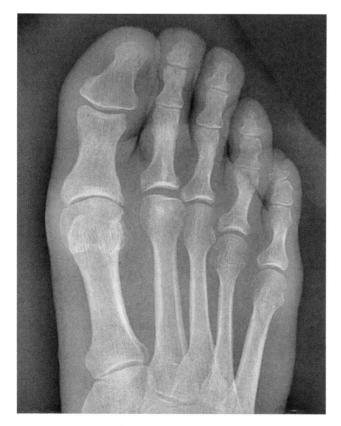

Figure 6H.6. Radiographs of the patient with hallux rigidus. AP view demonstrating joint space narrowing. (From Easley M, Wiesel SW, eds. *Operative Techniques in Foot and Ankle Surgery*. Philadelphia, PA: Wolters Kluwer Health, Lippincott Williams & Wilkins; 2011.)

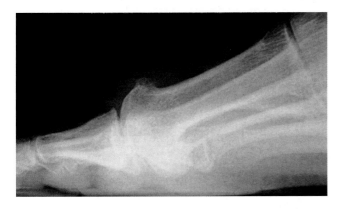

Figure 6H.7. Radiographs of the patient with hallux rigidus. Lateral view with dorsal osteophyte on the first metatarsal head. (From Easley M, Wiesel SW, eds. *Operative Techniques in Foot and Ankle Surgery*. Philadelphia, PA: Wolters Kluwer Health, Lippincott Williams & Wilkins; 2011.)

Hallux Rigidus

Plain Radiographs: Weight-Bearing AP and Lateral (Figure 6H.6)

- Lateral views demonstrate a prominent dorsal osteophyte at the metatarsal head and proximal phalanx (Figure 6H.7)
- A fractured osteophyte may present as a loose body in the joint
- Joint space is narrowed, often dorsal > plantar, along with degenerative changes such as subchondral cyst formation and sclerosis
- When related to gout, periarticular erosions will typically be seen

REFERENCES

1. Coughlin MJ. Hallux valgus. *J Bone Joint Surg*. 1997;78-A:932-966.
2. Easley ME, Trnka H-J. Current concepts review: hallux valgus Part 1: pathomechanics, clinical assessment, and nonoperative management. *Foot Ankle*. 2007;28(5):654-659.
3. Perera AM, Mason L, Stephens MM. The pathogenesis of hallux valgus. *J Bone Joint Surg Am*. 2011;93(17):1650-1661.
4. Shereff MJ, Baumhauer JF. Current concepts review: hallux rigidus and Osteoarthrosis of the first metatarsophalangeal joint. *J Bone Joint Surg Am*. 1998;80-A(6):898-908.
5. Yee G, Lau J. Current concepts review: hallux rigidus. *Foot Ankle Int*. 2008;29(6):637-646.

SECTION I
Morton Neuroma, Metatarsalgia, Lesser MTP Synovitis

Timothy Maxwell Hoggard

HISTORY

Morton Neuroma

- Named after Thomas George Morton, an American orthopedic surgeon
- Compressive neuropathy classically involving the third common digital nerve between the third and fourth metatarsals (75%-80%) but may also affect the second common digital nerve
- "Pebble in the shoe" or feeling that a "sock is bunched up under the toes"
- Patients report burning pain on the plantar surface of the web space that can radiate distally to the toes or rarely proximally to the midfoot
- Less than half of patients endorse numbness
- Pain is often worse with footwear that compresses medial-lateral

Metatarsalgia

- A general term referring to pain localized to 1 or more metatarsal head regions
- Often a "catch-all" diagnosis to describe forefoot pain
- The underlying cause is repetitive transfer of concentrated force through the forefoot during the gait cycle
- Many different etiologies: anatomic metatarsal deformities, soft tissue imbalances, hindfoot abnormalities, systemic inflammatory/neurologic disorders, or iatrogenic causes resulting in excessive shortening/elevation/depression of the metatarsals and shortened or incompetent first ray (idiopathic or iatrogenic)

Lesser MTP Synovitis

- Most frequently involves the second MTP joint
- Etiologies include repetitive trauma, restrictive footwear, hallux valgus, and elongated second metatarsal
- Chronic inflammation causes capsule and ligamentous laxity, leading to instability and eventual deformity
- Attenuation of the plantar plate causes dorsal subluxation of the second toe with associated sagittal plane instability

PHYSICAL EXAMINATION

Morton Neuroma

- **Thumb-Index Finger Squeeze** (Sensitivity: 0.96, Specificity: 1.00) (Figure 61.1)
  - Initial test maneuver described by Morton in 1876
  - Most sensitive and specific clinical test
  - **Maneuver:**
    - The examiner places the thumb and index finger between the affected web space just distal to the metatarsal heads
    - The area is then compressed between the thumb and index finger
    - The test is considered positive if there is recreation of pain during compression

- **Mulder Click Test** 🔊 (Sensitivity: 0.62-0.98, Specificity: 1.00) (Figure 61.2)
  - First described by Mulder[5] in 1951
  - **Maneuver:**
    - The examiner places the thumb on the dorsal surface and the index finger on the plantar surface in the affected web space and applies gentle pressure
    - With the opposite hand, the examiner applies a gentle squeeze to the forefoot in a mediolateral direction
    - A clicking sensation that reproduces the patient's pain will often be appreciated

- **Plantar Percussion Test** (Sensitivity: 0.36; Specificity: 1.00)
  - **Maneuver:**
    - The examiner percusses the web space in question plantarly
    - The test is considered a positive if localized pain or Tinel sign is produced

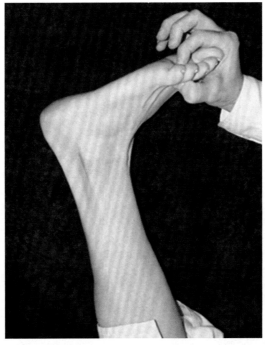

Figure 61.1. Thumb-index finger squeeze: The examiner places the thumb on the dorsal surface and the index finger on the plantar surface in the affected web space and applies gentle pressure. (From Wiesel SW, ed. *Operative Techniques in Orthopaedic Surgery - 4 Volumes*. Wolters Kluwer; 2011.)

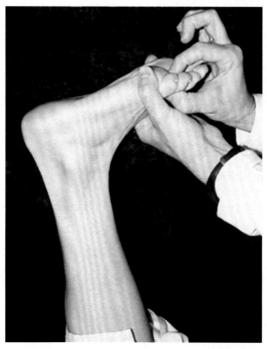

Figure 6I.2. Mulder click test: The examiner places the thumb on the dorsal surface and the index finger on the plantar surface in the affected web space and applies gentle pressure. With the opposite hand, the examiner applies a gentle squeeze to the forefoot in a mediolateral direction. A clicking sensation that reproduces the patient's pain will often be appreciated. (From Easley M, Wiesel SW, eds. *Operative Techniques in Foot and Ankle Surgery.* Philadelphia, PA: Wolters Kluwer Health, Lippincott Williams & Wilkins; 2011.)

Metatarsalgia

- **Observation**
  - Plantar keratosis may be noted underlying or adjacent to 1 or multiple MT heads (Figure 6I.3)
- **Gait analysis**
  - **"Rocker concept"** often used to identify etiology (Figure 6I.4)
    - "First-rocker": initial 10% of gait cycle between heel strike and forefoot contact
    - "Second-rocker" or "static" metatarsalgia: midstance phase from 10% to 30% of gait cycle with increasing metatarsal head loading
      - Painful in patients with plantar flexed or shortened MT
      - Keratosis strictly *plantar* to MT head
    - "Third-rocker" or "propulsive" metatarsalgia: 30% to 60% of cycle, which corresponds with heel rise
      - Painful in patients with excessive MT length
      - Keratosis plantar and *distal* to MT head

KEY EXAMINATION MANEUVERS

None specific to metatarsalgia

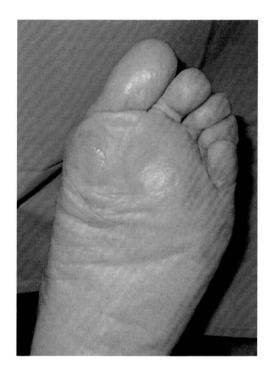

Figure 61.3. Plantar view of a case of metatarsalgia with plantar callosity underlying metatarsal heads. (From Easley M, Wiesel SW, eds. *Operative Techniques in Foot and Ankle Surgery*. Philadelphia, PA: Wolters Kluwer Health, Lippincott Williams & Wilkins; 2011.)

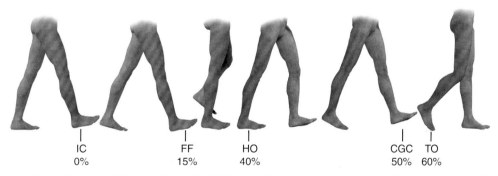

IC	FF	HO	CGC	TO
0%	15%	40%	50%	60%

Figure 61.4. Phases of the gait cycle. "First-rocker" corresponds to the phase from initial contact (IC) to forefoot contact (FF). "Second-rocker" includes midstance before heel-off (HO). "Third-rocker" corresponds to the phase from heel off, through contralateral ground contact (CGC), to toe-off (TO).

Lesser MTP Synovitis

- **Observation**
  - **"Crossover toe" deformity: most commonly** dorsomedial deviation of the second toe with an associated increased gap between the second and third toes (Figure 61.5)
    – As deformity progresses, the second toe may deviate up and over the hallux
- **Palpation**
  - Pain at the second MTP joint may be both dorsal and plantar (unlike a neuroma that is unlikely to cause tenderness dorsally)
  - May see warm and swollen second MTP joint in initial acute phase
- **Range of motion**
  - Decreased plantar flexion and painful motion decreased by traction

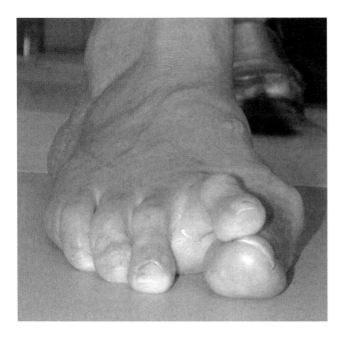

Figure 61.5. Multiplanar instability of the MTP joint causes a crossover toe deformity. (From Thordarson DB. *Foot and Ankle*. Philadelphia, PA: Kluwer/Lippincott Williams et Wilkins; 2013.)

KEY EXAMINATION MANEUVERS

- **Dorsal Drawer Test** (Figure 61.6)
  - First described by Thompson and Hamilton in 1987
  - **Maneuver:**
    - The examiner holds the MTP joint in a neutral position
    - A dorsal directed force is applied to the toe
    - A positive test causes pain at the MTP joint and in later stages subluxation of the proximal phalanx on the metatarsal head
    - Subluxation is indicative of plantar plate compromise

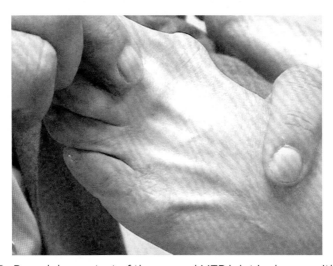

Figure 61.6. Dorsal drawer test of the second MTP joint is shown, with one hand securing the metatarsals and the other translating the phalanx dorsally. (From Kitaoka HB, ed. *Master Techniques in Orthopedic Surgery: The Foot and Ankle*. 3rd ed. Philadelphia, PA: Wolters Kluwer Health/Lippincott Williams & Wilkins; 2013.)

IMAGING

Morton Neuroma

- **Ultrasonography**
  - Uncompressible hypoechoic nodule is seen in the interdigital fat of the painful web space (Figure 6I.7)
  - Inexpensive and quick but operator-dependent
  - Easily used to confirm diagnosis if clinical findings are equivocal
- **MRI**
  - Used to confirm diagnosis if clinical findings and ultrasonography are equivocal
  - Expensive and time-consuming but not operator-dependent
  - Also allows for evaluation of other web spaces and overall forefoot anatomy (including second MTP joint plantar plate)

Metatarsalgia

- **Plain radiographs**
  - Standard weight-bearing radiographs of the bilateral foot, including anteroposterior, internal oblique, and lateral views
  - Evaluation of metatarsal morphology and length as well as overall relationship between the MT heads (Figure 6I.8)
  - Evaluate for cavus foot
- **Ultrasonography/MRI**
  - Can be used to rule out other causes

Lesser MTP Synovitis

- **Plain radiographs**
  - Standard weight-bearing radiographs of the foot
    - Widening of the interval between the second and third proximal phalanges with medial deviation of the second proximal phalanx (often very subtle)
    - Subluxation of the MTP joint may appear as narrowed or overlapping joint space (Figure 6I.9)

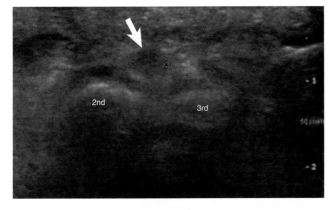

Figure 6I.7. Ultrasound image demonstrating a Morton neuroma in the second intermetatarsal space (arrow). (From Lee MJ, Kim S, Huh YM, et al. Morton neuroma: evaluated with ultrasonography and MR imaging. *Korean J Radiol.* 2007;8(2):148-155.)

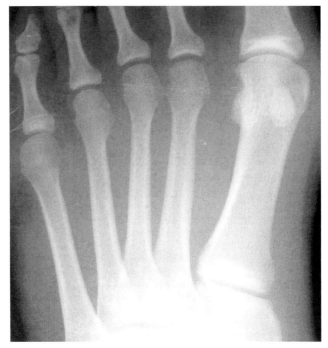

Figure 6I.8. Radiograph demonstrating variations of metatarsal length. This patient presents with a shortened second metatarsal. (From Christman RA. *Foot and Ankle Radiology*. Wolters Kluwer; 2015.)

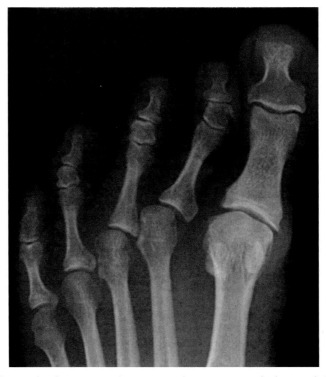

Figure 6I.9. Radiograph demonstrating second metatarsophalangeal joint subluxation. (From Easley M, Wiesel SW, eds. *Operative Techniques in Foot and Ankle Surgery*. Philadelphia, PA: Wolters Kluwer Health, Lippincott Williams & Wilkins; 2011.)

REFERENCES

1. Pastides P, El-Sallakh S, Charalambides C. Morton's neuroma: a clinical versus radiological diagnosis. *Foot Ankle Surg.* 2012;18(1):22-24.
2. Owens R, Gougoulias N, Guthrie H, Sakellariou A. Morton's neuroma: clinical testing and imaging in 76 feet, compared to a control group. *Foot Ankle Surg.* 2011;17(3):197-200.
3. Mahadevan D, Venkatesan M, Bhatt R, Bhatia M. Diagnostic accuracy of clinical tests for Morton's neuroma compared with ultrasonography. *J Foot Ankle Surg.* 2015;54(4):549-553.
4. Wu KK. Morton's interdigital neuroma: a clinical review of its etiology, treatment, and results. *J Foot Ankle Surg.* 1996;35(2):112-119.
5. Mulder JD. The causative mechanism in Morton's metatarsalgia. *J Bone Joint Surg Br.* 1951;33-B(1):94-95.
6. Espinosa N, Maceira E, Myerson MS. Current concept review: metatarsalgia. *Foot Ankle Int.* 2008;29(8):863-866.
7. Kaz AJ, Coughlin MJ. Crossover second toe: demographics, etiology, and radiographic assessment. *Foot Ankle Int.* 2007;28(12):1223-1237.

7

SECTION

The Spine

Section Editor
Hamid Hassanzadeh

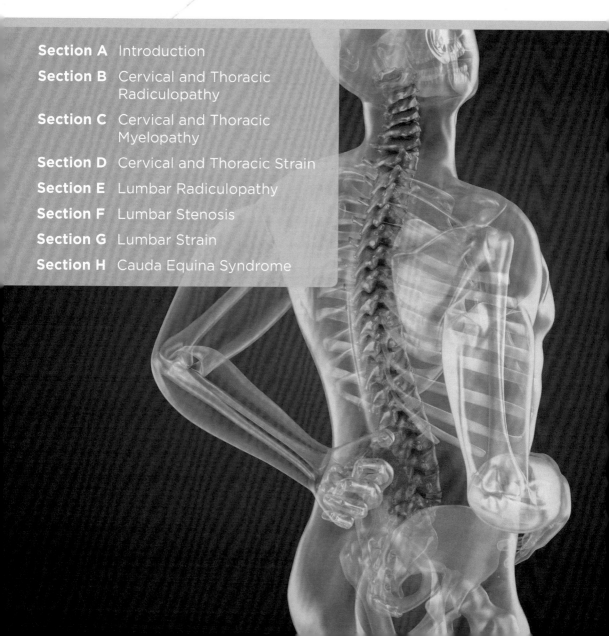

QUICK REFERENCE FLOW CHART

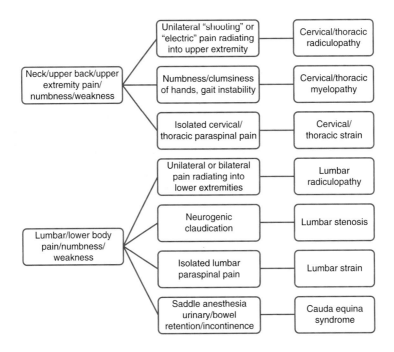

SECTION A
Introduction

Jason A. Horowitz, Dimitri S. Tahal, Bayan Aghadasi, and Hamid Hassanzadeh

HISTORY

It is important to consider the following parameters when a patient presents to the clinic with a spinal complaint:

- Patient description of pain
  - Location: may help to localize pathology
    - For example, lumbar paraspinal soreness may indicate a lumbar paraspinal muscle strain
  - Radiation
    - Unilateral or bilateral pain shooting through an upper extremity is a classic complaint associated with cervical radiculopathy
    - Unilateral or bilateral pain shooting through a lower extremity is more likely indicative of lumbar radiculopathy or stenosis
  - Quality
    - Soreness is a common patient description of a muscle or ligament strain
    - "Electric" or "shooting" pain is a classic description of radicular pain
  - Palliative and provocative positions
    - A brief inquiry into which body positions and movements exacerbate or relieve a patient's pain can quickly narrow down the diagnosis
    - For example, bilateral diffuse lower extremity pain provoked by standing and walking that is relieved by sitting is a classic description of neurogenic claudication, which greatly raises suspicion of lumbar stenosis
- Patient age
  - Older patients are more likely to suffer from insidious, degenerative conditions such as spinal stenosis
  - Younger patients are more likely to present with sudden onset symptoms caused by an acute injury, such as sudden onset back pain and radiculopathy caused by disk herniation following an attempt to lift a heavy object
- Onset of symptoms
  - Acute onset of symptoms may result from acute injuries, including muscle and ligament strains, disk herniation, and fractures
  - Insidious onset of symptoms more likely represents a gradually progressive, degenerative pathology, such as spinal stenosis
- Mechanism of injury (if any)
  - Heavy lifting may result in lumbar strain or disk herniation
  - Poor neck posture during sleep may provoke a cervical strain
  - Significant trauma, such as a motor vehicle accident, may cause sudden stenosis with radiculopathy or spinal cord injury
  - If no obvious mechanism of injury is apparent, a gradually progressive, degenerative pathology may be the culprit

- Neurologic symptoms
  - Sensory
    - Numbness
      - Numbness in a dermatomal distribution may be indicative of radiculopathy
      - Saddle anesthesia should raise suspicion of cauda equina syndrome
    - Impaired gait and balance may indicate diminished lower extremity proprioception stemming from cervical myelopathy or lumbar stenosis
  - Motor
    - Diminished strength—for example, unilateral upper extremity weakness—may be a sign of cervical radiculopathy
    - Diminished hand dexterity—for example, difficulty manipulating shirt buttons—is a classic complaint associated with cervical myelopathy
  - Bladder, bowel, and sexual dysfunction
    - Bladder and/or bowel retention/incontinence with or without associated sexual dysfunction should raise suspicion of spinal cord injury or cauda equina syndrome (CES)
- Prior spinal pathology or injury
  - Symptoms may represent worsening of a progressive degenerative condition
  - With a history of previous spinal injury, reinjury should be considered a possible etiology of new or recurrent symptoms
- Prior spinal surgery
  - In a patient with a history of spinal surgery, it is essential to obtain prior operative reports and images; patient reports are often incomplete or inaccurate. Imaging may reveal postoperative complications that could be contributing to the patient's current complaint, including pseudoarthrosis, construct failure, screw failure, and proximal junctional disease
- Prior treatment
  - The success or failure of previous treatments may provide crucial evidence for pinpointing a diagnosis
  - A history of an appropriate trial of nonsurgical treatment modalities is often necessary before proceeding to surgical intervention for many spinal pathologies
- Current medications

PHYSICAL EXAMINATION

Observation

- Observe the patient's posture, how they get onto the examination table and how they describe their pain
  - If the patient is relying on holding onto objects, such as counters and the examination table, for balance, they may have myelopathy
- Assess the patient's sagittal and coronal spinal alignment (Figure 7A.1)
- Evaluate the patient's gait pattern and posture
  - A wide-based gait may indicate myelopathy or lumbar stenosis

Palpation

- Paraspinal muscles
  - Tenderness to palpation of the paraspinal muscles may be present in a patient with a paraspinal muscle strain
  - A palpable paraspinal muscle spasm may also be present in a patient suffering from a paraspinal strain

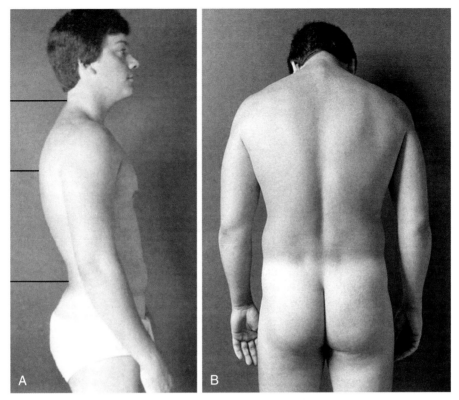

Figure 7A.1. Inspection and evaluation of patient's (A) sagittal and (B) coronal spinal alignment. (From Bickley LS, Szilagyi P. *Bates' Guide to Physical Examination and History Taking*. 8th ed. Philadelphia: Lippincott Williams & Wilkins; 2003.)

Range of Motion ▶ (Figure 7A.2)

- Cervical
  - Range restriction and/or painful movement may be present in a patient suffering from a muscle strain or a more severe neck injury
  - Average healthy range of motion:
    - Flexion = 58°
    - Extension = 56°
    - Lateral flexion = 45°
    - Axial rotation = 71°
- Lumbar
  - Range restriction and/or painful movement may be present in a patient suffering from a muscle strain or a more severe back injury
  - Average healthy range of motion:
    - Flexion = 52°
    - Extension = 20°
    - Lateral flexion = 30°
    - Axial rotation = 33°

Muscular Strength

- Normally graded 0 to 5 as follows:
  - Grade 0: no muscle contraction or movement
  - Grade 1: contraction of muscle but no movement at joint
  - Grade 2: movement at the joint with gravity eliminated

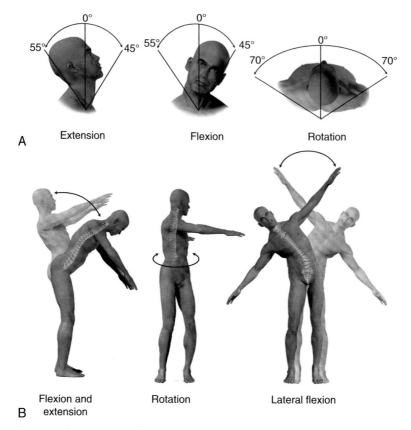

Figure 7A.2. Range of motion of the (A) cervical and (B) lumbar spine.

- • Grade 3: movement against gravity but not against added resistance
- • Grade 4: movement against added resistance but less strength than normal
- • Grade 5: normal strength
- Unilateral upper extremity weakness may represent cervical radiculopathy
- Unilateral lower extremity weakness may represent lumbar radiculopathy

Sensation

- Numbness/tingling
  - • Upper or lower extremity numbness/tingling may be unilateral or bilateral and may stem from myelopathic or radicular pathologies

KEY EXAMINATION MANEUVERS

- **Cervical and Thoracic Radiculopathy**
  - • Spurling maneuver
  - • Shoulder abduction relief test
  - • Manual neck distraction test
  - • Elvey upper limb tension test
  - • Valsalva maneuver

- **Cervical and Thoracic Myelopathy**
  - • Lhermitte sign
  - • Hoffman sign

- Plantar reflex
- Inverted brachioradialis reflex
- Ankle clonus

- **Cervical and Thoracic Strain**
  - Cervical range of motion
  - Paraspinal muscle palpation

- **Lumbar Radiculopathy**
  - Straight leg raise
  - Crossed straight leg raise
  - Muscle strength testing
  - Forward flexion
  - Achilles tendon reflex
  - Patellar tendon reflex

- **Lumbar Stenosis**
  - Romberg test
  - Gait evaluation
  - Spinal flexion
  - Spinal extension
  - Achilles tendon reflex
  - Pinprick test
  - Vibration test

- **Lumbar Strain**
  - Palpation of paraspinal musculature
  - Range of motion

- **Cauda Equina Syndrome**
  - Sensation testing
  - Anal sphincter tone
  - Anal wink reflex
  - Bulbocavernosus reflex
  - Lower extremity muscle strength testing
  - Achilles tendon reflex
  - Patellar tendon reflex

IMAGING

Plain Radiographs

- AP view (Figure 7A.3)
  - Coronal alignment
  - Fractures
  - Intervertebral disk space
  - Osteophytes
- Lateral view (Figure 7A.4)
  - Sagittal alignment
  - Fractures
  - Intervertebral disk space
  - Osteophytes
  - Spondylolisthesis

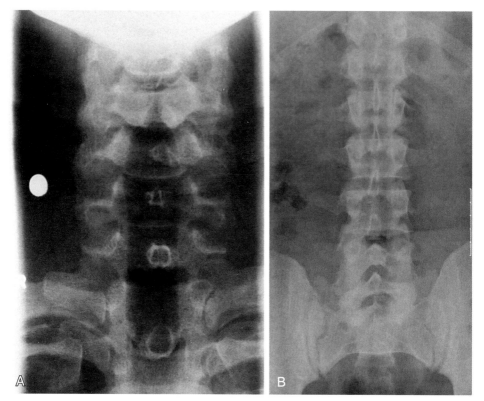

Figure 7A.3. Plain radiographs showing AP views of (A) cervical and (B) lumbar spine. ((A) Courtesy of Silzeski JC, DC, Denver, Colorado. (B) From Pope TL, Harris JH. *Harris & Harris' Radiology of Emergency Medicine.* Philadelphia: Wolters Kluwer; 2013.)

- Cervical flexion/extension views
  - Cervical spine instability

Magnetic Resonance Imaging

- Sagittal (Figure 7A.5A) and axial views (Figure 7A.5B)
  - Central canal stenosis
    - A classic "waist or "hourglass" figure on sagittal magnetic resonance imaging (MRI) is associated with cervical myelopathy and lumbar stenosis
  - Foraminal narrowing
    - Possible etiology of radiculopathy
  - Herniated disk
    - Classic finding with radiculopathy

Computed Tomography Myelography

- Computed tomography myelography (CTM) is indicated when evaluation with MRI is not possible or contraindicated
- CTM is superior to MRI for detecting bony abnormalities (Figure 7A.6)
  - For a symptomatic patient with no apparent pathology on MRI, further investigation with CTM may reveal an abnormality not previously detected on MRI
  - CTM provides a greater ability to distinguish narrowing due to soft tissue protrusion from narrowing due to osteophyte development

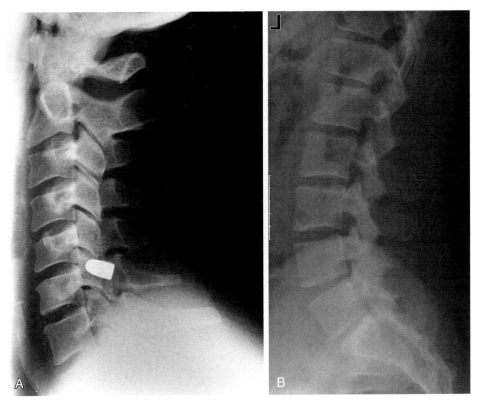

Figure 7A.4. Plain radiographs showing lateral views of (A) cervical and (B) lumbar spine. ((A) Courtesy of Silzeski JC, DC, Denver, Colorado. (B) From Pope TL, Harris JH. *Harris & Harris' Radiology of Emergency Medicine*. Philadelphia: Wolters Kluwer; 2013.)

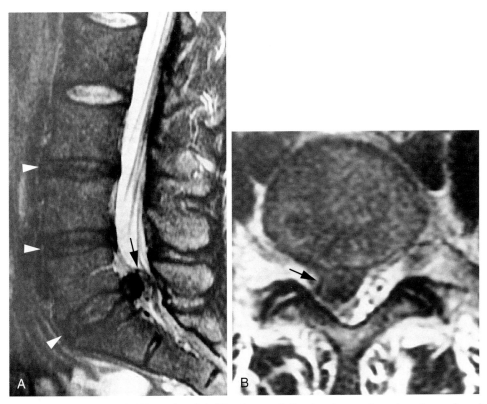

Figure 7A.5. MRI sagittal (A) and axial (B) views of the lumbar spine showing a herniated disk. Anterior bulging lumbar intervertebral disk (white arrowheads). Posterior Paracentral L5-S1 disk herniation (black arrows) (Courtesy of Alan ML. Las Vegas: Nevada.)

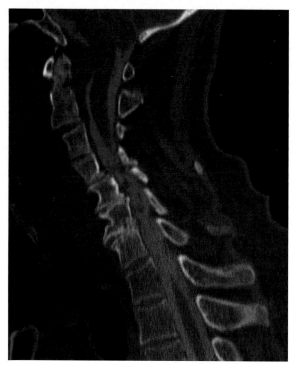

Figure 7A.6. CT myelogram of cervical spine showing spinal cord compression. (From Swiontkowski MF. *Manual of Orthopaedics*. Philadelphia: Wolters Kluwer; 2015.)

SECTION B
Cervical and Thoracic Radiculopathy

Jason A. Horowitz, Dimitri S. Tahal, Bayan Aghadasi, and Hamid Hassanzadeh

HISTORY

- Patients with cervical radiculopathy typically present with arm and neck pain
  - A classic presentation is "electric" or "shooting" pain radiating from the neck into the shoulder and down the upper extremity[1]
- 🔵 Upper extremity muscle weakness is also common
- Onset of symptoms may be acute or insidious depending on etiology
  - Disk herniation or trauma may present with acute onset of symptoms
  - Spondylosis usually presents with an insidious onset of symptoms

PHYSICAL EXAMINATION

KEY EXAMINATION MANEUVERS

- **Spurling Maneuver** 🔵 (Sensitivity: 0.47 acute, 0.15 chronic, Specificity: 0.85) (Figure 7B.1)
  - First described in the literature in 1944 by Spurling and Scoville[2]
  - There have been no significant modifications
  - **Maneuver:**
    - The patient is seated on the examination table
    - The examiner extends and rotates the patient's neck toward the affected side and applies downward pressure on the patient's head
    - If pain radiates into the upper limb the head is rotated toward, the test is positive
  - **Limitations of Maneuver:**
    - The Spurling maneuver should be avoided in patients who may have cervical instability to avoid further injury to the spine

- **Shoulder Abduction Relief Test** 🔵 (Sensitivity: 0.56 acute, 0.21 chronic, Specificity: 0.85) (Figure 7B.2)
  - First alluded to in a monograph published by Spurling in 1956[3]
  - Described in the literature by Davidson et al in 1981[3]
  - **Maneuver:**
    - The patient is seated on the examination table
    - The patient's shoulder is passively or actively abducted until the patient's hand rests on the top of the head
    - Ipsilateral relief or reduction of cervical radicular symptoms is a positive result

- **Manual Neck Distraction Test** 🔵 (Sensitivity: 0.43, Specificity: 1.00) (Figure 7B.3)
  - The origin of this maneuver is unknown[4]
  - There have been no significant modifications
  - **Maneuver:**
    - The patient is seated on the examination table

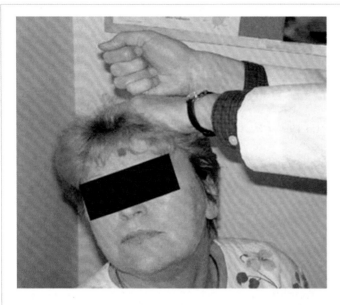

Figure 7B.1. Spurling maneuver. (From Lotke PA, Abboud JA, Ende J, Ovid Technologies I. *Lippincott's Primary Care Orthopaedics*. Philadelphia: Wolters Kluwer/Lippincott Williams & Wilkins Health; 2008.)

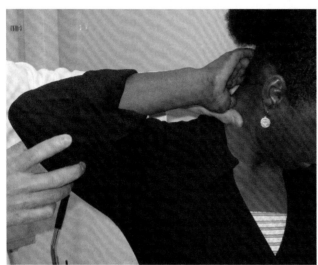

Figure 7B.2. Shoulder abduction relief test. (From Bridwell KH, DeWald RL, eds. *The Textbook of Spinal Surgery (2 Volumes)*. 3rd ed. Philadelphia: Wolters Kluwer/ Lippincott Williams & Wilkins Health; 2008.)

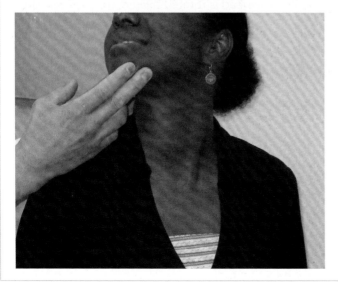

Figure 7B.3. Manual neck distraction test. (From Bridwell KH, DeWald RL, eds. *The Textbook of Spinal Surgery (2 Volumes)*. 3rd ed. Philadelphia: Wolters Kluwer/ Lippincott Williams & Wilkins Health; 2008.)

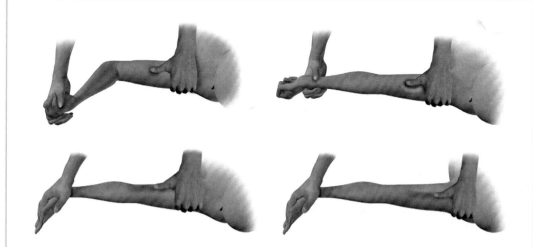

Figure 7B.4. Elvey upper limb tension test.

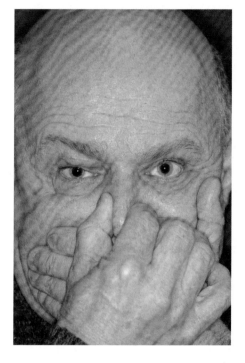

Figure 7B.5. Valsalva maneuver. (From Shields JA, Shields CL. *Eyelid, Conjunctival, and Orbital Tumors: An Atlas and Textbook.* 3rd ed. Philadelphia: Wolters Kluwer; 2016.)

  - The examiner grasps the patient's head beneath the mandible and occiput and applies axial traction
  - Relief or reduction of cervical radicular symptoms is a positive result

- **Elvey Upper Limb Tension Test** (Sensitivity: 0.60 acute, 0.35 chronic, Specificity: 0.85) (Figure 7B.4)
  - First described in the literature in 1979 by Elvey[5]
  - There have been no significant modifications
  - **Maneuver:**
    - The patient lies supine with the hand resting on the chest with the shoulder adducted, elbow flexed, and forearm pronated
    - One step at a time, the examiner abducts the patient's shoulder, then, extends the patient's elbow, and, lastly, supinates the patient's forearm.
    - Reproduction of radicular symptoms at any step in the maneuver is a positive result

- **Valsalva Maneuver** 🔊 (Figure 7B.5)
  - First described by an Italian anatomist Antonio Valsalva in 1704[6]

- **Maneuver:**
  - The patient is asked to attempt moderately forceful exhalation against a closed glottis
  - The test is positive if radicular symptoms are exacerbated

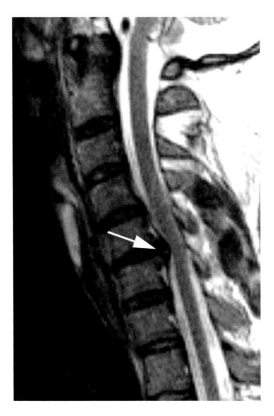

Figure 7B.6. T2-weighted, sagittal MRI showing the patient with a herniated disk (arrow) in the cervical spine resulting in cervical radiculopathy. (From Daffner RH, Hartman MS. *Clinical Radiology: The Essentials*. Philadelphia: Wolters Kluwer Health/Lippincott Williams & Wilkins; 2014.)

IMAGING

Magnetic Resonance Imaging

- MRI is the initial study of choice for evaluating patients with symptoms suggestive of cervical radiculopathy (Figure 7B.6)
  - Noninvasive
    - Contrast is generally not needed
    - No radiation exposure
  - MRI has similar sensitivity to CTM for identifying presence of narrowing

Computed Tomography Myelography

- CTM is indicated when evaluation with MRI is not possible or contraindicated
- CTM is superior to MRI for detecting bony abnormalities
  - For a symptomatic patient with no apparent pathology on MRI, further investigation with CTM may reveal an abnormality not previously detected on MRI[7]
  - CTM provides a greater ability to distinguish narrowing due to soft tissue protrusion from narrowing due to osteophyte development[8]

Plain Radiographs

- Rarely diagnostic of cervical radiculopathy in the absence of cervical trauma

REFERENCES

1. Woods BI, Hilibrand AS. Cervical radiculopathy: epidemiology, etiology, diagnosis, and treatment. *J Spinal Disord Tech*. 2015;28(5):E251-E259.
2. Spurling RG. Rupture of the cervical intervertebral disks. *J Int Coll Surg*. 1947;10(5):502-509.
3. Davidson RI, Dunn EJ, Metzmaker JN. The shoulder abduction test in the diagnosis of radicular pain in cervical extradural compressive monoradiculopathies. *Spine*. 1981;6(5):441-446.
4. Malanga GA, Landes P, Nadler SF. Provocative tests in cervical spine examination: historical basis and scientific analyses. *Pain Physician*. 2003;6(2):199-205.
5. Ghasemi M, Golabchi K, Mousavi SA, et al. The value of provocative tests in diagnosis of cervical radiculopathy. *J Res Med Sci*. 2013;18(suppl 1):S35-S38.
6. Jellinek EH. The Valsalva manoeuvre and Antonio Valsalva (1666-1723). *J R Soc Med*. 2006;99(9).
7. Modic MT, Masaryk TJ, Mulopulos GP, Bundschuh C, Han JS, Bohlman H. Cervical radiculopathy: prospective evaluation with surface coil MR imaging, CT with metrizamide, and metrizamide myelography. *Radiology*. 1986;161(3):753-759.
8. Yousem DM, Atlas SW, Goldberg HI, Grossman RI. Degenerative narrowing of the cervical spine neural foramina: evaluation with high-resolution 3DFT gradient-echo MR imaging. *AJNR*. 1991;12(2):229-236.

SECTION C
Cervical and Thoracic Myelopathy

Jason A. Horowitz, Dimitri S. Tahal, Nicolas Shen, Bayan Aghadasi, and Hamid Hassanzadeh

HISTORY

- Insidious onset of motor and/or sensory loss in the extremities, which may include the following:
  - Loss of dexterity
    - A classic patient complaint is clumsiness of the hands
    - Difficulty manipulating shirt buttons
    - Dropping items
  - Gait and balance problems
    - Patients may exhibit broad-based gait and difficulty with tandem gait
    - Patients may rely on holding onto objects around them for balance
- Pain
  - Unilateral or bilateral arm pain and/or neck pain may be present[1]

PHYSICAL EXAMINATION

KEY EXAMINATION MANEUVERS

- **Lhermitte Sign** ▶ (Sensitivity: 0.03-0.17, Specificity: 0.97) (Figure 7C.1)
  - First described in the literature in 1917 by Marie and Chatelin[2]
  - Elaborated on and linked to multiple sclerosis by Lhermitte et al in 1924[3]
  - **Maneuver:**
    - The patient is seated on the examination table
    - The examiner flexes the patient's neck anteriorly
    - Electrical sensations shooting down the spine or into the extremities on flexion is a positive result
  - **Limitations of Maneuver:**
    - Cervical flexion may be contraindicated in patients with history of cervical pathology or possible cervical injury

- **Hoffman Sign** ▶ (Sensitivity: 0.59, Specificity: 0.84) (Figure 7C.2)
  - First described in the literature in 1911 by Curschmann, a former pupil of Hoffman[4]
  - There have been no significant modifications
  - **Maneuver:**
    - The patient is seated on the examination table
    - The patient's hand is pronated
    - The patient is asked to completely relax the hand with fingers partially flexed
    - The examiner grasps the middle phalanx of the patient's third digit between the examiner's first and second digits

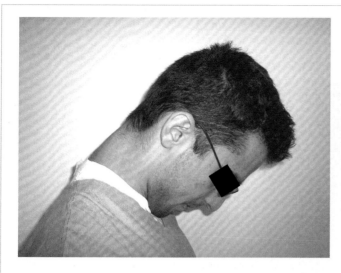

Figure 7C.1. Lhermitte sign. (From Lotke PA, Abboud JA, Ende J, Ovid Technologies I. *Lippincott's Primary Care Orthopaedics*. Philadelphia: Wolters Kluwer/Lippincott Williams & Wilkins Health; 2008.)

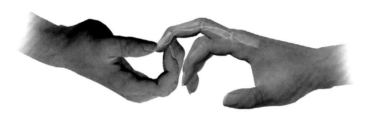

Figure 7C.2. Hoffman sign.

- The examiner flicks or snaps the nail or the distal end of the terminal phalanx of the patient's third digit
- Flexion of the ipsilateral first and second digits is a positive result, indicating upper motor neuron pathology

- **Plantar Reflex** 🎥 (Sensitivity: 0.13, Specificity: 1.00) (Figure 7C.3)
  - First reported after spinal cord transection in rabbits by Grainger in 1837[5]
  - Described in humans in 1896 and then linked to disturbances of the pyramidal tract in 1898 by Babinski[5]
  - **Maneuver:**
    - The patient is seated on the examination table
    - The examiner strokes the lateral side of the sole of the patient's foot from heel to toes with a narrow, blunt instrument
    - Extension of the hallux and abduction of the toes, known as Babinski sign, is a positive result

- **Inverted Brachioradialis Reflex** 🎥 (Sensitivity: 0.51, Specificity: 0.81) (Figure 7C.4)
  - First described in the literature by Babinski in 1910[6]
  - There have been no significant modifications
  - **Maneuver:**
    - The patient is seated on the examination table
    - With the patient's hand relaxed, the examiner strikes the patient's brachioradialis tendon just proximal to its insertion into the radial styloid process
    - Flexion of the fingers is a positive result

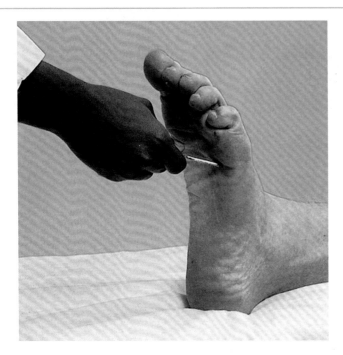

Figure 7C.3. Plantar reflex. (From Bickley LS, Szilagyi P. *Bates' Guide to Physical Examination and History Taking.* 8th ed. Philadelphia: Lippincott Williams & Wilkins; 2003.)

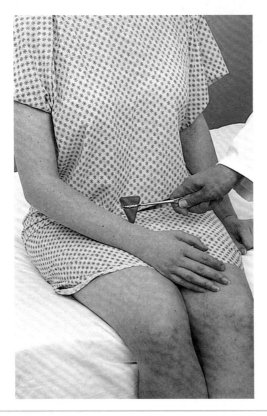

Figure 7C.4. Inverted brachioradialis reflex. (From Weber J, Kelley J. *Health Assessment in Nursing.* Wolters Kluwer Health; 2014.)

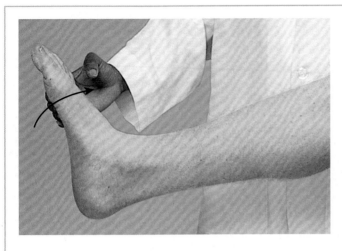

Figure 7C.5. Ankle clonus. (From Bickley LS, Szilagyi PG, Hoffman RM, Bickley LS. *Bates' Pocket Guide to Physical Examination and History Taking*. Wolters Kluwer Health; 2017.)

- **Ankle Clonus** 🔘 (Sensitivity: 0.13, Specificity: 1.00) (Figure 7C.5)
  - **Maneuver:**
    - The patient is seated on the examination table
    - The patient is asked to completely relax the leg, ankle, and foot
    - The examiner rapidly and forcefully dorsiflexes the patient's foot
    - Rhythmic beating of the ankle, alternating between flexion and extension, is a positive result

IMAGING

Magnetic Resonance Imaging

- MRI is the initial study of choice for evaluating patients with symptoms suggestive of cervical myelopathy (Figure 7C.6)
  - Noninvasive
    - Contrast is generally not needed
    - No radiation exposure
  - Allows for measurement of the anterior-posterior diameter of the cervical canal[7]
    - Normal AP canal diameter is approximately 17 mm
      - for >16 mm, cervical spondylotic myelopathy is unlikely
    - 10 to 13 mm represents relative stenosis
      - for 10 to 13 mm, the risk of cervical spondylotic myelopathy is increased
    - <10 mm is absolute stenosis
      - for <10 mm, cervical spondylotic myelopathy is probable
  - Greater intramedullary spinal cord detail than CTM
    - Areas of spinal cord hypointensity on T1-weighted and hyperintensity on T2-weighted images can indicate disease
    - High incidence of MRI abnormalities in the asymptomatic elderly population
      - MRI abnormalities in the elderly need to be viewed in the context of the patient's clinical presentation[8]

Computed Tomography Myelography

- Indicated for patients for whom MRI is contraindicated
- Superior to MRI in detecting bony abnormalities

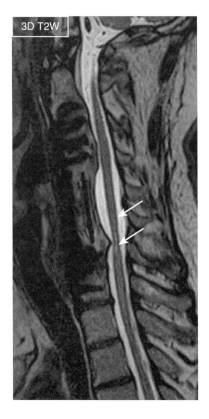

3D T2W

Figure 7C.6. T2-weighted, sagittal MRI showing cervical myelomalacia. Arrows showing areas white color change within the spinal cord signifying myelomalacia from stenosis, trauma, bruising, hemorrhage or edema of the spinal cord. (From Chhabra A, Soldatos T. *Musculoskeletal MRI Structured Evaluation: How to Practically Fill the Reporting Checklist.* Wolters Kluwer Health; 2015.)

- For a symptomatic patient with a normal MRI, further investigation with CTM may detect an abnormality not seen on MRI
- Better ability to distinguish narrowing due to soft tissue protrusion from narrowing due to osteophyte development

REFERENCES

1. Toledano M, Bartleson JD. Cervical spondylotic myelopathy. *Neurol Clin.* 2013;31(1):287-305.
2. Cuellar JM, Passias PG. Cervical spondylotic myelopathy a review of clinical diagnosis and treatment. *Bull Hosp Jt Dis.* 2017;75:21-19.
3. Lhermitte J, Bollak A, Nicholas M. Les douleurs a type de decharge electrique consecutives a la Flexion cephalique dans la sclerose en plaques. Un cas de forme sensitive de la sclerose multiple. *Revue Neurologique.* 1924;2:56-62.
4. Malanga GA, Landes P, Nadler SF. Provocative tests in cervical spine examination: historical basis and scientific analyses. *Pain Physician.* 2003;6(2):199-205.
5. Bassetti C. Babinski and Babinski sign. *Spine.* 1995;20(23):2591-2594.
6. Babinski J. Inversion du reflexe du radius. *Bulletin et Memoires de la Societe de Medecine des H6pitaux de Paris.* 1910;30:185-186.
7. Edwards WC, LaRocca H. The developmental segmental sagittal diameter of the cervical spinal canal in patients with cervical spondylosis. *Spine.* 1983;8(1):20-27.
8. Teresi LM, Lufkin RB, Reicher MA, et al. Asymptomatic degenerative disk disease and spondylosis of the cervical spine: MR imaging. *Radiology.* 1987;164:83-88.

SECTION D
Cervical and Thoracic Strain

Bayan Aghadasi, Jason A. Horowitz, Dimitri S. Tahal, Nicholas Shen, and Hamid Hassanzadeh

HISTORY

- Patients with cervical or thoracic strain often complain of pain, stiffness, and/or tightness in the neck, upper back, or shoulder
- No associated signs of symptoms of neurologic dysfunction should be present[1]
- There may be an inciting incident
  - Often the underlying cause is nontraumatic, such as poor posture or sleeping position

PHYSICAL EXAMINATION

KEY EXAMINATION MANEUVERS

- **Cervical Range of Motion** (Figure 7D.1)
  - **Maneuver:**
    - Assess active and passive flexion, extension, lateral bending, and rotation of the neck
      - Average healthy range of motion[2]
        - Flexion = 58°
        - Extension = 56°
        - Lateral flexion = 45°
        - Axial rotation = 71°
    - Range restriction and/or painful movement may be present in a patient with cervical strain
  - **Limitations of Maneuver:**
    - Cervical range of motion restriction and painful movement are not specific to cervical strain and may be present in a number of other more serious injuries
    - Movement of the cervical spine is contraindicated if there is any reason to suspect cervical instability

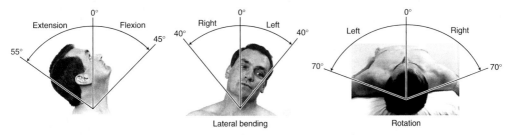

Figure 7D.1. Cervical range of motion. (From Jones RM, Jones RM. *Patient Assessment in Pharmacy Practice.* Wolters Kluwer Health; 2016.)

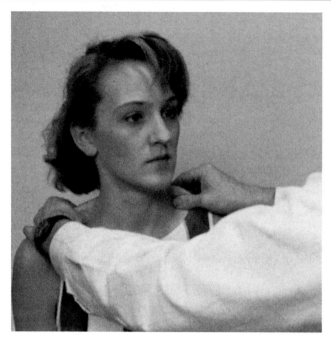

Figure 7D.2. Paraspinal muscle palpation. (From Hertling D, Kessler RM. *Management of Common Musculoskeletal Disorders: Physical Therapy Principles and Methods.* Philadelphia: Lippincott Williams & Wilkins; 2006.)

- **Paraspinal Muscle Palpation** (Figure 7D.2)
  - **Maneuver:**
    - Firmly palpate the paraspinal muscles of the neck and the trapezius
    - Findings of tenderness to palpation and/or palpable muscle spasm are supportive of a diagnosis of cervical strain
  - **Limitations of Maneuver:**
    - Findings of paraspinal tenderness to palpation and/or muscle spasm are not specific to cervical strain and may be present in a number of more serious injuries

IMAGING

- Imaging is not indicated for acute nontraumatic neck pain without neurologic symptoms[1]
- If trauma or neurologic symptoms are present, other diagnoses should be considered

REFERENCES

1. Cohen SP. Epidemiology, diagnosis, and treatment of neck pain. *Mayo Clin Proc.* 2015;90:284-299.
2. Cobian DG, Daehn NS, Anderson PA, Heiderscheit BC. Active cervical and lumbar range of motion during performance of activities of daily living in healthy young adults. *Spine.* 2013;38:1754-1763.

SECTION E
Lumbar Radiculopathy

Dimitri S. Tahal, Jason A. Horowitz, Bayan Aghadasi, and Hamid Hassanzadeh

HISTORY

- Lumbar disk herniation is the most common cause of an irritated nerve root causing radiculopathy
- Other causes include degenerative changes, tumors, and spinal stenosis
- Patients will present with low-back pain radiating unilaterally or bilaterally into the lower extremity with or without weakness, motor dysfunction, and sensory alteration in a dermatomal distribution[1]
- The associated pain is usually provoked by standing and activity and relieved by sitting
- Radiculopathy due to lumbar disk herniation can present acutely in younger patients, as well as in older patients, with a history of heavy lifting or significant trauma
- Radiculopathy due to degenerative osteoarthritic changes in older patients may or may not be associated with a specific inciting event

PHYSICAL EXAMINATION

KEY EXAMINATION MANEUVERS

- **Straight Leg Raise (Lasègue Sign)** (Sensitivity: 64% [56%-71%], Specificity: 57% [47%-66%]) (Figure 7E.1)
  - First described in the literature in 1881 by JJ Forst, a student of Lasègue[2]
  - A number of variations have been described including the seated straight leg raise and the crossed straight leg raise[3]
  - **Maneuver:**
    - The patient is positioned lying supine
    - The examiner lifts the patient's problematic leg by holding at the posterior ankle while the knee is kept in full extension
    - The examiner continues lifting the leg up the arc with passive flexion of the hip
    - If positive, the patient feels pain in the lower back or posterior aspect of the ipsilateral leg between 30° to 70° of hip flexion
  - **Limitations of Maneuver:**
    - The seated variation of this examination involves the examiner lifting the patient's leg while the patient is sitting, instead of supine, but this reduces the sensitivity of the test

- **Crossed Straight Leg Raise** (Sensitivity: 28% [22%-35%], Specificity: 90% [85%-94%]) (Figure 7E.2)
  - First described in the literature in 1901 by Fajersztajn[4]
  - There have been no significant modifications

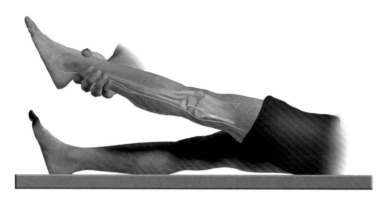

Figure 7E.1. Straight leg raise (Lasègue sign).

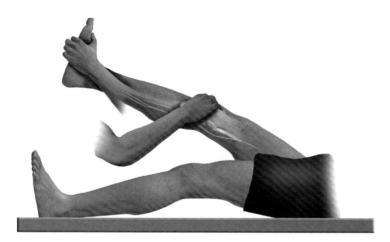

Figure 7E.2. Crossed straight leg raise.

- **Maneuver:**
  - The patient is positioned lying supine
  - The examiner lifts the patient's pain-free leg by holding at the posterior ankle while the knee is kept in full extension
  - The examiner continues lifting the leg up the arc with passive flexion of the hip
  - If positive, the patient feels pain in the lower back or posterior side of the problematic leg between 30° to 70° of hip flexion

- **Muscle Strength Testing** (Sensitivity: 27% [20%-37%], Specificity: 93% [88%-97%]) (Figure 7E.3)
  - First described in the literature in 1912 by Wright[5]
  - Expanded upon in 1916 by Lovett[6]
  - Significant modifications, including refinement of testing positions, in 1946 by Daniels and Worthington and in 1949 by F. Kendall and H. Kendall[7,8]
  - **Maneuver:**
    - Assess strength of dorsiflexion and extension of the great toe on the problematic side and compare with the strength of the contralateral side
    - If positive, weakness will be noted on the problematic side

- **Forward Flexion** (Sensitivity: 45% [37%-53%], Specificity: 74% [65%-81%]) (Figure 7E.4)
  - **Maneuver:**
    - From a standing position, ask the patient to bend forward
    - If positive, pain will be elicited

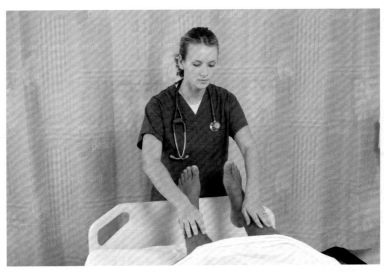

Figure 7E.3. Muscle strength testing. (From Springhouse. *Lippincott's Visual Encyclopedia of Clinical Skills*. Philadelphia: Wolters Kluwer Health; 2009.)

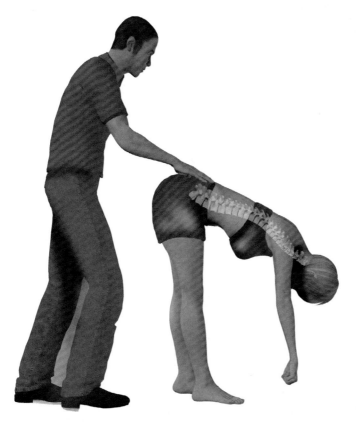

Figure 7E.4. Forward flexion.

● **Achilles Tendon Reflex** (Sensitivity: 15% [9%-21%], Specificity: 93% [88%-97%]) (Figure 7E.5)
  • Deep tendon reflexes were first described in the literature in 1875 by Erb and Westphal.[9] However, they were already well known and in wide use at the time of publication
  • There have been no significant modifications

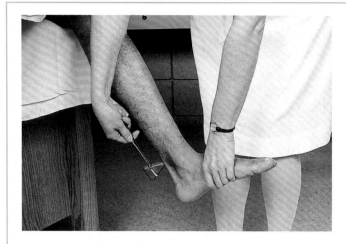

Figure 7E.5. Achilles tendon reflex. (From Taylor CR, Lillis C, LeMone P, et al. *Fundamentals of Nursing, The Art And Science Of Nursing Care*. 6th ed. Philadelphia: Lippincott Williams & Wilkins; 2008.)

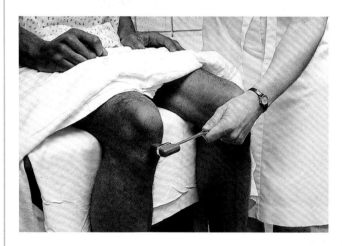

Figure 7E.6. Patellar tendon reflex. (From Taylor CR, Lillis C, LeMone P, et al. *Fundamentals of Nursing, The Art And Science Of Nursing Care*. 6th ed. Philadelphia: Lippincott Williams & Wilkins; 2008.)

- **Maneuver:**
  - The patient should be sitting with the leg hanging freely
  - The Achilles tendon is struck with a reflex hammer while holding the relaxed foot to elicit the reflex contraction of the calf muscles
  - The test should be performed on the contralateral leg for comparison
  - An impaired reflex is positive
- **Patellar Tendon Reflex** 🔘 (Sensitivity: 15% [9%-21%], Specificity: 75% [55%-89%]) (Figure 7E.6)
  - Deep tendon reflexes were first described in the literature in 1875 by Erb and Westphal. However, they were already well known and in wide use at the time of publication
  - There have been no significant modifications
  - **Maneuver:**
    - The patient should be sitting with the leg hanging freely
    - The patellar tendon is struck with a reflex hammer to elicit the reflex contraction of the quadriceps
    - The test should be performed on the contralateral leg for comparison
    - An impaired reflex is positive

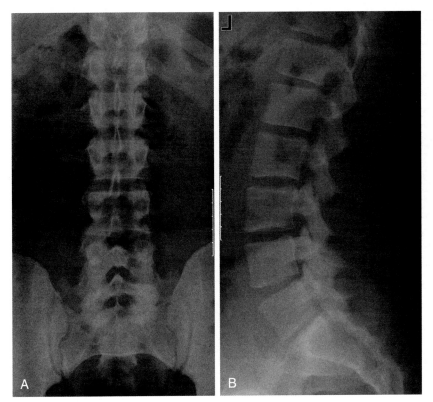

Figure 7E.7. Plain radiographs: AP (A) and lateral (B) views of the lumbar spine. (From Pope TL, Harris JH, Harris JH. *Harris & Harris' Radiology of Emergency Medicine.* Wolters Kluwer Health; 2013.)

IMAGING

- It is acceptable to forego imaging initially and undergo a trial of conservative management, unless the patient presents with symptoms concerning for a more serious injury. In the absence of these concerns, it is possible for the radiculopathy to resolve with conservative management. However, abnormal neurologic signs or symptoms without improvement for more than 4 to 6 weeks should be evaluated with imaging[10]

Plain Radiographs

- Initial imaging choice
- AP (Figure 7E.7A) and lateral (Figure 7E.7B) views are recommended to assess overall alignment of the spine, fractures, bone quality, intervertebral disk space, and osteophytes
- Flexion and extension views to demonstrate instability[11]

Magnetic Resonance Imaging

- Follow-up imaging to further assess the soft tissue surrounding the spinal cord and nerves
- Classic disk herniation:
  - Typically, central or posterolateral causing nerve compression (Figure 7E.8)
    - Better seen on axial images
  - Sagittal images are useful to narrow down the affected levels

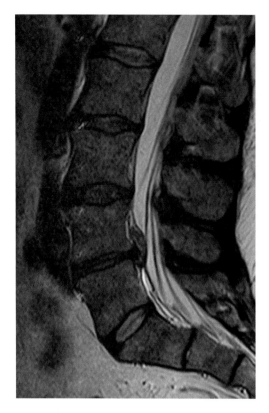

Figure 7E.8. T2-weighted, sagittal MRI showing lumbar disk herniation at the L4-L5 level resulting in radiculopathy. (From Greenspan A, Gershwin ME. *Imaging in Rheumatology: A Clinical Approach.* Wolters Kluwer Health; 2018.)

- Herniated disks usually appear as follows:
  - Intermediate intensity on T1W images
  - If acute, high intensity on T2W images
  - If chronic, low intensity on T2W images
- Lateral disk herniation:
  - Extraforaminal nerve compression is best seen on axial images
- Other findings associated with radiculopathy include the following:
  - Facet joint hypertrophy/arthropathy
  - Spine lesions
  - Cysts
  - Epidural abscesses (Figure 7E.9)
  - Tumors

Computed Tomography Myelography

- CTM is indicated when evaluation with MRI is not possible or contraindicated
  - CTM is superior to MRI for detecting bony abnormalities
    - For a symptomatic patient with no apparent pathology on MRI, further investigation with CTM may reveal an abnormality not previously detected on MRI[12]
    - CTM provides a greater ability to distinguish narrowing due to soft tissue protrusion from narrowing due to osteophyte development (Figure 7E.10)

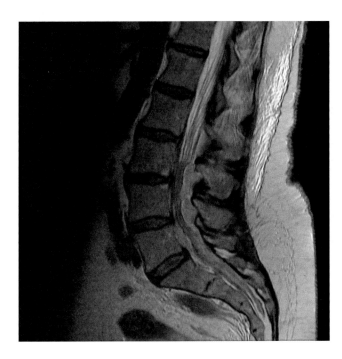

Figure 7E.9. T2-weighted, sagittal MRI showing large epidural abscess. (From Rathmell JP, Nelson GJ. *Atlas of Image-Guided Intervention in Regional Anesthesia and Pain Medicine: Incl. Fully Searchable Text and Image Bank.* 2nd ed. Philadelphia: Wolters Kluwer, Lippincott Williams & Wilkins; 2012.)

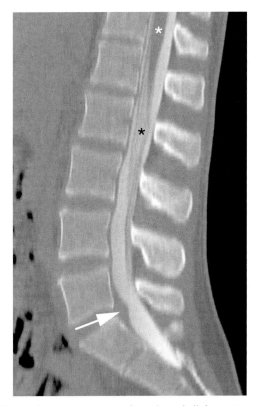

Figure 7E.10. Sagittal CT myelogram shows a herniated disk compressing the contrast-filled thecal sac (arrow). Conus medullaris (white asterisk). Cauda equina in CSF (black asterisk). (From Daffner RH. *Clinical Radiology: The Essentials.* 3rd ed. Philadelphia: Wolters Kluwer/Lippincott Williams & Wilkins; 2007.)

REFERENCES

1. Vroomen PC, de Krom MC, Knottnerus JA. Diagnostic value of history and physical examination in patients suspected of sciatica due to disc herniation: a systematic review. *J Neurol.* 1999;246(10):899-906.
2. Forst JJ, Contribution à l'étude clinique de La sciatique. *Paris These.* 1881;33.
3. van der Windt DA, Simons E, Riphagen II, et al. Physical examination for lumbar radiculopathy due to disc herniation in patients with low-back pain. *Cochrane Database Syst Rev.* 2010;(2):CD007431.
4. Fajersztajn J. Ueber das gekreuzte Ischiasph#{228}nomen. *Wiener klinische Wochenschrift.* 1901;14:41-47.
5. Wright W. Muscle training in the treatment of infantile paralysis. *Boston Med Surg J.* 1912;167(17):567-574.
6. Lovett R. Certain aspects of infantile paralysis. *JAMA.* 1916;LXVI(10):729.
7. Daniels L, Williams M, Worthington C. *Muscle Testing Techniques of Manual Examination.* Philadelphia: W. B. Saunders Company; 1946.
8. Kendall HO, Kendall FP, Wadsworth G. *Muscles: Testing and Function.* 1st ed. Baltimore: Williams and Wilkins; 1949.
9. Louis E. Erb and Westphal: simultaneous discovery of the deep tendon reflexes. *Semin Neurol.* 2002;22(4):385-390.
10. Hooten WM, Cohen SP. Evaluation and treatment of low back pain: a clinically focused review for primary care specialists. *Mayo Clin Proc.* 2015;90(12):1699-1718.
11. DeFroda SF, Daniels AH, Deren ME. Differentiating radiculopathy from lower extremity arthropathy. *Am J Med.* 2016;129(10):1124.
12. Chou R, Fu R, Carrino JA, Deyo RA. Imaging strategies for low-back pain: systematic review and meta-analysis. *Lancet.* 2009;373(9662):463-472.

SECTION F
Lumbar Stenosis

*Dimitri S. Tahal, Jason A. Horowitz, Bayan Aghadasi, and
Hamid Hassanzadeh*

HISTORY

- Lumbar stenosis is most commonly due to degenerative changes in the elderly (age >65 years)
- Other causes are congenital/developmental, traumatic, postoperative, metabolic/endocrine, or skeletal diseases/disorders[1]
- The commonality is a narrowing of the lumbar central canal, the subarticular canal/lateral recess, and/or intervertebral foramen/nerve root canal
- Lumbar stenosis usually presents as low-back pain with radiculopathy to unilateral or bilateral buttocks or legs depending on the location of stenosis, but the definitive symptom is neurogenic claudication[1]
- Neurogenic claudication is characterized as a poorly localized leg pain, which is exacerbated by postures that maintain or increase the degree of lumbar lordosis, such as in standing or spinal extension, and which is relieved by postures that decrease the degree of lumbar lordosis, such as sitting or spinal flexion[1]
- There will be a progressive reduction in time walking before pain is brought on
- There may also be motor or sensory dysfunction likely located in the same anatomic distribution as the radicular pain
- Patients with more severe cases of stenosis are likely to walk bend forward with a wide-based gait

PHYSICAL EXAMINATION

KEY EXAMINATION MANEUVERS

- **Romberg Test** (Sensitivity: 39% [24%-54%], Specificity: 91% [81%-100%]) (Figure 7F.1)
  - First described in the literature in 1846 by Romberg[2]
  - Variations with semitandem and tandem feet positions have been described
  - **Maneuver:**
    - Stand near the patients to prevent them from falling if they lose their balance
    - Ask the patients to stand, bring their feet close together, and close their eyes
    - If positive, the patients become unsteady, have problems standing erect, and may lose their balance when they close their eyes

- **Gait Evaluation** 🔄 (Sensitivity: 43% [28%-58%], Specificity: 97% [91%-100%]) (Figure 7F.2)
  - Gait changes after injury were first described in the literature approximately 1600 bc in the ancient Egyptian medical text, Edwin Smith Papyrus
  - Over time, gait analysis has been elaborated on by Aristotle, Borelli, Parkinson, Trendelenburg, and many others

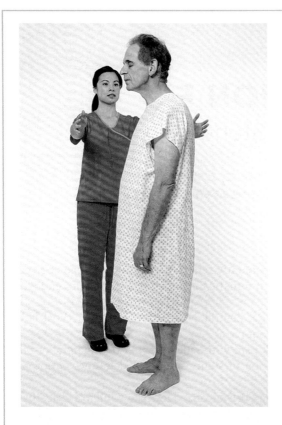

Figure 7F.1. Romberg test. (From Weber J, Kelley J. *Health Assessment in Nursing*. Wolters Kluwer Health; 2014.)

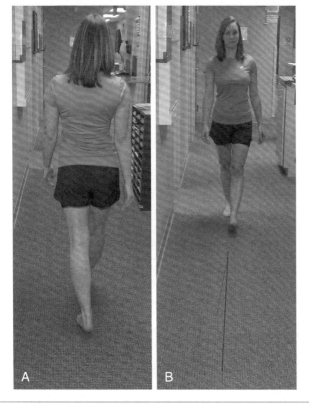

A

B

Figure 7F.2. Gait evaluation. A, Patient walking away from physician while her gait is assessed for antalgic gait, ataxia, and instability. B, Patient walking towards physician for the same evaluation. (From Callaghan JJ. *The Adult Hip: Hip Arthroplasty Surgery*. Wolters Kluwer Health; 2016.)

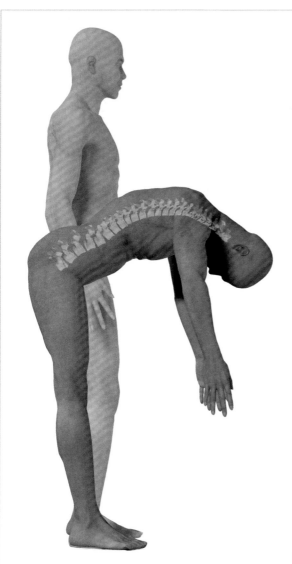

Figure 7F.3. Spinal flexion.

- **Maneuver:**
  - Ask the patients to walk a short distance and observe their gait
  - If positive, the patients will walk with a wide-based gait and may appear unsteady as they walk

- **Spinal Flexion** (Sensitivity: 79% [67%-91%], Specificity: 44% [27%-61%]) (Figure 7F.3)
  - **Maneuver:**
    - From a standing position, ask the patient to bend forward
    - If positive, the patient will have pain while standing, and forward flexion of the spine will relieve the pain to some extent causing the patient to feel better

- **Spinal Extension** (Sensitivity: 51% [36%-66%], Specificity: 69% [53%-85%]) (Figure 7F.4)
  - **Maneuver:**
    - From a standing position, ask the patient to bend backward
    - If positive, the patient will have pain while standing, and extension of the spine will exacerbate the pain to some extent causing the patient to feel worse

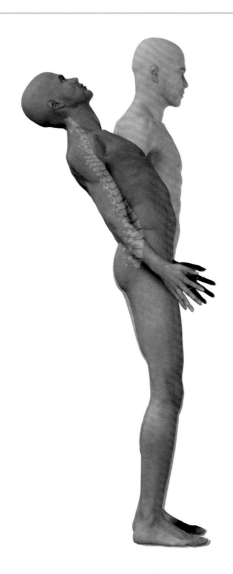

Figure 7F.4. Spinal extension.

- **Achilles Tendon Reflex** (Sensitivity: 46% [31%-61%], Specificity: 78% [64%-92%]) (Figure 7F.5)
  - Deep tendon reflexes were first described in the literature in 1875 by Erb and Westphal. However, they were already well known and in wide use at the time of publication[3]
  - There have been no significant modifications
  - **Maneuver:**
    - The patient should be sitting with the leg hanging freely
    - The Achilles tendon is struck with a reflex hammer while holding the relaxed foot to elicit the reflex contraction of the calf muscles
    - The test should be performed on the contralateral leg for comparison
    - An absent reflex is positive

- **Pinprick Test** (Sensitivity: 47% [32%-62%], Specificity: 81% [67%-95%]) (Figure 7F.6)
  - **Maneuver:**
    - Perform pinprick sensation testing bilaterally on the medial and lateral calves and feet
    - Reduced pinprick sensation compared with higher parts of the body is positive

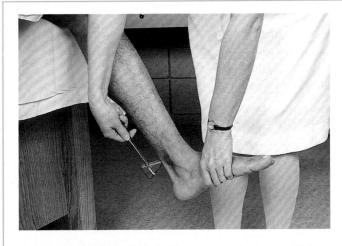

Figure 7F.5. Achilles tendon reflex. (From Taylor CR, Lillis C, LeMone P, et al. *Fundamentals of Nursing, The Art And Science Of Nursing Care*. 6th ed. Philadelphia: Lippincott Williams & Wilkins; 2008.)

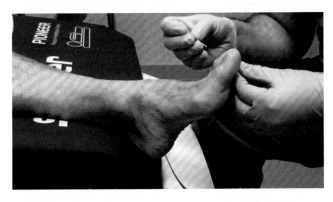

Figure 7F.6. Pinprick test.

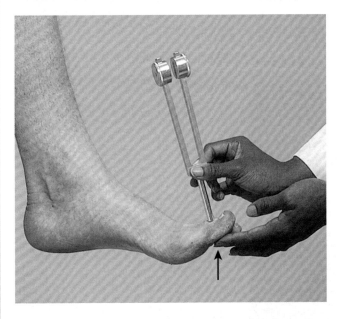

Figure 7F.7. Vibration test. (From Jensen S. *Nursing Health Assessment: A Best Practice Approach*. Philadelphia, Pennsylvania: Wolters Kluwer/Lippincott Williams & Wilkins Health; 2011.)

- **Vibration Test** (Sensitivity: 53% [38%-68%], Specificity: 81% [67%-95%]) (Figure 7F.7)
  - First described in the literature in 1889 by Rumpf[4]
  - There have been no significant modifications
  - **Maneuver:**
    - Perform vibration sensation testing using a tuning fork bilaterally on the lower extremities
    - Reduced vibration sensation compared with higher parts of the body is positive

IMAGING

Plain Radiographs

- MRI is first-line imaging, but plain radiographs are helpful for evaluation of gross bony changes[5]
  - Fractures
  - Bone quality
  - Intervertebral disk height
  - Osteophytes
  - Spinal instability
- Recommended views: lower lumbar centered, AP, lateral and flexion-extension views

Magnetic Resonance Imaging

- First-line imaging for lumbar stenosis (Figure 7F.8)
- Most frequent location is L4-L5 with the levels above and below the other main contributors
- Classic findings:
  - Smoothly marginated "waist" or "hourglass" configuration on sagittal images
  - Triangular or "trefoil" shape on axial images
- Central canal stenosis[6]:
  - Circumferentially narrowed canal on axial MRI images
  - Facet join hypertrophy appears as dark region of low signal on T1W and T2W images
  - Ligamentum flavum hypertrophy appears as an intermediate signal on T1W and T2W images
  - Epidural space fat loss appears as a loss of high T1 signal
- Lateral stenosis:
  - Bone encroachment and loss of fat signal best seen on T1W axial and sagittal images
- Other findings:
  - Multilevel disk degeneration
  - Spondylolisthesis

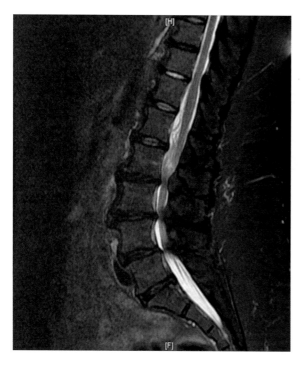

Figure 7F.8. T2-weighted, sagittal MRI showing lumbar stenosis with intervertebral disk protrusion. (From Lotke PA, Abboud JA, Ende J, Ovid Technologies I. *Lippincott's Primary Care Orthopaedics*. Philadelphia: Wolters Kluwer/Lippincott Williams & Wilkins Health; 2008.)

- Decreased ratio of CSF:nerve roots
- Nerve root enhancement is a sign of injury

Computed Tomography Myelography

- CTM is indicated when evaluation with MRI is not possible or contraindicated
- CTM is superior to MRI for detecting bony abnormalities
  - For a symptomatic patient with no apparent pathology on MRI, further investigation with CTM may reveal an abnormality not previously detected on MRI
  - CTM provides a greater ability to distinguish narrowing due to soft tissue protrusion from narrowing due to osteophyte development

REFERENCES

1. Issack PS, Cunningham ME, Pumberger M, Hughes AP, Cammisa Jr FP. Degenerative lumbar spinal stenosis: evaluation and management. *J Am Acad Orthop Surg.* 2012;20(8):527-535. doi:10.5435/JAAOS-20-08-527 [PMID:22855855].
2. Henoch E, Romberg HM. *Klinische Ergebnisse.* Berlin: A. Forstner (pub.); 1846:75-81.
3. Louis E. Erb and Westphal: simultaneous discovery of the deep tendon reflexes. *Semin Neurol.* 2002;22(4):385-390.
4. Rumpf H. *Uber einen Fall von Syringomyelie nebst Beitrag zur Untersuchung der Sensibilitat.* Neurologisches Zentralblatt; 1889.
5. Patrick N, Emanski E, Knaub MA. Acute and chronic low back pain. *Med Clin North Am.* 2016;100(1):169-181. doi:10.1016/j.mcna.2015.08.015 [PMID:26614726].
6. Katz JN, Harris MB. Clinical practice: lumbar spinal stenosis. *N Engl J Med.* 2008;358(8):818-825.

SECTION G
Lumbar Strain

Dimitri S. Tahal, Jason A. Horowitz, Nicholas Shen, Bayan Aghadasi, and Hamid Hassanzadeh

HISTORY

- Diffuse lumbosacral lower-back pain can present suddenly after an inciting incident or may be delayed by 1 to 2 days
- Commonly, the patient would report lifting a heavy object likely with poor form (excessive lower back curvature) or present with a history of trauma such as a fall or a motor vehicle accident
- Another common cause is participation in sport activities involving repetitive movements, pulling, pushing, or spinal torsion
- Pain is worse with activity or bending
- There is no radiation of pain to the lower extremities[1]
- Patients may present with tenderness to palpation of the lower back area with/without spasms[2]

PHYSICAL EXAMINATION

KEY EXAMINATION MANEUVERS

- **Palpation of Paraspinal Musculature** (Figure 7G.1)
  - **Maneuver:**
    - Firmly palpate the musculature on both sides of the lumbar spine to elicit signs of tenderness
    - Direct palpation of the spinous processes should not elicit or enhance pain unless a more serious pathology is present

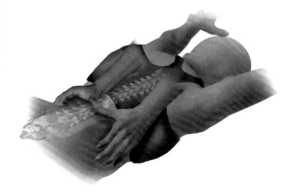

Figure 7G.1. Palpation of paraspinal musculature.

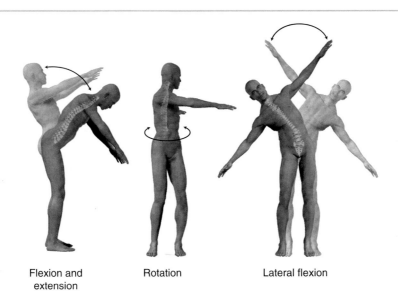

Flexion and
extension   Rotation   Lateral flexion

Figure 7G.2. Lumbar range of motion.

- **Assess Range of Motion** (Figure 7G.2)
  - **Maneuver:**
    - Assess active and passive flexion, extension, lateral bending, and rotation of the neck
      - Average healthy range of motion[4]:
        - Flexion = 52°
        - Extension = 20°
        - Lateral flexion = 30°
        - Axial rotation = 33°
    - Range restriction and/or painful movement may be present in a patient with lumbar strain

IMAGING

- Imaging is not usually indicated unless the patient presents with any red flag signs or experiences symptoms lasting for more than 4 to 6 weeks, which may indicate more serious pathology.[3] In the absence of these concerns, if imaging is undertaken, it is possible for it to show abnormal findings unrelated to the patient's symptoms

REFERENCES

1. Patrick N, Emanski E, Knaub MA. Acute and chronic low back pain. *Med Clin North Am.* 2016;100(1):169-181. doi:10.1016/j.mcna.2015.08.015 [PMID:26614726].
2. Hooten WM, Cohen SP. Evaluation and treatment of low back pain: a clinically focused review for primary care specialists. *Mayo Clin Proc.* 2015;90(12):1699-1718. doi:10.1016/j.mayocp.2015.10.009 [PMID:26653300].
3. Chou R, Fu R, Carrino JA, Deyo RA. Imaging strategies for low-back pain: systematic review and meta-analysis. *Lancet.* 2009;373(9662):463-472.
4. Cobian DG, Daehn NS, Anderson PA, Heiderscheit BC. Active cervical and lumbar range of motion during performance of activities of daily living in healthy young adults. *Spine.* 2013;38:1754-1763.

SECTION H
Cauda Equina Syndrome

Dimitri S. Tahal, Jason A. Horowitz, Bayan Aghadasi, and Hamid Hassanzadeh

HISTORY

- CES is characterized by bladder, bowel, and/or sexual dysfunction together with perianal and saddle numbness[1,3]
- CES can be classified into complete and incomplete:
  - Complete CES: saddle numbness plus retention/incontinence of bladder or bowel[1]
  - Incomplete CES: saddle numbness plus incomplete progression of bladder and bowel retention/incontinence[1]
- Other nondefining symptoms that may be present include back pain with or without radiculopathy, as well as lower limb sensory dysfunction and motor dysfunction
- The most common cause is disk herniation[2]
- Other common causes include spinal stenosis, tumors, and vascular occlusion
- Acute presentations are usually associated with significant trauma
- Delayed presentations are more likely with chronic stenosis and tumors among others

PHYSICAL EXAMINATION

KEY EXAMINATION MANEUVERS

- **Sensation Testing** (Figure 7H.1)
  - **Maneuver:**
    - Perform light touch, pinprick, and pressure sensation testing in the saddle, perineal, and perianal areas
    - Reduced or absent sensation in the saddle area is classic in CES

- **Anal Sphincter Tone** (Figure 7H.2)
  - **Maneuver:**
    - Observe anus and assess the tone of the anal sphincter

- **Anal Wink Reflex** (Figure 7H.3)
  - The origin of this maneuver is unknown
  - There have been no significant modifications
  - **Maneuver:**
    - Painful stimulus is applied to the perirectal region[4]
    - Normal response is an involuntary contraction of the anus[4]

- **Bulbocavernosus Reflex** (Figure 7H.4)
  - The origin of this maneuver is unknown
  - There have been no significant modifications

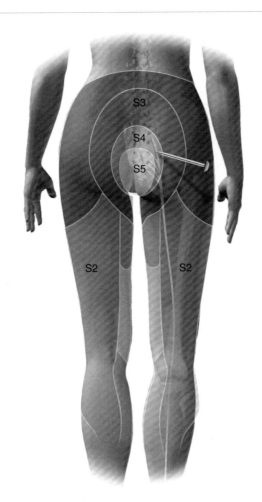

Figure 7H.1. Sensation testing.

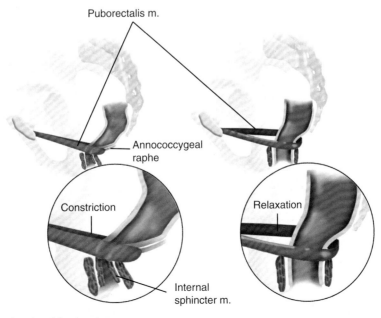

Figure 7H.2. Anal sphincter tone.

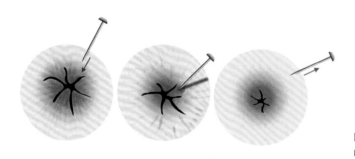

Figure 7H.3. Anal wink reflex.

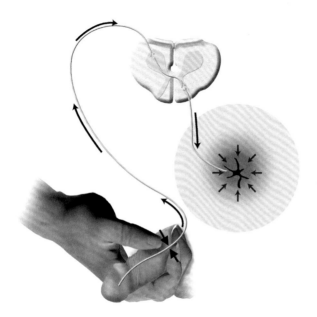

Figure 7H.4. Bulbocavernosus reflex.

- **Maneuver:**
  - Pressure is gently applied to the glans, penis, and clitoris, or an indwelling Foley catheter is gently pulled[4]
  - Normal response is an anal sphincter contraction[4]

- **Lower Extremity Muscle Strength Testing** 🔊 (Figure 7H.5)
  - First described in the literature in 1912 by Wright
  - Expanded upon in 1916 by Lovett
  - Significant modifications, including refinement of testing positions, in 1946 by Daniels and Worthington and in 1949 by F. Kendall and H. Kendall
  - **Maneuver:**
    - Assess strength of gluteal muscles, quadriceps, hamstrings, gastrocnemius, and soleus muscles bilaterally in lower extremities
    - Asymmetric weakness is likely to be noted

- **Achilles Tendon Reflex** (Figure 7H.6)
  - Deep tendon reflexes were first described in the literature in 1875 by Erb and Westphal. However, they were already well known and in wide use at the time of publication
  - There have been no significant modifications

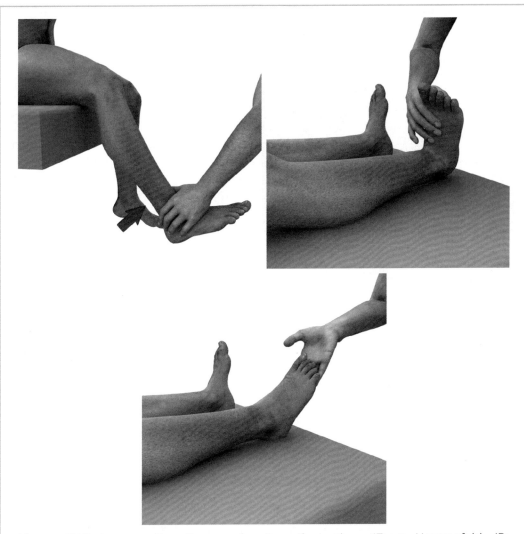

Figure 7H.5. Lower extremity muscle strength testing. (From Hoppenfeld JD. *Fundamentals of Pain Medicine How to Diagnose and Treat Your Patients*. Philadelphia: Wolters Kluwer Health; 2015.)

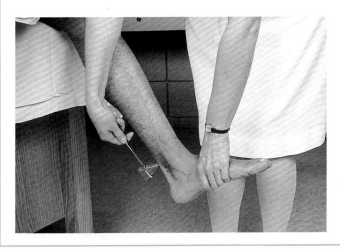

Figure 7H.6. Achilles tendon reflex. (From Taylor CR, Lillis C, LeMone P, et al. *Fundamentals of Nursing, The Art And Science Of Nursing Care*. 6th ed. Philadelphia: Lippincott Williams & Wilkins; 2008.)

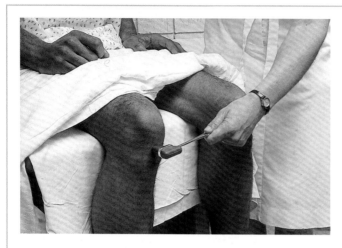

Figure 7H.7. Patellar tendon reflex. (From Taylor CR, Lillis C, LeMone P, et al. *Fundamentals of Nursing, The Art And Science Of Nursing Care.* 6th ed. Philadelphia: Lippincott Williams & Wilkins; 2008.)

- **Maneuver:**
  - The patient should be sitting with the leg hanging freely
  - The Achilles tendon is struck with a reflex hammer while holding the relaxed foot to elicit the reflex contraction of the calf muscles
  - The test should be performed on the contralateral leg for comparison
- **Patellar Tendon Reflex** (Figure 7H.7)
  - Deep tendon reflexes were first described in the literature in 1875 by Erb and Westphal. However, they were already well known and in wide use at the time of publication
  - There have been no significant modifications
  - **Maneuver:**
    - The patient should be sitting with the leg hanging freely
    - The patellar tendon is struck with a reflex hammer to elicit the reflex contraction of the quadriceps
    - The test should be performed on the contralateral leg for comparison

IMAGING

Plain Radiographs

- MRI is first-line imaging, but these are helpful for evaluation of gross bony changes
  - Fractures
  - Bone quality
  - Intervertebral disk height
  - Osteophytes
  - Spinal instability

Magnetic Resonance Imaging

- First-line choice
- Sagittal and axial views (Figure 7H.8) are recommended to evaluate compression of CES by one or a combination of some of the following[5]:
  - Major intervertebral disk pathology
  - Canal stenosis
  - Spondylolisthesis
  - Traumatic fractures and/or dislocations

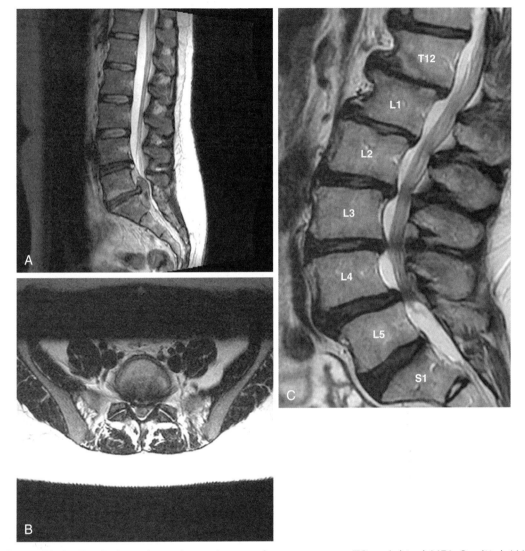

Figure 7H.8. Examples of cauda equina syndrome seen on T2-weighted MRI. Sagittal (A) and axial (B) views showing a large L5-S1 disk extrusion compressing the cauda equina. C, Sagittal view from another patient showing a combination of cauda equine compression, canal stenosis, and degenerative disk disease at multiple levels with retrolisthesis and anterolisthesis. ((A and B) From Hecht AC, American Academy of Orthopaedic Surgeons. *Spine Injuries in Athletes.* Wolters Kluwer Health; 2017 and (C) From Greenspan A, Gershwin ME. *Imaging in Rheumatology: A Clinical Approach.* Wolters Kluwer Health; 2018.)

- Cysts
- Epidural hematoma
- Epidural abscess
- Tumor, primary or metastatic
- Other space-occupying lesions

Computed Tomography Myelography

- CTM is indicated when evaluation with MRI is not possible or contraindicated
- CTM is superior to MRI for detecting bony abnormalities
  - For a symptomatic patient with no apparent pathology on MRI, further investigation with CTM may reveal an abnormality not previously detected on MRI

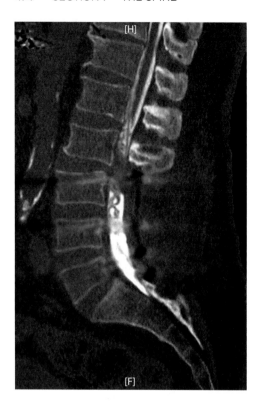

Figure 7H.9. CT myelogram. Lateral view showing severe cauda equina compression with die cut off at the L2-L3 level.

- CTM provides a greater ability to distinguish narrowing due to soft tissue protrusion from narrowing due to osteophyte development (Figure 7H.9)

REFERENCES

1. Fraser S, Roberts L, Murphy E. Cauda equina syndrome: a literature review of its definition and clinical presentation. *Arch Phys Med Rehabil.* 2009:90(11):1964-1968.
2. Gitelman A, Hishmeh S, Morelli BN, et al. Cauda equina syndrome: a comprehensive review. *Am J Orthop.* 2008;37(11):556-562.
3. Patrick N, Emanski E, Knaub MA. Acute and chronic low back pain. *Med Clin North Am.* 2016;100(1):169-181. doi:10.1016/j.mcna.2015.08.015 [PMID:26614726].
4. Radcliff KE, Kepler CK, Delasotta LA, et al. Current management review of thoracolumbar cord syndromes. *Spine J.* 2011;11(9):884-892. doi:10.1016/j.spinee.2011.07.022 [PMID:21889419].
5. Todd NV, Dickson RA. Standards of care in cauda equina syndrome. *Br J Neurosurg.* 2016;30(5):518-522. doi:10.1080/02688697.2016.1187254 [PMID:27240099].

8

SECTION

Pediatrics

Section Editors

Keith R. Bachmann, Dennis Chen, and Hakan C. Pehlivan

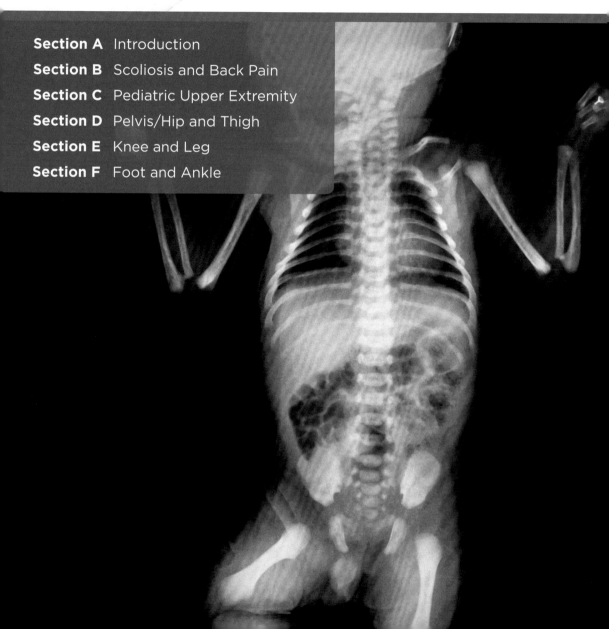

QUICK REFERENCE FLOW CHARTS (SECTION B)

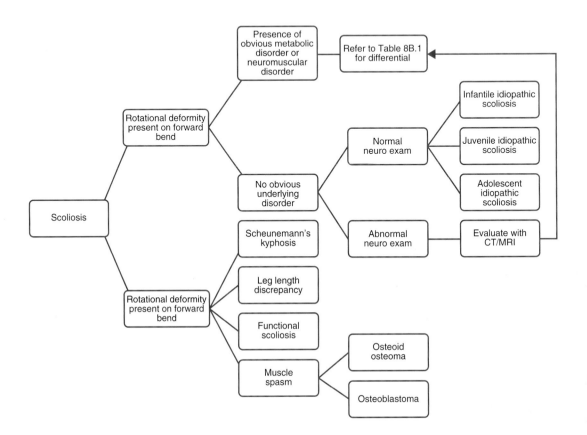

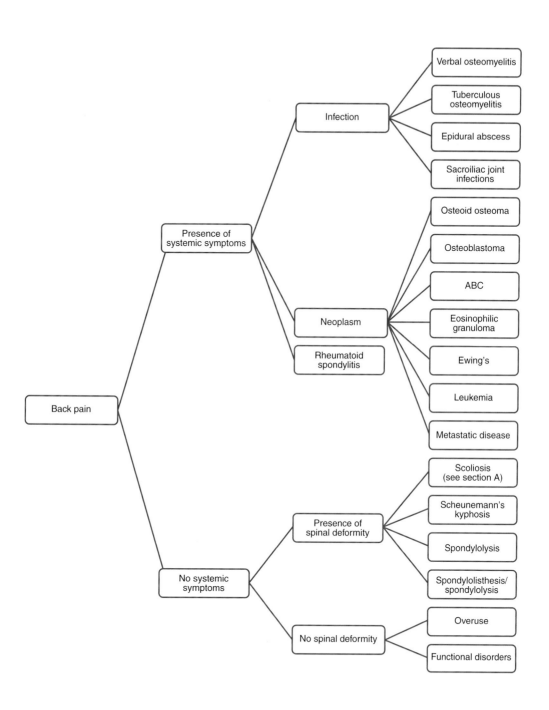

QUICK REFERENCE FLOW CHARTS (SECTION D)

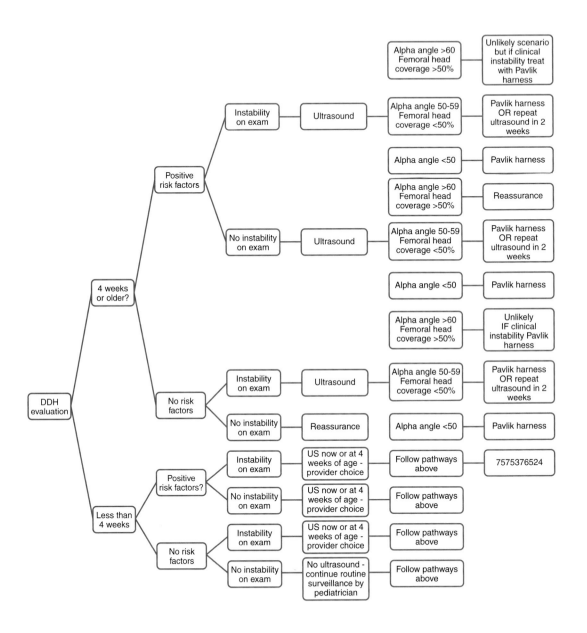

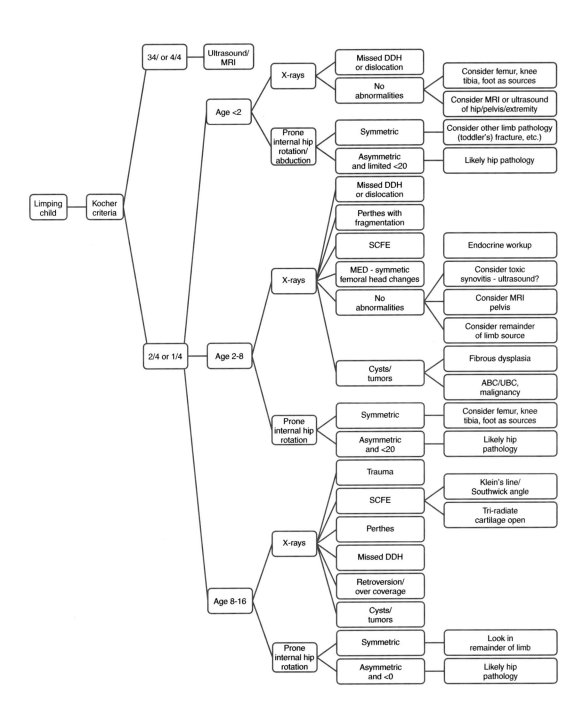

QUICK REFERENCE CHARTS (SECTION E)

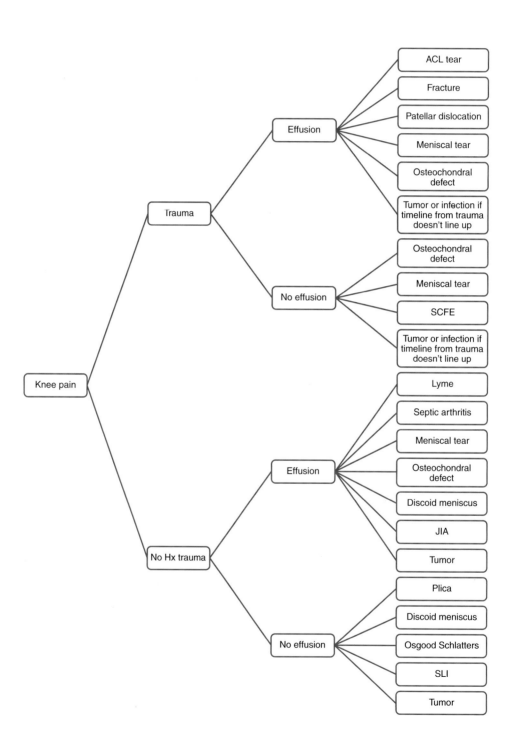

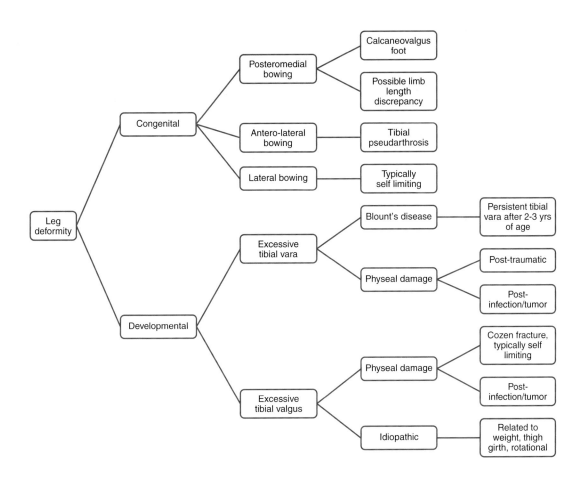

QUICK REFERENCE CHARTS (SECTION F)

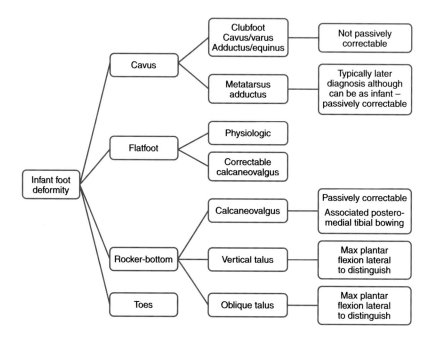

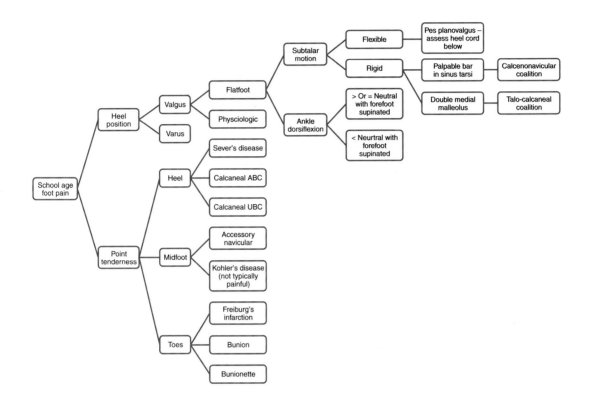

SECTION A
Introduction

Keith R. Bachmann

This chapter is organized slightly different, as there is a spectrum of conditions seen in a pediatric orthopedic clinic: congenital, developmental, traumatic, syndromic, autoimmune/autoinflammatory, neuromuscular, and overuse among others. The factors noted below help to narrow the differential diagnosis in each patient encounter. The sections are then divided into subsections with similar conditions. Examination maneuvers specific to pediatric patients are highlighted; however, especially in the teenage population, there is crossover with the more specific chapters preceding this one and those examinations are not duplicated here.

HISTORY

- Patient age
  - Infants tend to present with congenital or developmental conditions—clubfeet, hip dysplasia, congenital and infantile scoliosis, and congenital limb differences, among the most common
  - School-age children will present with developmental conditions, autoimmune/autoinflammatory, trauma, syndromic conditions, rotational profile complaints, genu valgum or vara, Perthes, flatfeet, and early onset scoliosis
  - Older patients present with traumatic injuries as well as overuse, and at times sequelae of conditions noted earlier in life: healed Perthes, scoliosis, and various overuse injuries
  - Growth spurts can lead to variance in muscle tension and apophysitis
  - Growth also factors into progression: limb length differences, scoliosis, limb alignment, etc
  - The age is not mutually exclusive of conditions but begins to frame an outline of a differential diagnosis
- Chronicity of symptoms
  - Acute issues or complaints tend to be traumatic or inflammatory such as septic arthritis, transient synovitis, fractures, and shoulder dislocation
  - Subacute issues are commonly overuse injuries; slipped capital femoral epiphysis (SCFE) often presents as subacute; apophysitis and chondritis present in a subacute to chronic manner
  - Chronic issues or complaints tend to be deformity either congenital or sequelae of prior trauma as well as features of syndromes or neuromuscular changes
  - Also important to ensure the timeline is spelled out. A child presenting with refusal to bear weight for the last day who suffered a fall 5 days ago and was willing to walk after the fall more likely has an infection than a delayed consequence of the fall
- Mechanism of injury
  - Trauma can be due to repetitive microtrauma or as a part of childhood play including falls or sports
  - Infection may be hematogenous, iatrogenic, or due to penetrating trauma
  - Deformity is usually a congenital issue and presents at birth but may not be noticeable until a more active lifestyle is achieved by the patient

- Consequences
  - Discuss with the family on how this has affected the child's life, as they may undersell the issues they are experiencing. Seeking the input from parents or guardians may also help develop rapport
  - It is not uncommon to see a patient regarding potential future impairment from an alignment issue or problem. How will these flatfeet, genu valgum, pigeon toes, etc, affect the child later in life? Will it lead to arthritis/back pain like Uncle Larry who has a similar problem? It is important to filter through the chief complaint to understand what is at the heart of the visit and most concerning to the family so that it can be appropriately addressed
- Prior treatment
  - Discuss with the family about what they have tried to do on their own or with any previous providers such as general pediatricians and other medical providers (podiatrists, chiropractors). If you are planning to repeat treatment, make sure you know how to differentiate it from what has already been done
- Family history
  - Having a sense of any familial conditions is important
  - At times a pattern can be recognized that may require genetic screening, and this referral should be made if needed
  - Learn on the knowledge of the family—if mom had scoliosis, she will view the treatment for her child differently depending on her outcome

PHYSICAL EXAMINATION

Again the physical examination is age-dependent. This requires a broad array of skills for the pediatric orthopedic surgeon.

- Newborns
  - No localization (point to the area that hurts) is possible from the patient
  - Parents may be able to implicate one limb but often that is all (pseudoparalysis)
  - More thorough examination is needed looking for cardinal signs of infection (rubor, dolor, calor, tumor)
  - Maintain comfort for the newborn and parents by examining while still in mother's arms (hip abduction) or while on a parent's lap
  - Don't forget the newborn reflexes
- Toddlers
  - Developmentally appropriate to have stranger-danger and avoidance/fear of health care situations (they are scheduled for a lot of vaccinations during this time)
  - May be able to point to a "boo-boo"
  - A lot of the examination should be obtained by observation—gait, favoring an arm while playing with toys. Chart as much as possible before attempting to lay hands on the child
  - Mimicry or having the child move toward parents can help ease the situation as well as small trinkets and toys as possible prizes or examination tools
- School-age children
  - Beginning to be able to elicit symptoms but corroborate history with the parents
  - Still would be well suited to observe a lot of the physical examination—strength can be tested with fun games
  - Do not forget simple screening tests (Gower maneuver, Adams forward bend)
- Teenager
  - Beginning to crest into adulthood
  - Examination and history can be obtained mostly with the patient, but keep in mind the parents are still guardians and in charge
  - Mostly adult maneuvers at this age still be sensitive to the awkward time: younger children may not need as much in the way of coverings and modesty, but teenagers certainly do

IMAGING

- Ultrasonography
  - A useful tool in children: provides for dynamic evaluation and structures that are perhaps too deep in an adult can be easily evaluated in the smaller soft tissue sleeve of a child (spine, hip)
  - No risk of radiation
  - Requires expertise from a technician and radiologist: harder for an orthopedist to accept deferring the interpretation of the study
- Plain radiographs
  - Be cognizant of radiation dosing, as the stochastic effect of radiation has more time to act on children
  - Still generally the first line and most interpretation is from X-ray
  - Extremity radiographs involve less radiation than chest, spine, pelvis—consider the area being imaged before ordering another test
  - Gonadal shielding, low-dose imaging, scanning slot imaging for anyone undergoing radiographic surveillance for a condition
- MRI
  - Similar utility to adults with the added inconvenience of often requiring sedation
  - Attempt to develop "fast" MRI protocols where possible to try to limit the anesthetic needs
  - Often children's imaging suites are capable of providing videos or music and distraction during the MRI: coupled with more limited sequences allows possible avoidance of anesthesia
  - Discuss with radiology whether sequences can be developed to replace CT scans: cartilage sensitive sequences to evaluate for bony bar, etc
- CT
  - Avoid if possible, especially body dosing (chest, pelvis, spine)
  - If needed for the bony detail and 3-dimensionality, then use sparingly
  - Attempt to avoid any protocols with CT scans for every patient—order on an as-needed basis
- Bone scan/nuclear medicine
  - Be cognizant of the radiation dose with these imaging modalities and consider the utility of the study before ordering

SECTION B
Scoliosis and Back Pain

Dennis Chen

HISTORY

Scoliosis

- Scoliosis is defined as a lateral curvature of the spine greater than 10°[6]
- In reality, it is a 3-dimensional structural deformity: lateral curvature in the coronal plane, typically lordosis in the sagittal plane, and rotation in the transverse plane (Figure 8B.1)
- Idiopathic scoliosis accounts for 80% of scoliosis in children and is a diagnosis of exclusion
- See classification of scoliosis in Table 8B.1
- Usual presenting complaint is positive screening based on Adams forward bend and/or scoliometer
- Parents or the patient may note chest wall or back asymmetry
- Adolescent girls may report breast asymmetry, unequal shoulders, uneven waistline, and difficulty with fitting clothes
- Scoliosis imitators
  - Nonstructural causes of spinal deformity, such as a leg length discrepancy, is monoplanar and resolves when the primary abnormality is treated
  - Scheuermann kyphosis is a rigid spinal deformity defined by >45° of hyperkyphosis in the thoracic spine[9]
    - May be mistaken for scoliosis by referring providers
    - 33% association with scoliosis

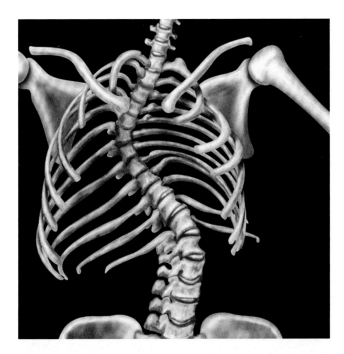

Figure 8B.1. Scoliosis: It is a 3-dimensional structural deformity with lateral curvature in the coronal plane, typically lordosis in the sagittal plane, and rotation in the transverse plane.

TABLE 8B.1 Differential Diagnosis

Secondary	● Muscle spasm/pain ● Leg length discrepancy ● Functional disorders
Congenital	● Failure of formation or segmentation ● Neural tissue disorders

Neuromuscular	● Upper motor neuron lesions
	 • Cerebral palsy
	 • Spinocerebellar degeneration
	  – Friedreich ataxia
	  – Charcot-Marie-Tooth
	● Lower motor neuron lesions
	 • Poliomyelitis
	 • Traumatic
	 • Spinal muscular atrophy
	 • Myelomeningocele
	● Myopathies
	 • Muscular dystrophy
	 • Arthrogryposis
	 • Congenital hypotonia

Constitutional	● Metabolic disorders • Rickets • Osteogenesis imperfecta • Homocystinuria ● Arthritis
Idiopathic	● Infantile ● Juvenile ● Adolescent
Miscellaneous	● Neurofibromatosis ● Connective tissue disorders • Marfan syndrome • Ehlers-Danlos syndrome ● Osteochondrodystrophies • Diastrophic dysplasia • Mucopolysaccharidosis • Spondyloepiphyseal dysplasia • Multiple epiphyseal dysplasia • Achondroplasia ● Tumors

- Sprengel deformity
  - Congenital high scapula
- Klippel-Feil syndrome
- Torticollis
- Pain-causing posture that results in an appearance of scoliosis
● Patient age and gender
  - Age of onset is particularly important in distinguishing between different types of scoliosis
    - Infantile idiopathic scoliosis: <3 years old; more common in boys (ratio, 3:2); most are apex left curves
    - Juvenile idiopathic scoliosis: 4 to 10 years old; more common in females; most are right main thoracic curves
    - Adolescent idiopathic scoliosis: 10 to 18 years old; most common type of scoliosis; 10:1 female to male ratios for curves >30; 1:1 ratio for smaller curves; most are right thoracic curves

- Chronicity of symptoms
  - Degree of curve/symptom progression over time is paramount
  - More worrisome if back pain persists >4 weeks and interferes with function
  - Nighttime pain is more concerning for tumor
- Mechanism of injury (if any)
  - Spondylolisthesis more common in children who participate in activities that involve hyperextension and rotation of the lumbar spine, such as gymnastics, diving, and weight lifting
- Prior treatment
  - Inflammatory pain from rheumatoid disorder and osteoid osteoma respond well to NSAIDs
- Associated pain
  - About a quarter of patients with adolescent idiopathic scoliosis (AIS) have back pain, which is usually benign and nonspecific. However, severe persistent back pain with associated red flag signs, such as fever and constitutional symptoms, may be related to infection/neoplasm and mandate further investigation
  - Back pain that is worse at night and relieved by NSAIDs suggest osteoid osteoma, which may be a secondary cause of scoliosis
- Family history/social history
  - Often a hereditary component to scoliosis
  - Children may learn about back pain from family members
  - Hereditary component to rheumatoid disorders
  - Psychosocial problems may contribute to back pain
- Presence of underlying disorder
  - Marfan syndrome, neurofibromatosis, osteochondrodystrophies, mucopolysaccharidoses, VACTERL

Back Pain[2]

- Back pain in children, compared with back pain in adults, is more likely to be a caused by an organic disease
- Most common cause of back pain are defects and stress reactions of the pars interarticularis (spondylolisthesis/spondylolysis)
- Other common causes include trauma, apophyseal ring fracture, Schmorl nodes, Scheuermann kyphosis, tumors, infection (vertebral osteomyelitis, tuberculous osteomyelitis, epidural abscess, sacroiliac joint infections) rheumatoid spondylitis, functional disorders, overuse syndromes, cervical disk calcification
- Risk factors include increasing age, female gender, increased height, family history, increased physical activity and competitive sport, psychologic distress, smoking, manual work, and carrying a heavy backpack

PHYSICAL EXAMINATION

- **Observation**
  - Observe the patient's posture and gait
  - Note any signs of truncal distortion, including rib or flank prominence, shoulder elevation, flank flattening or indentation, scapular rotation or elevation, and iliac crest prominence or elevation
  - Note any skin lesions that may hint at underlying pathology, for example, café au lait spots or axillary freckling associated with neurofibromatosis or midline hair tufts associated with spina bifida
  - Assess both coronal and sagittal balance evaluating for trunk shift, shoulder height imbalance, leg length discrepancy, and scapular asymmetry

- **Palpation**
  - Palpate spinous processes, paying attention to curve magnitude and rotation, as well as the presence of any step-offs
  - Palpate bilateral iliac crests, noting any asymmetry
- **Range of motion**
  - Perform Adams forward bend
  - Note any asymmetry with motion or limitation in motion
  - If the child is too young to perform forward bend, lay the child prone to help assess rotational deformity or suspended over the arm of the examiner
- **Neurologic examination**
  - In addition to routine assessment as detailed in section 7, The Spine, also assess abdominal reflexes. Asymmetry of the abdominal reflex or abnormalities in long tract signs (Babinski) or deep tendon reflexes may represent a neurologic abnormality that warrants MRI
- **Growth chart**
  - Patient's age and height should be documented on a growth chart to evaluate for peak growth velocity

KEY EXAMINATION MANEUVERS

- **Adams Forward Bend Test** (Sensitivity: 92%; Specificity: 60%; PPV: 70; NPV: 80 for detecting thoracic curves >20°) (Sensitivity: 73%; Specificity: 68%; PPV: 64; NPV: 77 for detecting lumbar curves >20°) (Figure 8B.2)
  - First described in the literature in 1865 by Dr William Adams[11]
  - "When rotation of the bodies of the vertebrae has taken place, in however slight a degree, the patient cannot stoop in a direct line and, at the same time, preserve the symmetrical form of the back. If rotation of the bodies of the vertebrae has occurred, the patient will always stoop in the oblique direction, and the angles of the ribs will be observed to project posteriorly and give a general prominence or fullness on the corresponding side; while on the opposite side a flattening—in slight cases not amounting to a depression—will be observed"[1]
  - No modifications
  - **Maneuver:**
    - The patient is standing next to the examination table with the examiner facing his/her back. The patient places the hands in front and bends forward with legs together and the head bent forward on the chest, as if to touch the toes. As the

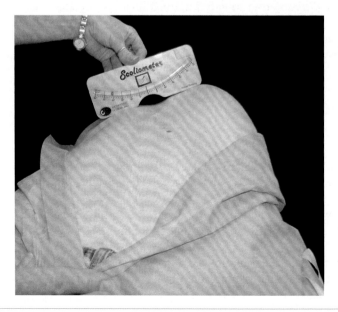

Figure 8B.2. Adams forward bend test and scoliometer measurement. In this patient, the angle of trunk rotation is 21° at T. (From Weinstein SL, Flynn JM. *Lovell and Winter's Pediatric Orthopaedics*. 7th ed. Philadelphia: Wolters Kluwer; 2014.)

patient bends forward, the examiner observes the spine to determine if it is supple and flexes symmetrically. Once the patient has bent forward so that the spine is parallel to the floor, the examiner looks for truncal asymmetry. This is often combined with scoliometer assessment
- **Limitations of Maneuver:**
  - Limited by observer errors; some patients were found to have a normal Adams test while having an abnormal scoliometer examination

- **Scoliometer** (Sensitivity: 71%-98%; Specificity: 29%-83%; PPV: 80; NPV: 75 for detecting thoracic curves >20°) (Sensitivity: 51%; Specificity: 83%; PPV: 70; NPV: 69 for detecting lumbar curves >20°) (Figure 8B.2)
  - First described in the literature in 1984 by Dr Bunnell[4]
  - Now also available as an application for smartphones
  - **Maneuver:**
    - Adams forward bend test is performed as described earlier. The scoliometer is placed on the patient's back by the examiner and used to measure the apex of the curve. The patient is then asked to continue bending until the curve in the lower back can be seen; the apex of this curve is then measured. The measurements are repeated twice, with the patient returning to a standing position between repetitions
    - A 5° to 7° measurement by the scoliometer is predictive of 20° or more of curvature depending on the patient body mass index. Higher BMI means lower threshold of positive test on the scoliometer
  - **Limitations of Maneuver:**
    - Variable sensitivity/specificity, high level of interexaminer error
    - Interrater error of 2.0° in the thoracic spine and 2.2° in the lumbar spine (ρ = 0.81 and ρ = 0.82 for the thoracic and lumbar regions, respectively)
    - Intrarater error of 1.5° in the thoracic spine and 1.9° in the lumbar spine (ρ = 0.995 and ρ = 0.998 for the thoracic and lumbar regions, respectively)[5,7,8]

- **Superficial Abdominal Reflex**
  - First described in the literature in 1876 by Rosenbach[3]
  - Georg Monrad-Krohn (1921)[3] recommended horizontal strokes toward the midline above, below, and at the level of the umbilicus, as well as a stroke above and along the costal margin
  - For overweight patients, he recommended a vertical stroke over the lateral abdomen
  - Wartenberg (1937)[3] recommended using a pinwheel to check superficial abdominal reflexes but noted that a dull pin, a pencil, a match, a key, a brush, the handle of the percussion hammer, a strip of paper, or fingernail could be used
  - **Maneuver:**
    - The abdomen is stroked in all 4 quadrants. This stimulation should cause the umbilicus to move toward the quadrant stimulated
    - In a set of 30 normal adolescents and 35 normal young adults, 60% had bilaterally equal abdominal reflexes, 14% had asymmetric reflexes, 11% had no reflex in at least 1 quadrant, 15% had absence of the abdominal reflexes in all quadrants, and 25% had extinguishing of the reflex in at least 1 quadrant as the test was repeated[10]
  - However, the finding of abdominal reflexes **consistently present on one side and consistently absent on the other side does not occur in normal subjects and should prompt further investigation of the neural axis**

LABORATORY FINDINGS

Back Pain

- **ESR and CRP**
  - Elevated in rheumatoid disorders and discitis
- **HLA-B27**
  - Strongly associated with spondyloarthropathies

IMAGING

Scoliosis

- **Plain radiographs**
  - 3-ft PA and lateral standing radiographs of the entire spine and including the hip joints limit radiation to sensitive organs—newer low radiation dose possible on a slot-scanning radiograph if available
    - A block should be used to level the pelvis if needed
    - A seated or supine radiograph may be performed instead of depending on patient limitations
    - In addition to evaluating the curve magnitudes by measuring the Cobb angle (Figure 8B.3), look for vertebral or rib malformations, which could suggest congenital scoliosis
    - Rib-vertebral angle difference (RVAD) of Mehta in early-onset patients (Figure 8B.4)
    - Note rotation of apical vertebrae
  - Lateral radiograph
    - Useful for assessment of sagittal balance
    - AIS creates lordosis or at least reduces kyphosis best visualized at the concave rib heads
    - Lack of vertebral rotation or lack of hypokyphosis at the apex may suggest a tumor or intraspinal abnormality as a cause of scoliosis
  - AP hand film: determination of bone age (Figure 8B.5)
- **CT**
  - Adjunct study to further define the anatomy for assessment of congenital abnormalities or suspected tumor (Figure 8B.6)

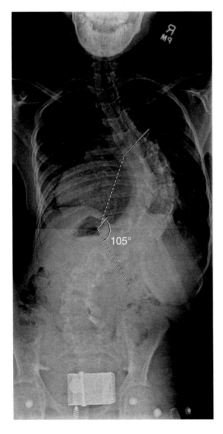

Figure 8B.3. PA radiograph of an 11-year-old female with adolescent idiopathic scoliosis and Cobb angle of 105°. (Used with permission of the Children's Orthopaedic Center, Los Angeles, CA.)

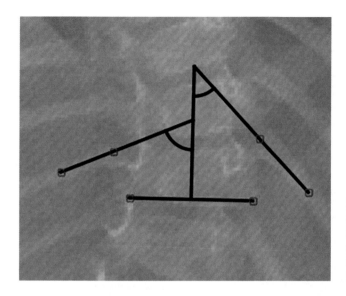

Figure 8B.4. Rib-vertebral angle difference: Measure the angle between the apical vertebral endplate and ribs. The rib angle of Mehta is the difference between the 2 rib-vertebral angles.

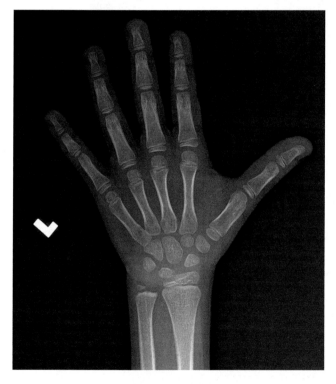

Figure 8B.5. AP left hand and wrist radiograph for bone age demonstrating a bone age of 6 y and 10 mo in a female based on comparison to the Greulich and Pyle atlas. (From Cordasco FA, Green DW. *Pediatric and Adolescent Knee Surgery*. Philadelphia: Wolters Kluwer; 2015.)

- **MRI**
  - Consider for all patients with early-onset scoliosis (<10 y old), persistent severe pain, atypical curve pattern (left thoracic), large curve on presentation, rapidly progressive curve, males with large curves, or an abnormal neurologic examination
  - Also may be obtained in surgical patients to rule out any unexpected intraspinal abnormality before surgery (Figure 8B.7)
- **Bone scan**
  - Pars stress reaction, infections, or tumors

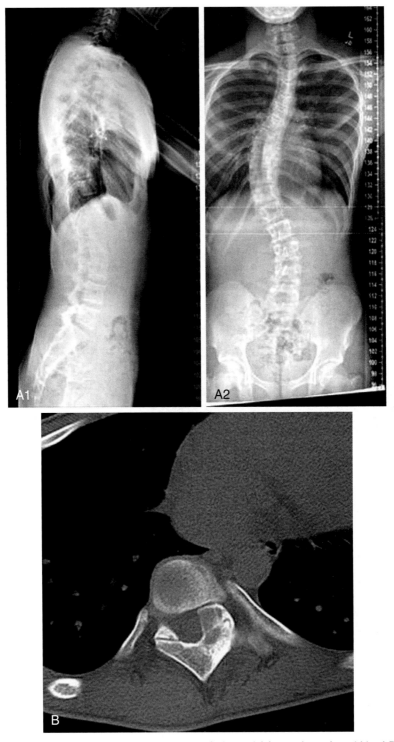

Figure 8B.6. Scoliosis due to osteoblastoma of the midthoracic spine (A). AP and lateral radiographs demonstrating scoliosis due to osteoblastoma of the midthoracic spine (A1 and A2). CT shows typical location in the posterior elements of the spine (B). (From Bridwell KH, DeWald RL, eds. *The Textbook of Spinal Surgery (2 Volumes)*. 3rd ed. Philadelphia: Wolters Kluwer; 2012.)

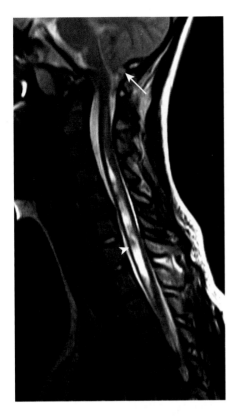

Figure 8B.7. Sagittal T2-weighted MRI sequence in a patient with thoracolumbar scoliosis reveals inferior cerebellar tonsillar ectopia (arrow), consistent with Chiari 1 malformation, associated with syrinx (arrowhead) in the upper cord. (From Iyer RS, Chapman T. *Pediatric Imaging: The Essentials.* Philadelphia: Wolters Kluwer; 2016.)

BACK PAIN

- **Plain radiographs**
  - Initial-focused AP and lateral radiographs of the region of spine that is in question (cervical, thoracic, or lumbar) or 3-ft standing radiograph if back pain is thought to be related to scoliosis or underlying structural alignment
  - Forward displacement of L4 or L5 on the lateral radiograph establishes diagnosis of spondylolisthesis
  - If no displacement is present, order oblique radiographs of the lumbar spine to better evaluate the pars (Figure 8B.8) although spondylolysis can be visualized on the lateral radiograph as well
  - Narrowing of disk space and endplate erosion seen on radiographs after discitis have been present for 2 to 4 weeks
    – If high clinical suspicion, order early MRI to avoid late detection and treatment
- **CT**
  - Most accurate method of diagnosing a spondylolysis (Figure 8B.9)
  - Allows for assessment of fracture pattern and gap
- **MRI**
  - Allows for detection of tumors, discitis, disc herniations, Schmorl nodes, subtle fractures not seen on radiographs, and evaluation of neural axis
  - Painful scoliosis should be further evaluated with MRI
- **Bone scan**
  - High-sensitivity scan in finding areas of inflammation or stress reaction
  - May show stress reaction in spondylolisthesis before the defect is seen on the radiograph
  - Increased signal intensity suggests increased osseous activity and healing potential, whereas decreased signal suggests nonunion
- **SPECT**: higher sensitivity scan in finding areas of inflammation or pars stress reaction

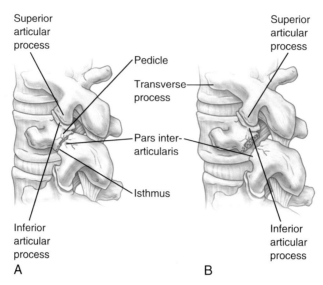

Figure 8B.8. Spondylolysis. Note disruption of the neck of the "Scottie dog" on oblique X-ray.   (From Anderson MK. *Foundations of Athletic Training.* LWW;October 12, 2012. ISBN:9781451116526.)

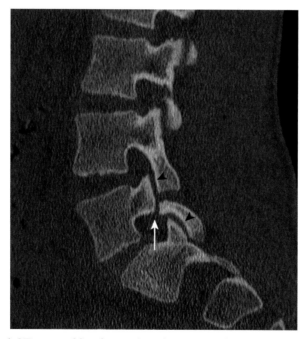

Figure 8B.9. Sagittal CT scan of lumbar spine demonstrating L5 pars interarticularis defect (white arrow). Normal L4-L5 and L5-S1 facet joints are indicated by black arrowheads. (From Iyer RS, Chapman T. *Pediatric Imaging: The Essentials.* Philadelphia: Wolters Kluwer; 2016.)

REFERENCES

1. Adams W. *Lectures on the Pathology and Treatment of Lateral and Other Forms of Curvature of the Spine, etc.* 2nd ed. London: J. & A. Churchill; 1882.
2. Altaf F, Heran MKS, Wilson LF. Back pain in children and adolescents. *Bone Joint Lett J.* 2014;96–B(6).
3. Boes CJ. The history of examination of reflexes. *J Neurol.* 2014;261(12):2264-2274. doi:10.1007/s00415-014-7326-7.
4. Bunnell WP. An objective criterion for scoliosis screening. *J Bone Joint Surg Am.* 1984;66(9):1381-1387.
5. Côté P, Kreitz BG, Cassidy JD, Dzus AK, Martel J. A study of the diagnostic accuracy and reliability of the Scoliometer and Adam's forward bend test. *Spine.* 1998;23(7):796-802 [discussion 803].
6. El-Hawary R, Chukwunyerenwa C. Update on evaluation and treatment of scoliosis. *Pediatr Clin North Am.* 2014;61(6):1223-1241. doi:10.1016/j.pcl.2014.08.007.
7. Grossman TW, Mazur JM, Cummings RJ. An evaluation of the Adams forward bend test and the scoliometer in a scoliosis school screening setting. *J Pediatr Orthop.* n.d.;15(4):535-538.
8. Murrell GA, Coonrad RW, Moorman CT, Fitch RD. An assessment of the reliability of the Scoliometer. *Spine.* 1993;18(6):709-712.
9. Staheli LT. *Practice of Pediatric Orthopedics.* Lippincott Williams & Wilkins; 2006.
10. Yngve D. Abdominal reflexes. *J Pediatr Orthop.* n.d.;17(1):105-108.
11. Fairbank J. Historical perspective: William Adams, the forward bending test, and the spine of Gideon Algernon Mantell. *Spine.* 2006;29(17):1953-1955.

SECTION C
Pediatric Upper Extremity

Dennis Chen

SECTION C1: NEONATAL BRACHIAL PLEXUS INJURY

History

- Occurs during delivery
- Risk factors include maternal diabetes, macrosomia, breech position, shoulder dystocia, forceps delivery, and clavicle fracture

Physical Examination

- **Observation**
  - Observe how the patient uses his/her upper extremities, noting any differences in spontaneous movement
  - Loss of movement may be due to true paralysis from a nerve injury or pseudoparalysis, which is a common sign of trauma/injury in an infant or small child
- Presentation differs depending on location of lesion
  - Erb palsy (C5, C6) (Figure 8C1.1)
    - Most common
    - Adducted and internally rotated shoulder, extended elbow, pronated forearm ("waiter's tip")

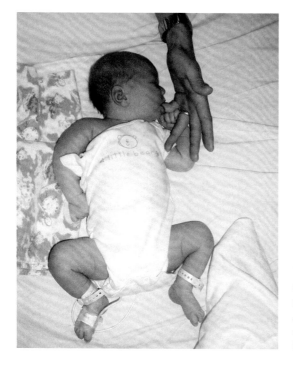

Figure 8C1.1. Right-sided Erb palsy with characteristic "waiter's tip" position. (From MacDonald MG, Seshia MMK, eds. *Avery's Neonatology: Pathophysiology and Management of the Newborn*. 7th ed. Philadelphia: Wolters Kluwer; 2015.)

- Best prognosis for spontaneous recovery[1]
- Moro reflex absent
- Hand grasp reflex present
- Extended Erb palsy (C5-C7)
  - Similar to the above, elbow may be flexed
  - Erb and extended Erb have a spontaneous recovery rate of 64% by 3 months in a meta-analysis[5]
- Klumpke palsy (C8, T1)
  - Wrist in extension, hyperextension at MCP, flexion at IP joints ("claw hand")
  - Poor prognosis for spontaneous recovery
  - Often associated with Horner syndrome (ptosis, anhidrosis, miosis)
- Total plexus palsy (C5-T1)
  - Flaccid arm with both motor and sensory deficits
  - Worst prognosis

KEY EXAMINATION MANEUVERS

- Return of biceps function at 3 months is a strong prognostic indicator for full recovery

- **Moro Reflex** (Figure 8C1.2)
  - First described by Dr Ernst Moro in 1918[2]
  - Present in all children up to 3 or 4 months of age as a response to a sudden loss of support
  - **Maneuver:**
    - To elicit, hold the infant with one hand behind the chest and the other supporting the head. Drop the head back a few centimeters

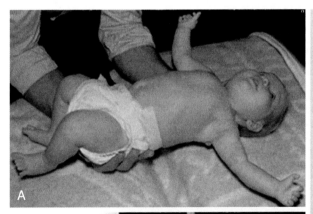
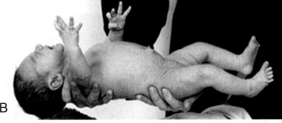
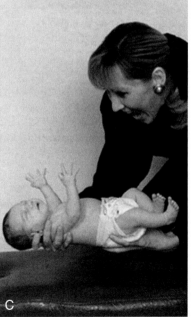

Figure 8C1.2. Moro reflex. A, First phase of symmetrical abduction and extension of the upper extremities with extension of the trunk and flexion of the lower extremities. B, Second phase illustrating the upper extremities returning to the thorax in adduction. C, An inappropriate Moro response would exhibit asymmetry of the upper extremities or lower extremities.

- It is important to ensure that both the infant's hands are open at the moment of elicitation of the reflex so as not to provoke an asymmetrical response
- The following should happen:
  - Abduction of the shoulders and extension of the elbows. The forearms are supinated and the digits extended, except for the semiflexed index fingers and thumbs, forming the shape of a "C"
  - Subsequently, the arms adduct at the shoulders and the forearms flex at the elbows, bringing the hands back to their original position
- Reflex should disappear by 6 months of age
- Absence or asymmetry of either abduction or adduction is abnormal, as is persistence of the reflex in older children

SECTION C2: CONGENITAL UPPER EXTREMITY DEFECTS

History

- Present at birth; may be isolated finding or part of a syndrome
- Two main types of conditions:
  - Structural deformities
    - Syndactyly
    - Cleft hand
    - Missing parts
    - Extra parts
  - Postural deformities
    - Normally formed hands but with contractures
- In addition to diagnosis of congenital upper extremity defects, it is also important to look for associated conditions[4]
  - Radial defects: Fanconi anemia (skin and hematologic defects), Holt-Oram (cardiovascular), Ladd (craniofacial), Nagar (craniofacial), TAR (thrombocytopenia), VACTERL association (Figure 8C2.1)
  - Ulnar defects: Goltz (bone, skin, eye, anus, mental handicap), mammary aplasia
  - Syndactyly: Apert, Carpenter, Poland, Waardenburg, etc (Figure 8C2.2)
  - Postaxial polydactyly (small finger duplication) (Figure 8C2.3)
    - 10× more common in African Americans
    - Inherited in autosomal dominant pattern in African Americans
    - More complex genetics and rarer in Caucasians, therefore mandates further genetics workup
- Sprengel deformity (Figure 8C2.4): congenital elevation of the scapula resulting in visible shoulder deformity and loss of abduction
  - Usually unilateral
  - Often associated with other abnormalities: hypoplastic parascapular musculature, abnormalities in the cervicothoracic vertebrae or thoracic rib cage, presence of an omovertebral bone, limited shoulder abduction, and shoulder instability
- Congenital pseudoarthrosis of the clavicle: presents as prominence over the clavicle (Figure 8C2.5)
  - Almost always right-sided
  - Slight ipsilateral shoulder weakness
- Poland syndrome (Figure 8C2.6)
  - Absence of sternal head of the pectoralis major
  - Usually unilateral, often associated with the ipsilateral finger or forearm abnormalities

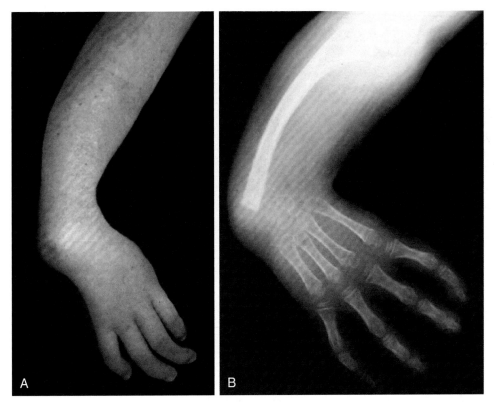

Figure 8C2.1. Radial dysplasia. Absence of radius produces a radial clubhand and a prominent end of ulna. (From Staheli LT. *Fundamentals of Pediatric Orthopedics.* 5th ed. Philadelphia: Wolters Kluwer; 2016.)

- Cleidocranial dysostosis: congenital disorder that presents with poorly developed or absent clavicles allowing the shoulders to narrow (Figure 8C2.7)
  - Associated with craniofacial defects and coxa vara

Physical Examination

- **Observation**: Upper limb deficiencies are usually apparent on physical examination, assess for symmetry, both of appearance and motion
- **Range of motion**
  - Assess forearm rotation with the elbow flexed to a right angle. Normal supination and pronation is 90°
  - Attempt to hyperextend elbow, wrist, and fingers to assess for joint laxity
- There are no pediatric-specific tests to diagnose congenital upper extremity defects. A careful physical examination as detailed in the section 5, Wrist/Hand, will allow the clinician to pick up on any clinically significant defects

IMAGING

Plain Radiographs

- Initial evaluation should begin with plain radiographs
- Although diagnosis of limb deficiency is often evident based on physical examination, radiographs are helpful for classification

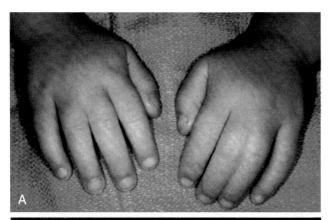

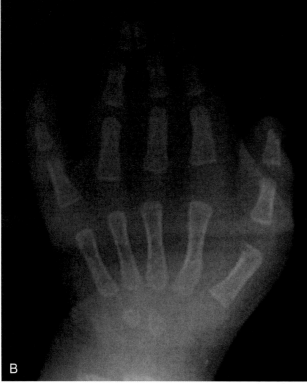

Figure 8C2.2. Simple complete syndactyly of the second and third web spaces. Observe the conjoined fingernail (synonychia) between the long and ring fingers. (From Flynn JM, Wiesel SW. *Operative Techniques in Orthopaedic Pediatric Surgery.* Philadelphia, PA, London: Lippincott Williams & Wilkins; 2010.)

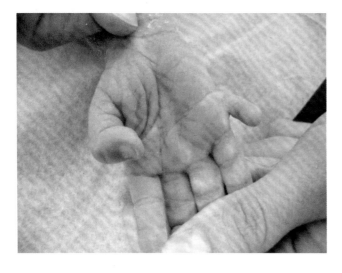

Figure 8C2.3. Postaxial polydactyly. A newborn with postaxial fifth finger duplication of the right hand. (Courtesy of Paul S. Matz, MD.)

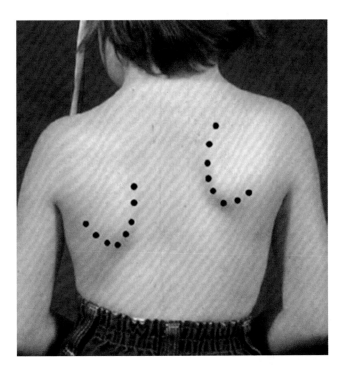

Figure 8C2.4. Sprengel deformity of the right shoulder. (From Wiesel SW, ed. *Operative Techniques in Orthopaedic Surgery - 4 Volumes*. Wolters Kluwer; 2011.)

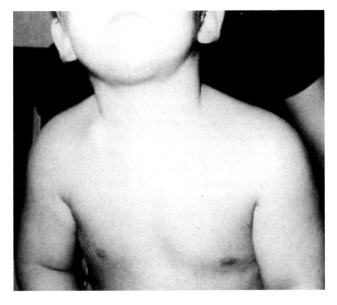

Figure 8C2.5. A 2-year-old child with congenital pseudoarthrosis of the right clavicle. (From MacDonald MG, Seshia MMK, eds. *Avery's Neonatology: Pathophysiology and Management of the Newborn*. 7th ed. Philadelphia: Wolters Kluwer; 2015.)

Ultrasonography

- Ultrasonography of heart and kidneys may be indicated for workup of associated syndromes

SECTION C3: OVERUSE AND TRAUMATIC INJURIES

History

- Little league shoulder[3]
  - Seen in adolescent throwing athletes
  - Salter-Harris type I physeal injury to proximal humerus (Figure 8C3.1)
  - Presents with shoulder and arm pain, worsened by throwing, decreased throwing speed

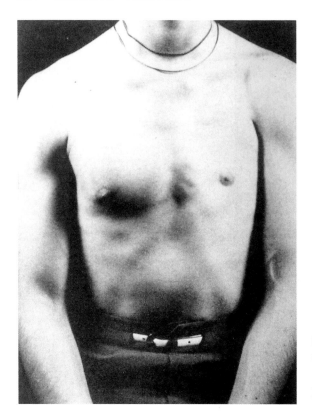

Figure 8C2.6. Poland syndrome. (From Shamberger RC. Chest wall deformities. In: Shields TW, ed. *General Thoracic Surgery*. 4th ed. Baltimore: Williams & Wilkins; 1994:529-557.)

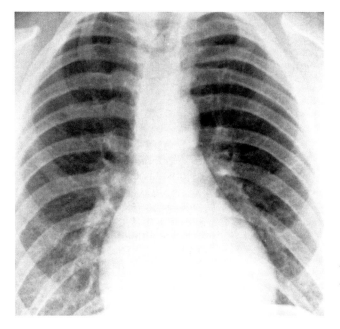

Figure 8C2.7. Cleidocranial dysostosis. (From Eisenberg RL. *An Atlas of Differential Diagnosis*. 4th ed. Philadelphia: Lippincott Williams & Wilkins; 2003.)

- Panner disease: spontaneous osteochondrosis of the capitellum (Figure 8C3.2)
  - Patients are usually younger than 10 years and have several weeks of pain and stiffness in the elbow with tenderness over the capitellum/lateral elbow
    - Limited range of motion is typically observed with approximately 20° of extension loss
  - Symptoms increased by activity and relieved by rest in most patients

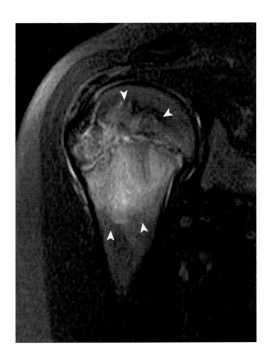

Figure 8C3.1. MRI of little league shoulder. Note the extensive metaphyseal edema extending into the epiphysis across the growth plate (arrowheads) in this 13-year-old pitcher. (From Greenspan A, Beltran J, Ovid Technologies I. *Orthopedic Imaging: A Practical Approach.* Philadelphia: Wolters Kluwer Health/Lippincott Williams & Wilkins; 2015.)

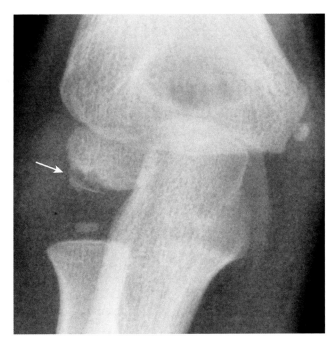

Figure 8C3.2. Panner disease: osteochondrosis of the capitellum. (From Chew FS, Ovid Technologies I. *Skeletal Radiology the Bare Bones.* Philadelphia: Wolters Kluwer/Lippincott Williams & Wilkins Health; 2010.)

- Presents in 90% of males (thought to be due to delayed appearance and maturation of the secondary growth centers)
- Self-limited disease process; most patients have a complete recovery within months
- Osteochondritis dissecans (OCD) of the capitellum (Figure 8C3.3)
  - Typically presents in adolescents, more frequently in males
  - Commonly seen in overhead athletes and gymnasts
    - Related to repetitive valgus loading of elbow (overhead athletes) or increased axial load (gymnasts) causing lateral compression injuries
  - Similar presentation to Panner disease but in older children (>10 y old)

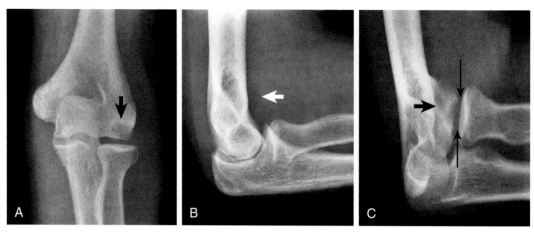

Figure 8C3.3. Osteochondritis dissecans of the capitellum. The anteroposterior radiograph of the elbow (A) reveals a radiolucent defect in the capitellum (arrow) suggesting osteochondritis dissecans; the lateral radiograph (B) shows only positive anterior fat-pad sign (arrow). The radial head-capitellum projection (C) demonstrates not only the full extent of the lesion in the capitellum (arrow) but also the osteochondral bodies in the joint (thin arrows)—a sign of advanced-stage osteochondritis dissecans. (From Greenspan A, Norman A, Rosen H. Radial head-capitellum view in elbow trauma: clinical application and radiographic-anatomic correlation. *Am J Roentgenol*. 1984;143:355-359.)

- Little league elbow[6]
  - Seen in adolescent throwing athletes
    - Related to repetitive valgus loading of elbow causing tension overload of medial structures
  - Spectrum of medial-sided elbow injuries that include medial epicondyle stress fractures, ulnar collateral ligament (UCL) injuries, and flexor-pronator mass strains
    - Younger patients: apophysitis
    - Older children: epicondylar avulsion fracture
  - Presents with medial-sided elbow pain, decreased throwing speed, possible effusion, possible flexion contracture
- Cubitus varus deformity (Figure 8C3.4)
  - Varus deformity of the elbow following a malunited supracondylar fracture
  - Inquire about history of injury
- Traumatic radial head subluxation
  - Subluxation of the radial head ("nursemaid's elbow") most commonly occurs in children aged 2 to 5 years and is caused by longitudinal traction applied to an extended arm, resulting in subluxation of the radial head and interposition of the annular ligament
  - The child holds the elbow in slight flexion with the forearm pronated
  - Reduce by manually supinating the forearm and maximally flexing the patient's elbow while the clinician's thumb applies pressure over the radial head (Figure 8C3.5)
- Traumatic radial head dislocation (Figure 8C3.6)
  - Isolated radial head dislocation is very rare
  - Look for plastic deformation of ulna (Monteggia variant)
  - More often anterior dislocation
- Atraumatic radial head dislocation (Figure 8C3.7)
  - Often congenital and bilateral
  - More often posterior dislocation
  - Congenital anterior dislocations are usually associated with other defects

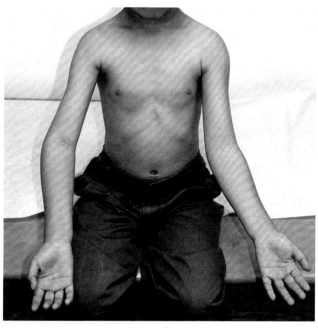

Figure 8C3.4. Right elbow cubitus varus following a supracondylar humerus fracture. (From Wenger D. Rang's Children's Fractures. 4th ed. Philadelphia, PA: LWW; 2017.)

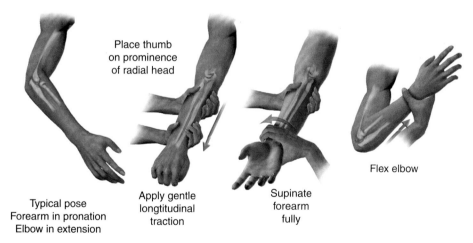

Place thumb on prominence of radial head

Typical pose
Forearm in pronation
Elbow in extension

Apply gentle longtitudinal traction

Supinate forearm fully

Flex elbow

Figure 8C3.5. Supination-flexion reduction maneuver for radial head subluxation, also known as nursemaid's elbow or a pulled elbow.

- Radioulnar synostosis (Figure 8C3.8)
  - Presents with decreased forearm rotation
  - May be unilateral or bilateral and congenital or following fractures of proximal forearm

Physical Examination

- There are no pediatric-specific tests. A careful physical examination as detailed in sections 2 and 4, The Shoulder and The Elbow, will help guide the clinician in making the diagnosis. The following are some key physical examination findings specific to the diseases outlined earlier

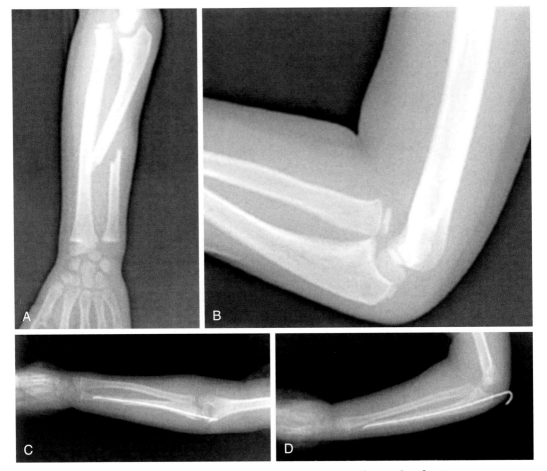

Figure 8C3.6. Traumatic radial head dislocation with concomitant ulna fracture.

- Because both Panner disease and OCD of the capitellum present with elbow stiffness and lateral-sided pain, age of patient and radiographic findings are key distinguishing features
  - Panner disease: <10 years
  - OCD: >10 years
- Little league elbow
  - Tenderness about the medial elbow
  - Pain with valgus stress, recreated with throwing motion
  - Possible instability with valgus stress
    - Check in both flexion and extension
- Little league shoulder
  - Point tenderness over proximal humeral physis/biceps groove
  - Pain reproducible with shoulder rotation, recreated with throwing motion
- Radial head dislocation
  - Palpable prominence over displaced radial head
  - Dislocation causes shortening of the radial side of the forearm, making the ulna more prominent at wrist
  - Difficult to maintain reduction of congenital radial head dislocation
- Radioulnar synostosis
  - Loss of forearm rotation

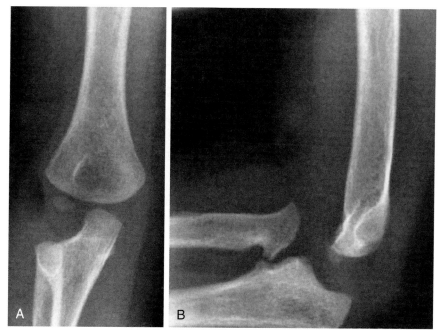

Figure 8C3.7. Congenital dislocation of the radial head in a 7-year-old boy. A, AP radiograph demonstrates an abnormal radiocapitellar line. B, Lateral elbow radiograph also demonstrates an abnormal radiocapitellar line with anterior dislocation of the radial head. The dysplasia of the radial head and hypoplastic appearance of the capitellum are consistent with a congenital etiology despite the anterior radial head dislocation, which is more frequently seen after trauma. (From Shah AS, Waters PM. Monteggia fracture-dislocation in children. In: *Rockwood and Wilkins' Fractures in Children*. 8th ed. Philadelphia: Lippincott Williams & Wilkins; 2014.

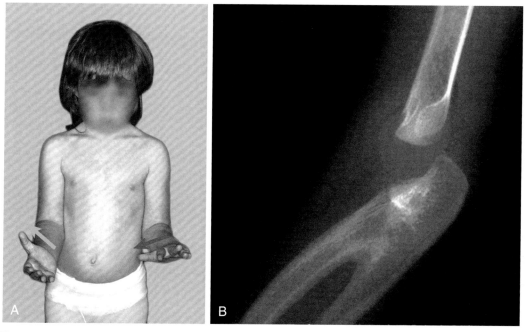

Figure 8C3.8. Radioulnar synostosis. The left forearm is fixed in pronation (red arrows). The right forearm rotates freely (green arrows). (From Staheli LT. *Fundamentals of Pediatric Orthopedics*. 5th ed. Philadelphia: Wolters Kluwer; 2016 and Chew FS, Ovid Technologies I. *Skeletal Radiology the Bare Bones*. Philadelphia: Wolters Kluwer/Lippincott Williams & Wilkins Health; 2010.)

IMAGING

- Plain radiographs
  - Evaluation should begin with plain radiographs
  - Anteroposterior shoulder radiograph with the arm in external rotation will demonstrate proximal humeral epiphyseal widening in little league shoulder
    – Finding may be relative and subtle; contralateral radiograph can be helpful
  - An irregular epiphysis is seen in Panner disease, whereas a well-defined subchondral lesion is seen in OCD of the capitellum
  - Physeal widening or fragmentation/avulsion of the medial epicondyle can be seen in little league elbow
  - Radiocapitellar line: the line down the shaft of radius should always pass through the center of capitellar ossification center unless there is pathology (Figure 8C3.9)
  - Forearm radiographs should be obtained for all radial head dislocations
  - In traumatic radial head dislocations, the radial head maintains a concave contour with normal capitellum and ulna
  - In atraumatic congenital radial head dislocations, the radial head has a round contour with a convex capitellum and ulna
  - Contralateral elbow films can help in delineating true pathology from normal or slightly variable development
- MRI
  - Useful for assessment of cartilage status in OCD of the capitellum as well as extent of injury (Figure 8C3.10)
  - Also useful for the spectrum of conditions that make up little league elbow

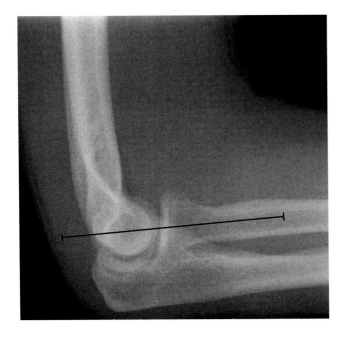

Figure 8C3.9. Radiocapitellar line.

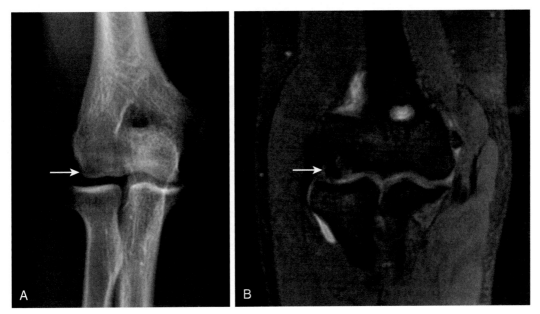

Figure 8C3.10. OCD lesion of the capitellum with subchondral separation.

REFERENCES

1. Foad SL, Mehlman CT, Foad MB, Lippert WC. Prognosis following neonatal brachial plexus palsy: an evidence-based review. *J Child Orthop.* 2009;3(6):459-463. doi:10.1007/s11832-009-0208-3.
2. Goldstein K, Landis C, Hunt WA, Clarke FM. Moro reflex and startle pattern. *Arch Neurol Psychiatr.* 1938;40(2):322. doi:10.1001/archneurpsyc.1938.02270080106006.
3. Osbahr DC, Kim HJ, Dugas JR. Little league shoulder. n.d. http://doi.org/10.1097/MOP.0b013e328334584c.
4. Staheli LT. *Practice of Pediatric Orthopedics.* Lippincott Williams & Wilkins; 2006.
5. Waters PM. Comparison of the natural history, the outcome of microsurgical repair, and the outcome of operative reconstruction in brachial plexus birth palsy. *J Bone Joint Surg Am.* 1999;81(5):649-659.
6. Wei AS, Khana S, Limpisvasti O, Crues J, Podesta L, Yocum LA. *Clinical and Magnetic Resonance Imaging Findings Associated with Little League Elbow.* n.d. Retrieved from: https://insights.ovid.com/pubmed?pmid=20864859.

SECTION D
Pelvis/Hip and Thigh

Hakan C. Pehlivan

- Many hip problems in adults are due to developmental issues as a child
- Up to 90% of total hip arthroplasty can be attributed to a structural deficit leading to abnormal loading of a hip, which in turn leads to cartilage degeneration

SECTION D1: DEVELOPMENTAL DYSPLASIA OF THE HIP

History

- Abnormalities of the hip that are congenital or develop in utero are referred to as developmental dysplasia of the hip (DDH)
  - Wide spectrum from subtle dysplasia to congenital dislocation of the hip
- It occurs in roughly 1 of 1000 pregnancies
- Diagnosis is usually during the neonatal examination
- Risk factors include a positive family history, breech position, and firstborn child
  - Presence of other abnormalities (clubfoot, torticollis) should lead to careful hip inspection
  - "Packaging disorders"
- Common reasons for referral: hip click felt in newborn examination or subsequent examination, thigh fold asymmetry, breech position, suspected leg length inequality

Physical Examination

- Perform a full-body examination to assess for any deformities of the upper and lower body
- Usually the newborn will not have any pain on examination
- Range the hips: the examiner may find more success with the child in the parent's lap, supine, legs facing you—a screaming child cannot give a good hip examination
  - Pay attention to hip abduction: asymmetric abduction is a relatively reliable finding in unilateral hip dislocation. Bilateral dislocations will also exhibit reduced abduction although it may appear symmetric. Also note any unequal skin folds on the lower extremities (Figure 8D1.1)
- Examine feet for clubfeet and limbs for any inequality; examine the back for hairy patches or dimples that may be a sign of myelomeningocele; and evaluate neck rotation and tilt
- If the child is of weight-bearing age, carefully pay attention to any limp or gait changes

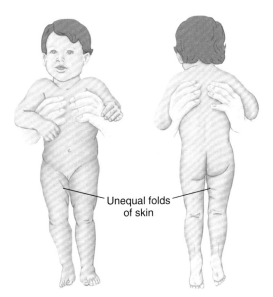

Figure 8D1.1. Image demonstrating an example of unequal skin folds in the event of a dislocated hip. (Used with permission from Anatomical Chart Co.)

KEY EXAMINATION MANEUVERS

- **Limited Hip Abduction Test** (Sensitivity 70%, Specificity 90%) to determine the unstable hip in an infant
  - Maneuver:
    - Passive abduction of the hips is evaluated as the infant is placed supine on an examination table. The examiner places one hand on each leg, grasping the knees to maneuver the legs. The examiner elevates the legs to flex the hip to 90°. The examiner measures abduction range of motion of the hip by slowly moving the leg with the hand out to the side. The abduction angle is determined by a perpendicular line from the table and the angle of the thigh; if abduction is 20° or greater on one side than it is on the other side, it is considered positive and further evaluation is warranted. Limited abduction is a common finding in a dislocated hip (Figure 8D1.2)

- **Barlow Technique** (combined with Ortolani, Sensitivity 67%, Specificity 96%)
  - Thomas Geoffrey Barlow developed this test in 1962[4]
  - **Maneuver:**
    - The test is performed by placing the infant supine on an examination table. The examiner grasps each leg at the level of the knee and proximal tibia and adducts

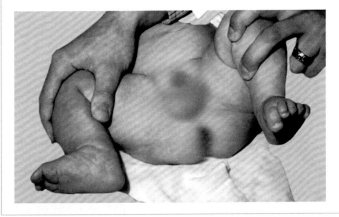

Figure 8D1.2. Example of difference in hip abduction with DDH. (From Staheli LT. *Fundamentals of Pediatric Orthopedics*. 5th ed. Philadelphia: Wolters Kluwer; 2016.)

the leg to midline while the hip is flexed to 90°. At this time the examiner directs a posterior force with the hand down the axis of the femur. If the hip comes out of the socket, it can be felt by the examiner and thus is positive. The examiner should perform one side at a time

- Ortolani Technique
  - Marino Ortolani developed this test in 1935[5] and is specific to posterior dislocation of the hip
  - **Maneuver:**
    - This test is performed by having the patient supine. The examiner grasps each leg at the level of the knee and proximal tibia and directs the knees midline and flexes the hips to 90°. The examiner gently abducts the hips by moving the leg away from the midline with the hand until a click is felt or heard. This is the femoral head relocating into the acetabulum. The examiner should perform one side at a time
  - **Limitations of Maneuver:**
    - Arguments stem as to whether a hip can have a "positive" finding on Barlow AND Ortolani tests. Suffice it to say if either is "positive," the hip is at risk and should receive treatment. Providers can figure out for documentation how they would like to reference a hip that presents in the acetabulum and can be dislocated or subluxated compared with the hip that presents dislocated and can be reduced. In both scenarios, the hip often resumes its initial presenting position (Figure 8D1.3)

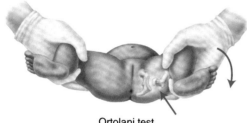

Ortolani test

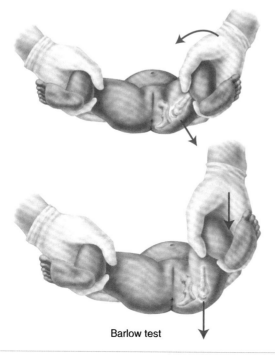

Barlow test

Figure 8D1.3. Examples of Barlow and Ortolani examination techniques and the demonstrated finding based on the femoral head and the acetabulum. (From Porth C, Gaspard KJ. *Essentials of Pathophysiology: Concepts of Altered Health States*. Philadelphia: Wolters Kluwer; 2015.)

- **Galeazzi Test** (Sensitivity: not available, Specificity: not available)
  - First described by Dr Riccardo Galeazzi in the early 1900s during his time at the Pius Institute for Crippled Children and the University of Milan[3]
  - **Maneuver:**
    - Limb length discrepancy is important to determine. While the patient is supine, the examiner levels the pelvis so that the upper body is perpendicular to the horizontal axis of the pelvis. With the legs out in full extension, the examiner grasps the hindfoot of each leg with the hands and can compare the limb lengths at the knee and at the ankle to determine a difference and where it could originate from

- Thomas Test
  - First described by Hugh Owen Thomas in his 1883 work "The Principles of the Treatment of Disease Joints"[2]
  - **Maneuver:**
    - Hip flexion contractures can be evaluated by the prone extension test. The patient is placed prone on the examination table at the level anterior fold of the pelvis, with the legs off the table. The examiner grasps and flexes the nonexamined hip while simultaneously the other leg is raised up until the pelvis rises off the table. This can be performed by cupping the anterior distal femur and raising the leg off the hip in question. At this position the examiner can use the horizontal-thigh angle to quantify the degree of flexion contracture. If contracture is not present, the examiner will note that the hip in question is extended beyond neutral

- **Trendelenburg Sign** (Sensitivity 23%-73%, Specificity 77%-94%)
  - Developed by Friedrich Trendelenburg at the University of Rostock in 1875.[1] Originally developed to assist in the evaluation of congenital hip dislocation and muscular atrophy
    - Can be used to assess abductor lurch. The patient stands on one leg and holds this position while the examiner observes from behind the patient. If there is weakness in the abductors, there will be uncontrolled movements, and the pelvis will drop to the opposite side of the weak abductors owing to the dislocated or displaced hip (Figure 8D1.4)

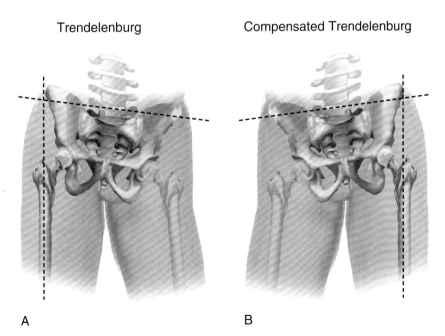

Trendelenburg   Compensated Trendelenburg

A   B

Figure 8D1.4. A drawing demonstrating the findings of the Trendelenburg sign.

IMAGING

- Ultrasonography has become the gold standard for imaging infants presenting with concern for hip dysplasia
  - Static measurements can be made (alpha angle, hip coverage)
  - Dynamic testing of the hip for stability can be made
  - Evaluation of the acetabulum, unossified femoral head, and soft tissue blocks to reduction with evaluation of the labrum and pulvinar
  - Progression over time with no need for sedation or radiation exposure (Figure 8D1.5)
- Plain radiographs
  - AP/frog-leg lateral view of the pelvis (age 6 mo or later on presentation)
    - Observe any differences in the femoral head ossification—smaller ossification center may indicate dysplasia
    - Shenton line: inferior border of superior pelvic ramus to the inferomedial border of the proximal femur; subluxation of the hip would disrupt this line
    - Various methods of quadrants to evaluate severity of subluxation/dislocation
      - The most recent methods developed by International Hip Dysplasia Institute:
        - Hilgenreiner line, Perkin line, and then 45° angle line in the inferior lateral quadrant
          - Location of medial metaphysis of the proximal femur determines severity
    - Acetabular index: the angle between Hilgenreiner line and a line drawn from the triradiate cartilage to the lateral edge of the sourcil (Figure 8D1.6)
    - Migration index: the percentage of the femoral head that falls medial to Perkin line
    - Lateral center-edge angle: a line is drawn vertically from the center of the femoral head, and then a second line is drawn from the same center of the femoral head to the lateral edge of the acetabulum; an angle less than 25° should be worrisome for subluxation and dysplasia
      - More useful in older patients once ossification has progressed
      - Standing films if at all possible
  - False profile: standing X-ray with the beam of the X-ray centered on a hip, pelvis rotated 60° with the hip being imaged more posterior
    - Allows for measurement of anterior coverage with the anterior center-edge angle

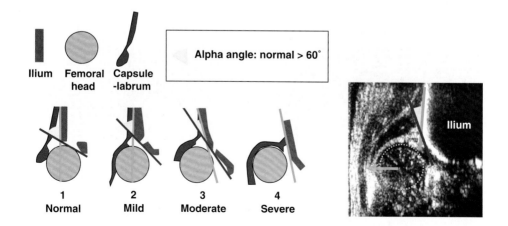

Figure 8D1.5. Drawing and representative image of the alpha angle in a hip and summary dysplasia grading. Alpha angle is described by Nötzli et al and is formed by the acetabular roof to the vertical cortex of the ilium. (From Staheli LT. *Fundamentals of Pediatric Orthopedics.* 5th ed. Philadelphia: Wolters Kluwer; 2016.)

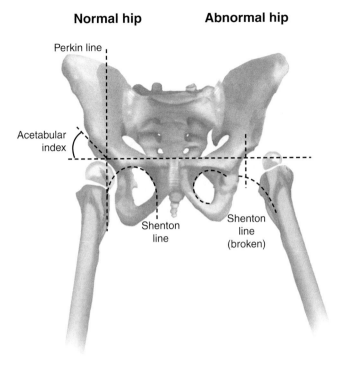

Figure 8D1.6. Radiographic landmarks in developmental dysplasia of the hip.

- MRI/CT
  - Not frequently used in infant DDH. May play a role in older adolescent DDH or in evaluation of avascular necrosis (AVN) typically due to treatment

SECTION D2: LEGG-CALVE-PERTHES DISEASE

History

- Also known as idiopathic AVN of the femoral head
- More commonly found in boys and can be bilateral in around 10% of patients
- Predisposition could be due to vascular variability of the femoral head, trauma, hypercoagulable state, and endocrine disorders
- Typical presentation is a hyperactive early school-age boy (4-8 y of age) who presents with a "funny run" or limp during activities or at the end of a day
- Less common to present with complaints of pain although a recurrent theme in this chapter is to evaluate the hips in the setting of knee complaints in any age group
- As infarcts occur in the femoral head, pathologic fractures then follow, leading to a collapse or flattening. Younger patients tend to have a better prognosis than older patients, as their remodeling potential is greater. Should it occur in an older patient or growth arrest occurs, disability will ensue usually due to osteoarthritis
- If imaging were to demonstrate physeal bridging, where bone fills in across the growth plate, this will lead to increasing deformity and a poorer prognosis
- Four stages of the disease include initial or necrosis, fragmentation, reossification, and healed
- Several classification schemes exist, with Catterall classification focusing on the extent of involvement of the epiphysis and the Herring lateral pillar classification focusing on the extent of collapse of the lateral third of the femoral head

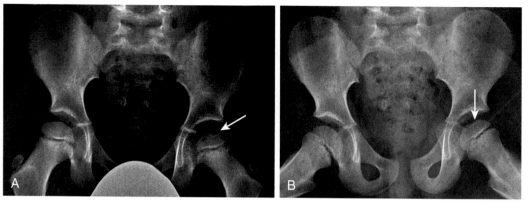

Figure 8D2.1. Radiographs demonstrating (A) AP and (B) frog-leg lateral view to visualize a crescent sign in Legg-Calve-Perthes disease. (From Iyer RS, Chapman T. *Pediatric Imaging: The Essentials*. Philadelphia: Wolters Kluwer; 2016.)

Physical Examination

- Begin with gait evaluation
  - Often avoidance or antalgia can be subtle
  - Look for subtle Trendelenburg gait as noted in the section D1, Developmental Dysplasia of the Hip
- Hip range of motion similar to DDH evaluation
  - Limitation in supine frog abduction is common due to synovitis
- Limitations in hip internal rotation supine with the hip in flexion or on prone evaluation
- Disease can be bilateral although typically at different stages
  - This may make comparative examination difficult
- Atypical to have tenderness to palpation

IMAGING

- Radiographs of the hip are used to stage the disease. AP/frog-leg lateral view of the pelvis is the typical series (Figure 8D2.1)
  - Most commonly used classification is the lateral pillar classification
    - The lateral third of the epiphysis is evaluated. Group A is with full height, group B is with >50% height but demonstrating changes, group B/C border is narrowed and with approximately 50% height, and group C is with <50% height. The order from A to C is from a relatively good outcome to a poor outcome
    - Staging often cannot happen until later in the disease process on plain radiograph evaluation, hence the push for more advanced imaging (Figure 8D2.2)
- MRI can be used to evaluate the marrow and growth plate and to assess the extent of necrosis
  - How to use perfusion MRI as a prognosticator is still in early phases/proprietary phases (Figure 8D2.3)
- CT scans are not commonly used but can provide detailed bony anatomy of the femoral head and acetabulum

SECTION D3: SLIPPED CAPITAL FEMORAL EPIPHYSIS

History

- Most common in overweight children entering or in early second decade of life (8-12 years of age)
- Mechanical insufficiency of the proximal femoral physis (due to obesity or endocrinopathy) leads to settling of the epiphysis posterior and typically in varus relative to the metaphysis of the proximal femur

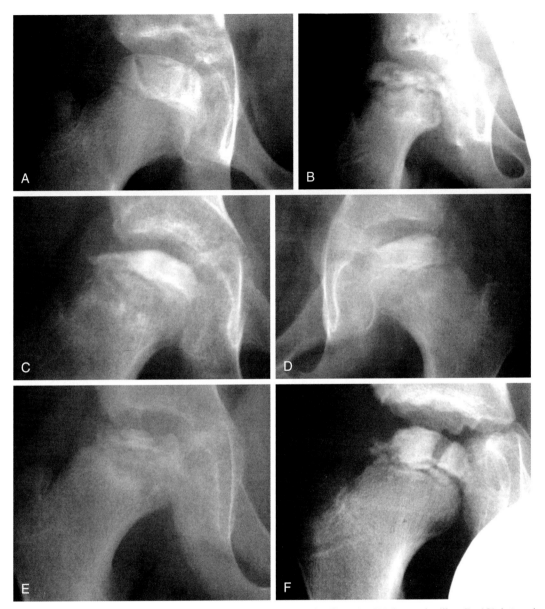

Figure 8D2.2. Radiographs demonstrating (A) lateral pillar A; (B) lateral pillar B; (C) lateral pillar C; (D-F) B/C border examples. (Reprinted from Herring JA, Kim HT, Browne R. Legg-Calvé-Perthes disease: part I: classification of radiographs with use of the modified lateral pillar and Stulberg classifications. *J Bone Joint Surg Am.* 2004;86(10):2103-2120, with permission.)

- The epiphysis stays in the hip joint, while the metaphysis displaces around it
- Can be acute, subacute, or chronic
  - Typically patients with acute worsening on questioning have had symptoms of groin or knee pain leading up to the acute change
- Key point: In a portion of the population, hip pain is interpreted as knee pain. SCFE is the entity that drives this point home in most orthopedic teaching. Normal knee radiographs should prompt evaluation of the hip, especially if knee symptoms are replicated with hip testing

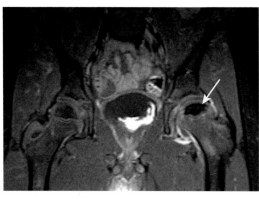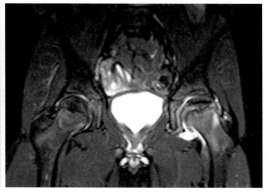

Figure 8D2.3. MRI sequences of LCP in a 5-year-old. (From Iyer RS, Chapman T. *Pediatric Imaging: The Essentials*. Philadelphia: Wolters Kluwer; 2016.)

- Also divided based on stability
  - Stable SCFE means the patient can bear weight on the affected side EVEN IF this requires the use of assistive device (crutches)
  - Unstable SCFE behaves like a femoral neck fracture—unable to bear weight EVEN WITH assistive device
  - Prognostic finding for the risk of AVN
- Do not fall into the trap of assuming only overweight children can have SCFE—many metabolic imbalances can lead to widening or "laxity" of the physis allowing for instability

Physical Examination

- Key findings on the physical examination for SCFE include decreased internal rotation due to the characteristic posterior-inferior displacement of the femoral head. This leads to increased retroversion and decreased internal rotation
  - In the acute setting with a child who is unwilling to bear weight, this will not be your first examination maneuver
- Often there is retroversion present at baseline even on a nonslip side of the hip, meaning relative change from a "good" limb can be useful to interpret severity
- Hip pain on examination and a limp may also be noted

IMAGING

- Radiographs of the hip are the main methods of radiographic diagnosis. An AP and frog-leg lateral views are best for visualizing the displacement of the epiphysis (Figure 8D3.1)
  - Southwick angle can be used to calculate severity
    - Difference between sides of an angle subtended by a perpendicular line connecting the medial and lateral points of the epiphysis and a line down the axis of the femur measured on a frog-leg lateral view: mild is 0° to 30°, moderate is 30° to 60°, and severe is 60° or greater (Figure 8D3.2)
- MRI
  - Can help establish baseline level of epiphyseal perfusion although most do not delay intervention to obtain images
  - In more subtle cases, MRI can distinguish the "sick physis" or "preslip" that may lead to SCFE if left untended (Figure 8D3.3)

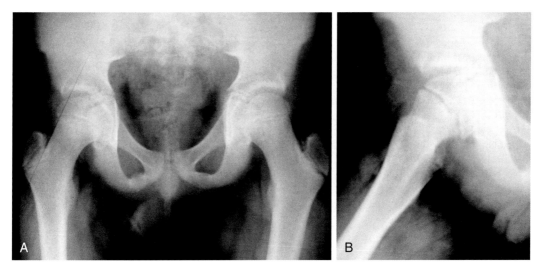

Figure 8D3.1. AP (A) and frog-leg lateral (B) radiographs of a child demonstrating the characteristic SCFE finding of the epiphysis translating posteromedially, best seen on the frog-leg lateral view. (From Frassica FJ. *The 5-Minute Orthopaedic Consult*. Philadelphia: Lippincott Williams & Wilkins; 2007.)

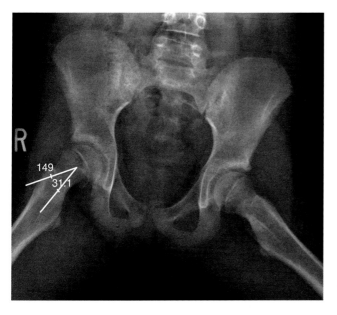

Figure 8D3.2. The Southwick slip angle: the angle between a line parallel to the femoral shaft and a line perpendicular to a line connecting the edges of the epiphysis. The slip angle is the angle as determined in the affected hip minus the angle in the unaffected hip. (From Clohisy JC. *The Adult Hip: Hip Preservation Surgery*. Wolters Kluwer Health; 2015.)

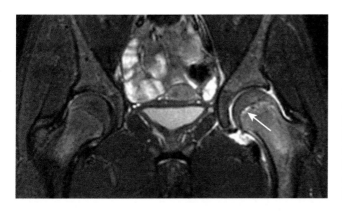

Figure 8D3.3. MRI of SCFE without obvious displacement; however, note the irregularity and increased signal of the physis. (From Greenspan A, Gershwin ME. *Imaging in Rheumatology: A Clinical Approach*. Wolters Kluwer Health; 2018.)

REFERENCES

1. Cassidy L, Bandela S, Wooten C, et al. Friedrich Trendelenburg: historical background and significant medical contributions. *Clin Anat*. 2014;27(6):815-820.
2. Macnab DS. Hugh Owen Thomas (1834-1891): the founder of orthopaedic surgery. *Can Med Assoc J*. 1941;45(5):448-452.
3. Galeazzi R. *Curriculum Vitae*. Milan: Archives, University of Milan; 1933:1-21.
4. Barlow TG. Early diagnosis and treatment of congenital dislocation of the hip. *J Bone Joint Surg Am*. 1962:44–B(2):92-301.
5. Ortolani M. A very little known sign and its importance in the early diagnosis of congenital hip predislocation. *Atti Accad Med*. 1936.
6. Nötzli HP, Wyss TF, Stoecklin CH, et al. The contour of the femoral head-neck junction as a predictor for the risk of anterior impingement. *J Bone Joint Surg Br*. 2002;84(4):556-560.
7. Stalehi L. *Practice of Pediatric Orthopaedics*. 2nd ed. Philadelphia, PA: LWW; 2006:159-193.

SECTION E
Knee and Leg

Hakan C. Pehlivan

- Knee problems account for more than 25% of all musculoskeletal complaints in pediatric patients, and the frequency of complaints increases in the teenage years
- Disorders more likely to be due to underlying dysplasia or congenital/developmental defect in a younger population
- Important to understand the natural alignment progresses from genu varum past neutral (~age 2 years) to overcorrect into too much valgus (ages 3-4 years) before settling into physiologic valgus around age 7 years (Figure 8E1.1)

SECTION E1: KNEE PAIN AND PATELLOFEMORAL DISORDERS

History

- Knee pain is a common presenting complaint and generally occurs after the child is active and weight-bearing. Self-limiting disorders of the bones and joints tend to occur, as the child is rapidly growing and remaining active
- Do not forget to rule out referred pain from the hip in a patient with knee pain with no other source
- Mostly present as anterior knee pain or a more generalized knee pain
- Generally the child falls onto one extreme or the other when it comes to collagen tension
- Tight collagen evidenced by limited joint range of motion
  - Osgood-Schlatter disease: apophysitis of the tibial tuberosity where the patellar tendon attaches to the tibia. Presenting complaint is pain/prominence of the tibial tuberosity, especially with jumping or stairs (Figures 8E1.2 and 8E1.3)

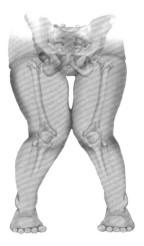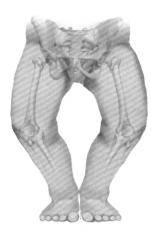

Figure 8E1.1. Genu varum and genu valgum with a demonstration of the differences between the Q-angle in each.

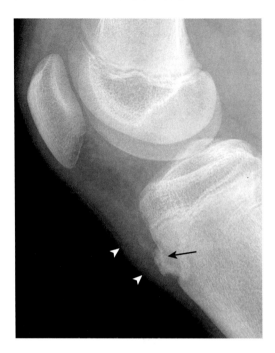

Figure 8E1.2. Lateral radiograph of the knee with Osgood-Schlatter disease. Black arrow demonstrating ossicle of the apophysis and white arrowheads demonstrating soft tissue thickening overlying the tubercle. (From Siegel MJ, Coley BD. *Pediatric Imaging*. Philadelphia: Lippincott Williams & Wilkins; 2006.)

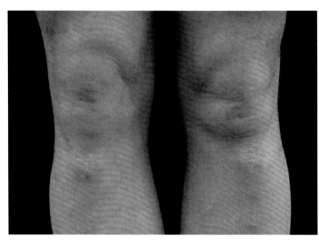

Figure 8E1.3. Clinical photo showing prominent tuberosities as seen with Osgood-Schlatter disease. (Courtesy of Julie A. Boom, MD.)

- Sinding-Larsen-Johansson (SLJ) disorder is an apophysitis of the distal pole of the patella and is less common than Osgood-Schlatter. Presenting history is pain at the inferior pole of the patella[1]
  - Both Osgood-Schlatter and SLJ can present as a referral for patellar tendonitis or patellar tendon rupture from providers less familiar with pediatric patients (Figures 8E1.4 and 8E1.5)
- Bursitis occurs most commonly over the insertion of the hamstring tendon insertions, known as the pes anserinus. Rest and conservative management is the mainstay of treatment
- Loose collagen evidenced by joint hypermobility:
  - See key examination maneuver for Beighton criteria below
  - Patellofemoral disorders generally come down to the lateralization of the patella in relation to the femur. Factors that can affect the position of the patella include torsion of the femur and tibia, genu valgum, hypoplasia of the distal femoral condyles, patella alta or

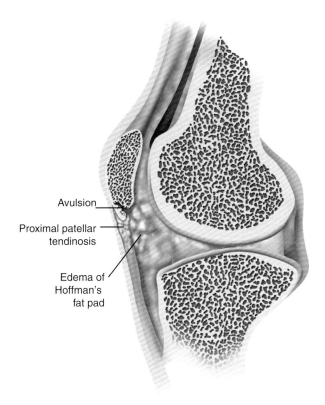

Figure 8E1.4. Illustration showing pathology of Sinding-Larsen-Johansson disorder at the distal patella and proximal portion of the patellar tendon.

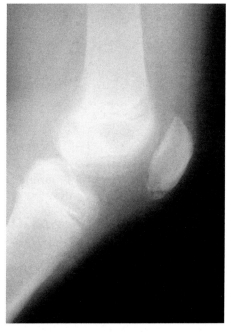

Figure 8E1.5. Lateral radiograph of a patient with painful Sinding-Larsen-Johansson disorder. (From Fleisher GR, Ludwig S. *Textbook of Pediatric Emergency Medicine*. Philadelphia: Lippincott Williams & Wilkins; 2010.)

baja, quadriceps weakness and insufficiency, and vastus lateralis contractures. All these conditions can lead to the patella subluxating or dislocating laterally
  – May not be hyperlax but need to consider hyperlaxity if there are no signs of improper torsion, coronal plane alignment, or traumatic event

Physical Examination

- See how the child stands with the knees extended, paying attention to rotational profile and long bone profiles. You can observe bowing of the long bones, knee angle, presence of recurvatum, tracking of the patella, or muscular hypoplasia, which can clue you in to a diagnosis
- Ask the child to point to where it hurts the most and then palpate to determine the point of maximal tenderness
- Gait assessment
  - Foot progression angle
  - Recurvatum
  - Antalgia
  - Heel strike to toe off or any avoidance of a rocker
- Assess ROM
  - Prone assessment of hip internal and external rotation to evaluate anteversion of the femur (Figure 8E1.6)
  - Thigh foot axis to assess for tibial torsion (Figure 8E1.7)
  - While prone, evaluate the passive knee ROM as well as quadriceps tone—should be able to passive flex the knee until the heel can contact buttock without pelvic tilt
  - While supine, evaluate the popliteal angle to assess hamstring tone
- Evaluate patellar tracking, as the knee is taken from flexion into extension. If the patella deviates laterally once it is superior to the trochlear groove, this is a positive J-sign
- Patellar apprehension is tested out in extension and is performed by applying a lateralizing force to the patella.[2] The patient becomes uncomfortable as you attempt to displace laterally in the extended position. See if this improves with engagement of the patella in the trochlea with knee flexion around 30°
  - Also document patellar translation by a number of quadrants of the patella that end lateral to the lateral aspect of the trochlea

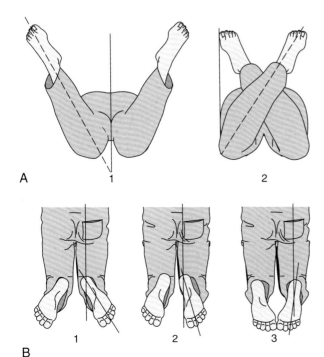

Figure 8E1.6. Illustrations demonstrating prone evaluation of rotational profile. A, Hip internal rotation (1, medial rotation) and external rotation (2, lateral rotation). B, Thigh foot axis with (1) external rotation, (2) less severe external rotation, and (3) internal tibial rotation. (Adapted from Staheli LT. Torsional deformity. *Pediatr Clin North Am.* 1986;33:1378 and Kliegman RM, Neider MI, Super DM, eds. *Practical Strategies in Pediatric Diagnosis and Therapy.* Philadelphia: W.B. Saunders; 1996.)

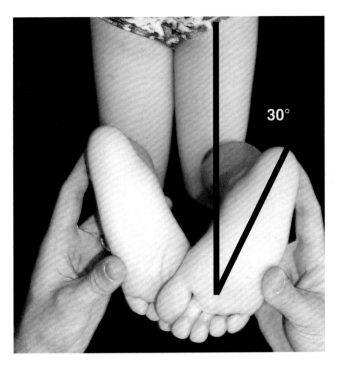

Figure 8E1.7. Thigh foot angle measurement in a child demonstrating 30°. (From Weinstein SL, Flynn JM. *Lovell and Winter's Pediatric Orthopaedics.* Vol 1. Wolters Kluwer Health; 2014.)

KEY EXAMINATION MANEUVERS

- See the adult knee section for special examination maneuvers of the knee

- **Assessment of general laxity—Beighton criteria**
  - First described in the literature in 1964 by Carter and Wilkinson;[3] it was modified in 1973 by Beighton et al[4]
  - **Maneuver:**
    - Components of Beighton scale
      - Passive dorsiflexion of fifth MCP beyond 90°
      - Passive apposition of the thumb to flexor aspect of the forearm
      - Passive hyperextension of the elbow beyond 10°
      - Passive hyperextension of the knee beyond 10°
      - Active forward flexion of the trunk with knees extended so that palms rest flat on the floor
    - The examiner should have the patient become comfortable on the examination table. Starting proximally, you would take the little finger of each hand and extend maximally without causing pain and note the angle of the MCP joint. The next criteria are by the examiner grasping the thumb while simultaneously flexing the wrist and allowing it to lay on the volar surface of the forearm. After both hands are examined, the patient can then place both arms forward and extend the elbows. The examiner should then place one hand on the posterior distal humerus as support while the other hand gently hyperextends the forearm, noting the angle of the elbow. The same examination can be performed for the knees; however, one hand of the examiner should be on the anterior distal femur while the other hand gently hyperextends the knee. Lastly, ask the patient to stand and touch the palms to the floor with the legs shoulder-width apart
  - **Limitations of Maneuver:**
    - Many patients may have general ligamentous joint laxity without pathologic motion

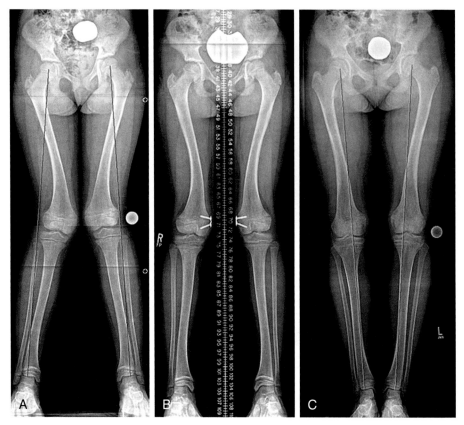

Figure 8E1.8. Genu valgum standing leg films with subsequent treatment and follow-up imaging. (From Cordasco FA, Green DW. *Pediatric and Adolescent Knee Surgery*. Philadelphia: Wolters Kluwer; 2015.)

IMAGING

- Radiographs can be helpful in the assessment of knee pain and patellofemoral disorders
  - An AP, lateral, tunnel (PA flexion), and sunrise view will demonstrate the position of the patella relative to the trochlea of the femur
  - Concern for pathologic varus or valgus at the knee should be evaluated with a standing long leg alignment film (Figure 8E1.8)
  - Q-angle is formed by a line drawn from the anterior superior iliac spine to the center of the patella and a second line drawn from the center of the patella to the tibial tuberosity (Figure 8E1.9)
- CT can be used to assess for hypoplasia of the condyles, dysplasia of the trochlea or patella, and torsional deformities of the distal femur and proximal tibia
- MRI is useful to evaluate the tendon insertions of the patella and the hamstrings. It can also demonstrate any intra-articular pathology if there is concern for a loose body after patellar dislocation

SECTION E2: INTRA-ARTICULAR DISORDERS

History

- Commonly a sporting event or acute change in symptoms although discoid meniscus and OCD lesions may not have an acute change
- When the patient presents with swelling/effusion, complaints of giving way need to ensure there is no intra-articular pathology

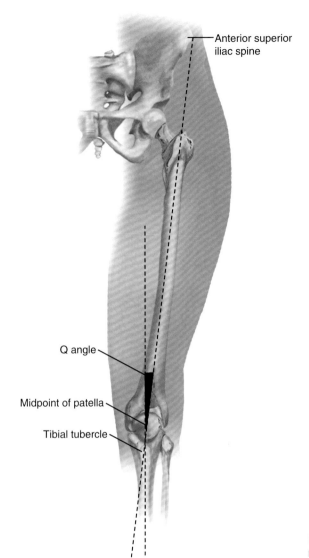

Figure 8E1.9. Illustration of the Q-angle measurement.

- Traumatic sports injuries can include meniscal tears and ligament tears such as the anterior cruciate ligament or the medial collateral ligament. Refer to the adult knee section for information on these injuries
- Ask patients about feeling of a "pop," immediate pain onset, whether any "reduction maneuver" had to be performed and what it was, presence and resolution of any swelling (effusion or soft tissues), and whether they were able to return immediately to sport
  - Pop, immediate swelling, and inability to return are concerning for ACL rupture or patellofemoral dislocation
  - More specific to children, these may be presenting complaints of a Salter-Harris fracture of the distal femur or a tibial eminence or tibial tubercle avulsion fracture
    – Depending on suspicion (weight-bearing?), may want to start with non–weight-bearing X-rays before any stress testing for ligamentous injury
  - ACL tear and patellofemoral dislocation are still more likely causes of traumatic effusion in children
- Discoid meniscus is a congenital problem that presents in younger children as catching, locking, pain with activity, and the knee "giving out." The meniscus can be more mobile than a

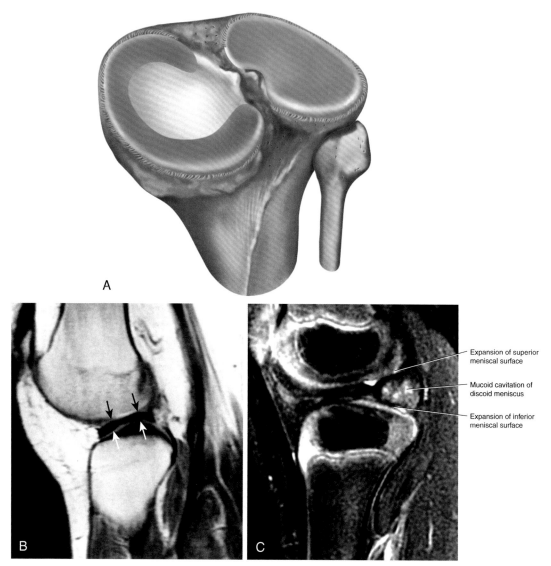

A

B

C

Expansion of superior
meniscal surface

Mucoid cavitation of
discoid meniscus

Expansion of inferior
meniscal surface

Figure 8E2.1. Illustration (A) and MRI findings (B and C) that demonstrate a discoid meniscus.

normal meniscus and thus is more likely to be compressed between the condyles and receive damage (Figures 8E2.1 and 8E2.2)

- Ligament insufficiency can also be congenital and does not present until ambulation is achieved. Vague complaints of knee instability and occasionally "giving out" with pain after activity are common

Physical Examination

- A complete physical examination of the knee and its ligaments should be performed when a traumatic intra-articular diagnosis is suspected or there is concern for ligament insufficiency. Assess for an effusion and area of maximal pain and tenderness. Refer section 1, The Knee, in this book as a guide
- Discoid meniscus may have tenderness and a fullness over the lateral joint line. Motion of the knee between flexion and extension may reveal crepitus and snapping
  - They may exhibit an inability to obtain a deep squat

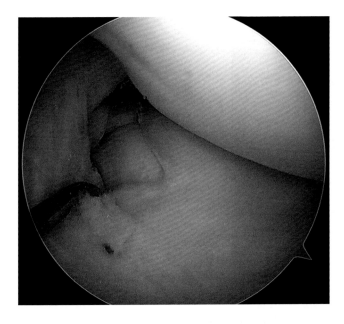

Figure 8E2.2. Arthroscopic image of a discoid meniscus before partial resection. (From Skaggs DL, Kocher MS. *Master Techniques in Orthopaedic Surgery*: Pediatrics. Wolters Kluwer Health; 2016.)

- OCD lesions may behave like a meniscus injury with catching due to loose body, joint line tenderness, and effusion
- Special examination maneuvers
  - See the adult knee section for special examination maneuvers of the knee

IMAGING

- Standard radiographs of the knee: standing AP, tunnel, lateral, sunrise
  - Weight-bearing is possible, but exercise caution in the child who is unable to bear weight, given the possibility of a physeal injury or avulsion fracture[5]
  - OCD is more likely to be present on tunnel view and lateral view owing to the most common location in the posterolateral aspect of the medial femoral condyle but can be present in the lateral condyle and patella
  - Discoid meniscus may demonstrate a widened lateral joint line and blunting of the lateral femoral condyle
- CT is used for evaluation of joint involvement with a tibial eminence fracture or tibial tubercle fracture with extension to the plateau
- MRI remains the gold standard for confirmatory diagnostic imaging when it comes to intra-articular disorders
  - ACL tear, meniscal injury, PCL injury as in adult patients
  - Evaluate for entrapment of meniscus in tibial eminence fractures and also assess at the time of diagnostic arthroscopy for repair
  - OCD: evaluate for fluid signal behind the lesion to indicate instability
  - Discoid meniscus: presence of complete lateral meniscal tissue on 3 consecutive slices diagnostic of discoid meniscus, as seen in Figure 8E2.1

SECTION E3: LEG DEFORMITIES

History

- Wide range of causes can lead to deformities of the knee and leg, which can include contractures, bony dysplasia, neuromuscular disorders, trauma, and infection
- Can present during the newborn period due to contractures and neuromuscular disorders, which can lead to deformity over time due to a continuous force applied to growing extremity

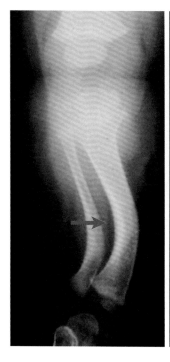
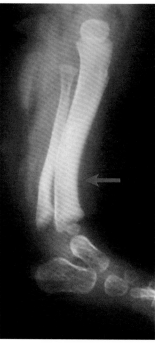

Figure 8E3.1. AP and lateral radiographs of posteromedial bowing. (From Staheli LT. *Fundamentals of Pediatric Orthopedics*. 5th ed. Philadelphia: Wolters Kluwer;2016.)

- Deformities due to trauma and infection are generally due to bony destruction or damage to the growth plate of the involved bone
  - Should have a history of trauma or infection even if remote
    – Some pediatric joint infections can go unnoticed other than a period where the child was ill with no other known source—more common in missed hip septic arthritis due to intra-articular metaphysis of the hip
- Recurvatum can occur after trauma to the proximal tibia, as the anterior tibial tuberosity is vulnerable to arrest
- Tibial bowing is common and the direction of the bowing dictates management. It is often noticeable before ambulation begins in the child
  - Lateral tibial bowing is common and generally self-limiting
  - Posteromedial bowing improves with growth but may require surgical correction when limb length discrepancy exists—history of associated calcaneovalgus foot (Figure 8E3.1)
  - Anterolateral bowing is more rare and has a worse prognosis, as this is most commonly associated with tibial pseudoarthrosis
    – May be treated with bracing, but generally surgical correction is necessary (Figure 8E3.2)
- May also present as genu varum or valgus
  - Understanding natural history of knee alignment is important to evaluate when a child has fallen off the expected progression
  - Infantile Blount disease is persistent genu varum typically in an obese child who was an early ambulator (before 1 y of age)
- History of other medical problems or need for supplementation can be present
  - Renal disorders leading to rickets
- Family history might also be pertinent
  - Dysplasias (multiple epiphyseal dysplasia, spondyloepiphyseal dysplasia, achondroplasia, etc)

Physical Examination

- Observe the overall alignment of the knee joint and the tibia
- Rotational profile as previously mentioned

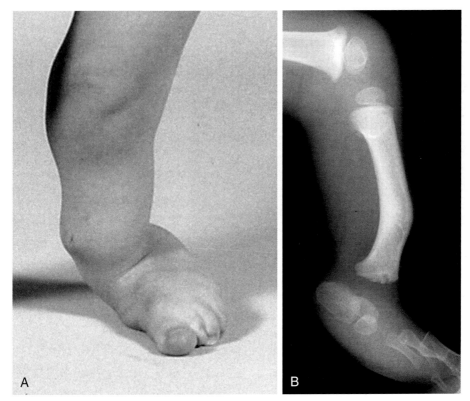

Figure 8E3.2. Clinical photograph (A) and radiograph (B) of pathologic anterolateral bowing. (From McCarthy JJ, Drennan JC. *Drennan's the Child's Foot and Ankle*. Philadelphia, PA: Lippincott Williams & Wilkins; 2010.)

- In extension with the patella facing forward, evaluate for intercondylar distance at the knee and intermalleolar distance at the ankle
  - May not be useful as absolute values but can be useful as serial evaluations of the child
- Complete knee examination as previously covered
- Special examination maneuvers
  - **Popliteal angle** (Figure 8E3.3)
    - Used frequently in the literature but not associated with one specific person
    - **Maneuver:**
      - This examination maneuver is used to measure tightness of the hamstring muscle group. The examiner places the patient in the supine position on the examination table. While stabilizing the pelvis with one hand, the examiner grasps the ankle of the extremity to be examined and flexes the hip up to 90°. The examiner continues to extend the knee while the hip is maintained at 90°. Once maximum extension of the knee is obtained, the examiner should document the angle formed by the tibia and femur at the knee. This is helpful in determining any contracture or neuromuscular disorders of the leg

IMAGING

- True AP and lateral radiographs of the leg will allow for assessment of alignment
- Standing alignment films must be obtained with the patella facing forward and without the legs touching
  - At times this means the individual legs must be imaged separately as both legs may not fit on 1 cassette unless they are placed together at the thigh, knee, or ankle
    - Look for soft tissue overlap if both legs are visible on 1 cassette
  - EOS imaging can reduce the radiation dose

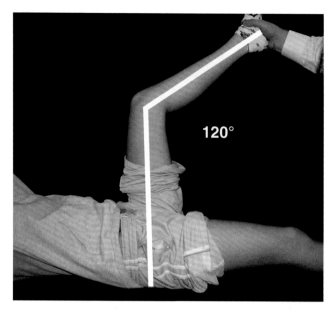

Figure 8E3.3. Clinical example of the popliteal angle examination. (From Weinstein SL, Flynn JM. *Lovell and Winter's Pediatric Orthopaedics*. Vol 1. Wolters Kluwer Health; 2014.)

TABLE 8E4.1 Pediatric Tumors and Malignancies of the Lower Extremity

Popliteal cyst
Lipoma
Pigmented villonodular synovitis
Unicameral bone cyst
Aneurysmal bone cyst
Nonossifying fibroma
Osteochondroma
Enchondroma
Neurofibroma
Fibrous dysplasia
Ewing sarcoma
Rhabdomyosarcoma
Osteosarcoma
Chondroblastoma

- Radiographs of pseudoarthrosis will show an area of nonunion
- CT is used to evaluate for suspected bony bar or changes associated with Blount disease
- MRI sequences can also help delineate articular involvement
  - Better able to demonstrate not yet ossified aspects of the proximal tibia and distal femur

SECTION E4: TUMORS

History

- Tumors of the distal femur or proximal tibia generally present as pain at the site of the tumor and a gradually developing limp that does not resolve[6]
- Differential is broad and is dependent on a variety of factors
- A complete history is important; ask about appetite changes, fevers and episodes of diaphoresis, nighttime pain or changes in sleep habits, and weight-loss that is unintentional
- Do not be fooled by a history of trauma—often present in all children
  - Do not skip radiographic surveillance because of relatively mild presenting signs and symptoms that are attributed to a "sprain" or Salter-Harris type I injury (Table 8E4.1; Figures 8E4.1-8E4.5)

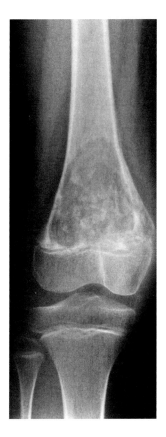

Figure 8E4.1. Osteosarcoma in an 8-year-old girl. (Courtesy of Dr M. M. Lewis, Santa Barbara, California.)

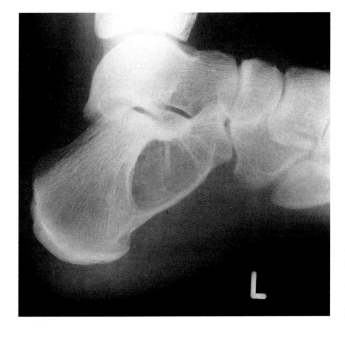

Figure 8E4.2. Bone cyst in a 13-year-old boy. (From Brant WE, Helms CA. *Fundamentals of Diagnostic Radiology*. Philadelphia, PA: Lippincott Williams & Wilkins; 2007.)

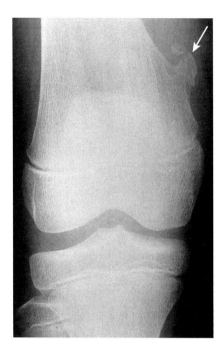

Figure 8E4.3. Osteochondroma of the distal femur. (From Yochum TR, Rowe LJ. *Yochum and Rowe's Essentials of Skeletal Radiology*. 3rd ed. Philadelphia: Lippincott Williams & Wilkins; 2004.)

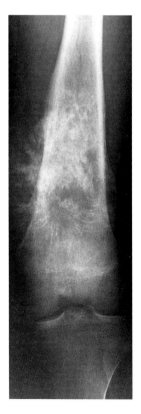

Figure 8E4.4. Radiograph demonstrating Ewing sarcoma in a 17-year-old male. (From Greenspan A, Steinbach LS, Borys D, Wolters Kluwer Health. *Radiology and Pathology Correlation of Bone Tumors: A Quick Reference and Review*. Philadelphia [etc.]: Wolters Kluwer; 2016.)

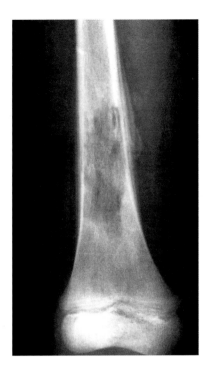

Figure 8E4.5. Radiograph of osteomyelitis mimicking Ewing sarcoma in a 7-year-old boy. (From Greenspan A, Beltran J, Ovid Technologies I. *Orthopedic Imaging*: *A Practical Approach*. Philadelphia: Wolters Kluwer Health/ Lippincott Williams & Wilkins; 2015.)

Physical Examination

- Examination will generally indicate pain over the site of the tumor or malignancy. ROM and stability are variably affected. Palpable masses may be present, so be sure to evaluate the entire leg
- Other workup would include laboratory findings such as a complete blood count, comprehensive metabolic panel, alkaline phosphatase, C-reactive protein, erythrocyte sedimentation rate, and lactate dehydrogenase

IMAGING

- Radiographs of the affected area coupled with MRI are usually indicated for further diagnostic data. Discuss findings with musculoskeletal radiologist and consider consultation with orthopedic oncologists if necessary
- Use Enneking's 4 questions: Assess the location of the pathology, what it is doing to the bone, what the bone is doing to it, and what the tumor is producing

REFERENCES

1. Stalehi L. *Practice of Pediatric Orthopaedics*. 2nd ed. Philadelphia, PA: LWW; 2006:143-158.
2. Cleland JA, Koppenhaver S, Su J, et al. *Netter's Orthopaedic Clinical Examination*. 3rd ed. Philadelphia, PA. Elsevier; 2016:323-395.
3. Carter C, Wilkinson J. Persistent joint laxity and congenital dislocation of the hip. *J Bone Joint Surg (Br)*. 1964;46:40-45.
4. Beighton P. Articular mobility in an African population. *Ann Rheum Dis*. 1973;32(5):413-418.
5. Vijayasankar D, Boyle AA, Atkinson P, et al. Can the Ottawa knee rule be applied to children? A systematic review and meta-analysis of observational studies. *Emerg Med J*. 2009;26(4):250-253.
6. Arndt CA, Crist WM. Common musculoskeletal tumors of childhood and adolescence. *N Engl J Med*. 1999;341:342-352.

SECTION F
Foot and Ankle

Hakan C. Pehlivan

- Developmental variations in feet are common and are a major reason for referral. The more extreme variations may benefit from orthopedic management
- The foot achieves adult length early; around half of the terminal length is achieved by 12 to 18 months
- Accessory ossification centers are common and may or may not be symptomatic
- Parents typically pass on to their children the shape of their feet

SECTION F1: CONGENITAL FOOT DEFORMITIES/PACKAGING DISORDERS

History

- Congenital foot problems are present at birth and are typically noticed by the family or perhaps on a prenatal ultrasonography. The most likely encountered conditions include clubfoot, metatarsus adductus, skewfoot, polydactyly/syndactyly, calcaneovalgus foot, and vertical/oblique talus
- They can be associated with other congenital abnormalities
- These conditions can be mild or self-limiting; however, some require interventions such as serial casting or corrective surgery. Clubfoot, skewfoot, and vertical talus can go on to cause significant deformity if left untreated
- Presentation
  - Often referral from pediatrician or even from obstetrician with prenatal diagnosis or nursery diagnosis
  - Clubfoot: cavus, adductus, varus, equinus—consult from ultrasonography or in newborn nursery (Figure 8F1.1)
  - Metatarsus adductus: forefoot adduction—usually presents later; "pigeon-toed"; combined with midfoot abduction and hindfoot valgus in skewfoot
  - Polydactyly: more than 5 digits in varying attachments to the foot
  - Syndactyly: webbing to varying degrees between toes
  - Calcaneovalgus foot: extreme dorsiflexion with the dorsum of the foot nearly meeting the tibia; also associated with posteromedial tibial bowing
  - Vertical/oblique talus: rocker bottom foot

Physical Examination

- As most congenital foot deformities will present before ambulation, it is important to note the resting position of the foot
  - Hindfoot position: varus—deviation of calcaneus toward the midline of body; valgus—deviation of calcaneus away from the midline of body
  - Hindfoot position: calcaneus—deviation of the anterior process dorsal (dorsiflexion); equinus—deviation of the anterior process plantar (plantar flexion)

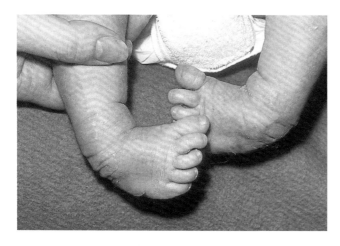

Figure 8F1.1. Clinical photograph demonstrating the characteristic position of foot with clubfoot. (From Ricci SS. *Essentials of Maternity, Newborn & Women's Health Nursing*. Philadelphia: Wolters Kluwer/Lippincott Williams & Wilkins; 2013.)

- Midfoot position: adductus—toward the midline of the body; abducted—away from the midline of the body
- Midfoot position: cavus—relative elevation of the midfoot with plantar flexion of the forefoot; planus—relative sag of the midfoot with dorsiflexion of the forefoot
- Forefoot position: adductus—toward the midline of the body; abducted—away from the midline of the body
- Forefoot position: supination—internal rotation/elevation of the forefoot in relation to the midfoot; pronation—external rotation/plantar flexion of the forefoot in relation to the midfoot
- Combined position: inversion—varus, adductus, supination; eversion—valgus, abduction, pronation
- Be sure to note the flexibility of the deformity and document range of motion of the affected joints of the hindfoot, midfoot, and forefoot; also note contractures
  - Calcaneovalgus foot flexible and completely correctable passively, similar in some cases of metatarsus adductus. Clubfoot and vertical talus not completely passively correctable on the first evaluation
- Pirani classification can be useful in determining severity of clubfoot, based on features of the midfoot and hindfoot. Dimeglio classification characterizes the stiffness of equinus, varus, rotation, and adduction (Figure 8F1.2)
- Vertical talus manifests as rocker bottom feet, with a convex plantar surface (Figure 8F1.3)
- Most foot conditions considered some form of packaging disorder; therefore, there is high incidence of associated packaging disorders (~10% association with DDH, 10% association with torticollis). Be sure to complete a hip and neck examination

IMAGING

- Clubfoot X-rays are rarely needed. Later in treatment, one may need to assess parallelism (or lack thereof) between talus and calcaneus or tibiocalcaneal angle on the lateral view and talus-first metatarsal angle on the lateral and AP views. In early presentation, no imaging is needed
- To differentiate between the metatarsus adductus and skewfoot on an AP of the foot, the alignment of the forefoot and midfoot should be keenly observed (Figure 8F1.4)
- Vertical vs oblique talus is diagnosed based on maximum plantar flexion lateral radiograph, which demonstrates a vertically oriented talus with no congruity between talus and navicular (if ossified) (Figure 8F1.5). Typically the navicular is not yet ossified and uses the first ray as proxy

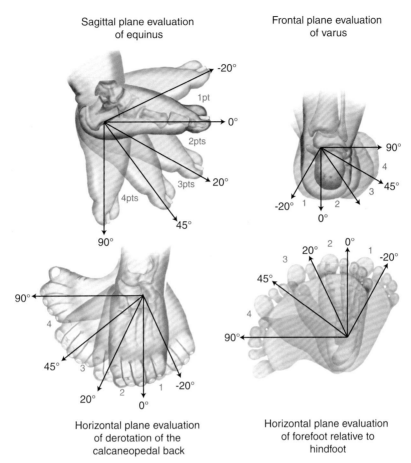

Sagittal plane evaluation
of equinus

Frontal plane evaluation
of varus

Horizontal plane evaluation
of derotation of the
calcaneopedal back

Horizontal plane evaluation
of forefoot relative to
hindfoot

Figure 8F1.2. Dimeglio classification with a scoring system 0 to 20, higher score correlating with severity of the clubfoot. The position of the foot relative to equinus, varus, foot rotation, and forefoot medial deviation and then 4 special scoring points.

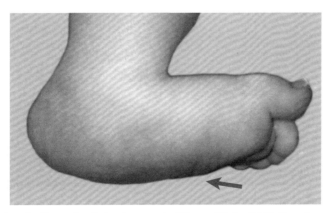

Figure 8F1.3. Rocker bottom foot (red arrow). (From Staheli LT. *Fundamentals of Pediatric Orthopedics*. 5th ed. Philadelphia: Wolters Kluwer; 2016.)

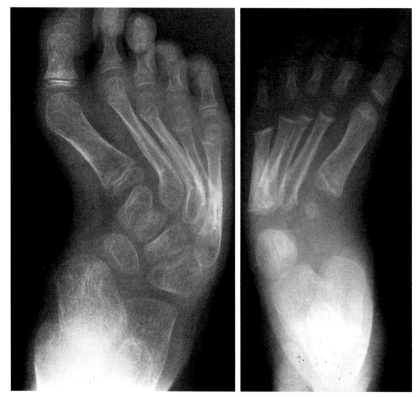

Figure 8F1.4. Metatarsus adductus and skewfoot side by side; note the "Z" deformity on the right consistent with skewfoot involving hindfoot valgus in addition to the forefoot adductus. (From Berquist TH, ed. *Imaging of the Foot and Ankle*. 3rd ed. Philadelphia: Wolters Kluwer/ Lippincott Williams & Wilkins; 2011.)

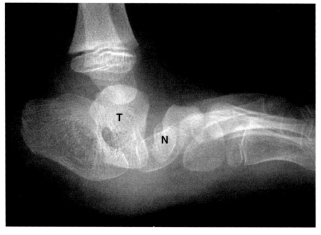

Figure 8F1.5. Lateral radiograph of vertical talus. T, talus; N, navicular. (From Siegel MJ. *Pediatric Sonography*. Philadelphia: Wolters Kluwer/Lippincott Williams & Wilkins; 2011.)

SECTION F2: FLATFOOT, CAVUS DEFORMITIES, TOE-WALKING, AND COALITIONS

History

- Walking age through school ages
  - Sometimes driven by foot pain, often simply concerned parents (or grandparents) wishing to establish best foundation for the child
  - When presenting with foot pain, establish the site of pain: arch (rigid flatfoot, tarsal coalition), toes (cavus), metatarsal heads (cavus, toe-walking), sinus tarsi (flatfoot, tarsal coalition)
- Flexible flatfoot is a normal physiologic finding in infants and is very common in patients with joint laxity or a family history
- Cavus foot requires that you obtain family and personal history of progressive or nonprogressive neurologic disorders such as Charcot-Marie-Tooth and Friedreich ataxia
- Tarsal coalitions often have a familial component
- Toe-walking is typically associated with a neurologic or behavioral condition

Physical Examination

- With physiologic deformities, typically patients have full ROM of the foot and ankle. Normal ranges include 23° to 48° of plantar flexion and 10° to 23° of dorsiflexion
- Limited subtalar inversion and eversion may be present in tarsal coalitions. Pretend to "shake the foot" like you are shaking a hand. This will allow control of the forefoot and hindfoot to evaluate for subtalar motion
- Make note of the position of the foot when the child is sitting and standing, things to pay attention to include the position of the hindfoot, midfoot, forefoot. Observe what happens with gait. Evaluate what happens to the arch, especially when transitioning from resting to walking
- Being a "shoe reader" can be important—often they will have breakdown of the inner aspect of the shoe. Either the tread is worn or the wall of the shoe and heel have broken down due to the foot position. Cavus feet may present with a lateral shoe wear pattern
- Have the child walk, heel walk, toe walk, and squat. This will give an overview of neurologic capabilities with strength (heel-walking requires strong dorsiflexion at the ankle, toe-walking requires strong plantar flexion). Also pay attention to the arch of the foot with toe-walking
- Calcaneonavicular coalitions may have a palpable bony bar distal to the sinus tarsi on the lateral aspect of the foot. Talocalcaneal coalitions may have a "double medial malleolus sign" as described by Mubarak with the prominence of the coalition representing a more distal malleolus

---

KEY EXAMINATION MANEUVERS

- **Coleman Block Test** (Figure 8F2.1)
  - Developed by Sherman Coleman; first published in 1977[2]
  - **Maneuver:**
    - A wooden block is placed on the floor, and the patient with cavus stands on the block with the heel and lateral edge of the foot on the block. When observed from behind, the examiner should note if the deformity of the hindfoot is flexible allowing correction to neutral or valgus at the heel. The heel should correct to a neutral position and the first ray should be in contact with the floor. This may suggest an issue with the first ray being overly plantar flexed. If the hindfoot deformity remains in varus, the deformity is considered rigid

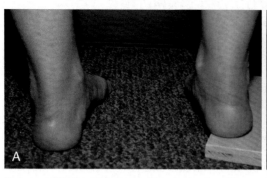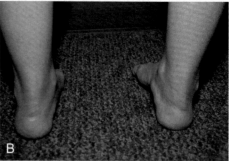

Figure 8F2.1. Coleman block test. (From Wiesel SW. *Operative Techniques in Orthopaedic Surgery. Sports Medicine; Pelvis and Lower Extremity Trauma; Adult Reconstruction 11*. Philadelphia: Wolters Kluwer; 2016.)

- Silfverskiold Test
  - Described by Nils Silfverskiold in 1924[4] regarding his work on children with neuromuscular disorders
  - **Maneuver:**
    - The patient is lying supine on the examination table. The examiner measures ankle dorsiflexion while the knee is extended. Then the examiner remeasures ankle dorsiflexion when the knee is flexed to 90°. If the issue lies in the gastrocnemius/soleus muscle complex, the dorsiflexion will significantly improve with knee flexion due to relaxation of the gastrocnemius as it crosses the knee joint. If the issue lies in the Achilles tendon, there will not be significant change in ankle dorsiflexion with knee extension or flexion

IMAGING

- All nontrauma foot X-rays should be obtained standing
- Typical X-rays include standing AP ankle and standing AP and lateral foot X-rays. Concerns for calcaneonavicular coalition, talocalcaneal coalition, and accessory navicular should include internal oblique foot X-ray, Harris heel view, and external oblique view, respectively (Figure 8F2.2)
- Talus-first metatarsal angles measured on standing films can help to reveal the center of rotation of angulation of foot deformity, a concept popularized in limb deformity by Paley et al and translated to the pediatric foot by Mosca (Figure 8F2.3)

SECTION F3: OSTEOCHONDRITIS, IMPINGEMENT SYNDROMES

History

- Osteochondritis and impingement syndromes present typically in the second decade of life, as the child begins to become more active
- Pain is generally during or after activity and resolves with rest
- OCD patients present with chronic pain, swelling after activity, and stiffness. Most commonly the lesion is located on the medial side of the talus in children,[5] as opposed to the lateral side in adults, and may be associated with ankle laxity (Figure 8F3.1)
- Kohler disease is an osteochondritis of the navicular and is more common in young males presenting with arch pain (Figure 8F3.2)

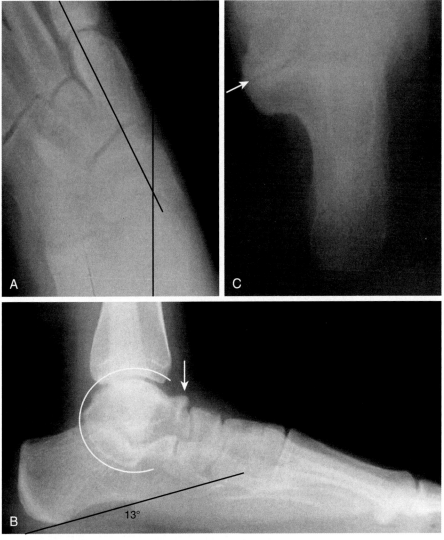

Figure 8F2.2. Talocalcaneal coalition. Flatfoot associated with coalition. Note the lateral position of the navicular. B, C-sign of lateral and dorsal talar beaking. C, Harris view showing irregular middle facet with coalition. (From Mosca VS. *Principles and Management of Pediatric Foot and Ankle Deformities and Malformations*. Wolters Kluwer; 2014.)

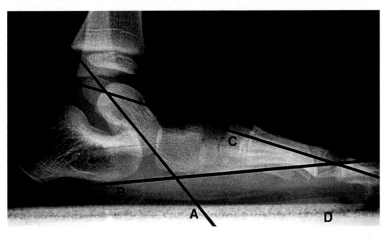

Figure 8F2.3. Talar axis (A); calcaneal axis (B); first metatarsal axis (C); plane of support (D). Talocalcaneal angle (AB); talar-first metatarsal angle (AC); talar declination angle (AD); calcaneal inclination angle (BD); Hibb angle (BC). (From Christman RA. *Foot and Ankle Radiology*. Wolters Kluwer; 2015.)

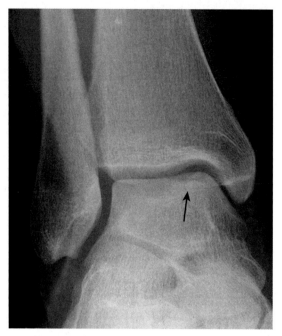

Figure 8F3.1. Radiograph demonstrating talar osteochondral lesion. (From Christman RA. *Foot and Ankle Radiology*. Wolters Kluwer; 2015.)

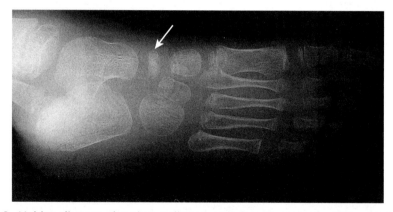

Figure 8F3.2. Kohler disease showing collapse and fragmentation of the navicular. (From Fleisher GR, Ludwig S, Baskin MN. *Atlas of Pediatric Emergency Medicine*. Philadelphia: Lippincott Williams & Wilkins; 2004.)

- Freiberg infraction is an osteochondritis/necrosis of the metatarsal head, more specifically the second metatarsal head. It is most common in adolescent females; rarely disabling or requires surgical intervention; and presents as forefoot pain (Figure 8F3.3)
- Sever disease is an osteochondritis/apophysitis of the calcaneal apophysitis and typically presents as heel pain in active young children
- Impingement syndromes can occur when accessory bones or excess tissue becomes compressed during specific motion. Commonly associated with an os trigonum posteriorly, which can be painful in deep plantar flexion, or anterior impingement due to an osteophyte or excess capsule anteriorly

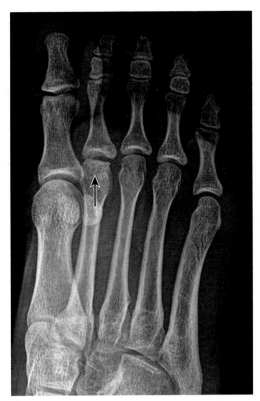

Figure 8F3.3. Freiberg infraction in a 15-year-old girl. (From Lee EY. *Pediatric Radiology: Practical Imaging Evaluation of Infants and Children.* Wolters Kluwer Health; 2018.)

TABLE 8F3.1 Summary of Osteochondritis Conditions of the Foot

Köhler disease, accessory navicular	Navicular tenderness
Freiberg infraction	Second metatarsal head tenderness
Sever disease	Calcaneal apophysitis tenderness/pain with heel squeeze

Physical Examination

- For OCD lesions, an ankle effusion may be present. Generally, ROM is full but may be limited due to pain. Point of maximal tenderness over the OCD can occur and is more readily accessible when the ankle is plantar flexed
- Tenderness typically correlates with the location of the osteochondritis/apophysitis (Table 8F3.1)
- For impingement syndromes, clinically correlate area of pain and tenderness with radiographic findings. Generally, the point of maximal tenderness and pain with ROM is the area of impingement

Special Examination Maneuvers

- **Anterior drawer test** (sensitivity 58%, specificity 100%)
  - Used to assess laxity
  - First appears in the literature described by Nilsonne in 1932[7], who described a ligament reconstruction of a 13-year-old girl who had a ruptured calcaneofibular ligament

- **Maneuver:**
  - The examiner grasps the calcaneus and imparts an anteriorly directed force to move the talus of the patient and notes movement of the talus within the mortise. This examination can help determine if there is congenital laxity of the ankle joint or injury to the lateral stabilizers
- **Anterior or anterolateral ankle impingement exam** (sensitivity 90%, specificity 88%)
  - Described as a "footballer's ankle" by McMurray in 1950,[3] a common condition involving symptomatic anterior osteophytes
  - **Maneuver:**
    - The examiner grasps the calcaneus with one hand and uses the other hand to plantar flex the foot of the patient. The examiner then places the thumb over the area of concern anteriorly and applies pressure, while bringing the foot up from plantar flexion to dorsiflexion. Note if there are any changes in the level of pain
- **Posterior impingement examination**
  - Similar to anterior examination except with a posterior directed force
  - **Maneuver:**
    - The examiner applies pressure to the posterior ankle and retrocalcaneal space from both sides by grasping with the thumb and index, while simultaneously plantar flexing the ankle with the other hand. Note any change in the level of pain

IMAGING

- Plain radiographs
  - Obtain 3 view ankle (AP, mortise, lateral) or 3 view foot (AP ankle, AP foot, lateral foot) as workhorse imaging. Special views as discussed in section 6, The Foot and Ankle, can include Harris view for talocalcaneal coalition, sesamoid views, and internal and external oblique views for calcaneonavicular coalition and accessory navicular, respectively
    - Obtain standing films whenever possible
    - Useful to assess overall foot architecture
    - Tibocalcaneal angle (normal 70°-90°)
    - Kite angle between the talus and calcaneus (normal 25°-40°)
    - Meary angle between the longitudinal axis of the talus and first metatarsal
    - Calcaneal pitch angle (average between 20° and 30°, lower can indicate pes planus and higher can indicate pes cavus)
    - Be mindful on standing lateral of the amount of subtalar joint visible. Cavus hindfoot means more of the middle subtalar joint is visible
- CT scans
  - Useful in evaluating for coalitions or injury to accessory ossicles or sesamoids
- MRI
  - Can be used to evaluate for OCD, ligament and tendon pathology, or cysts and tumors
- Bone scans
  - Can be useful for sites of inflammation such as infection or osteochondrosis as seen in Freiberg disease[6]

REFERENCES

1. Di Matteo B, Tarabella V, Filardo G, et al. A historical perspective on ankle ligaments reconstructive surgery. *Knee Surg Sports Traumatol Arthrosc.* 2016;24(4):971-977.
2. Coleman SS, Chesnut WJ. A simple test for hindfoot flexibility in the cavovarus foot. *Clin Orthop Relat Res.* 1977;123:60-62.
3. McMurray TP. Footballer's Ankle. *Bone Joint J.* 1955;32-B,1
4. Silfverskild N. Reduction of the uncrossed two-joints muscles of the leg to one-joint muscles in spastic conditions. *Acta Chir Scand.* 1924;56:315-330.
5. Zanon G, DI Vico G, Marullo M, et al. Osteochondritis dissecans of the talus. *Joints.* 2014;2(3):115-123.
6. Stalehi L. *Practice of Pediatric Orthopaedics.* 2nd ed. Philadelphia, PA: LWW; 2006:105-140.
7. Nilsonne H. Making a New Ligament in Ankle Sprain. *J Bone Joint Surg.* 1932;14:380.

Index

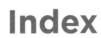

Note: Page numbers followed by "f" indicate figures, "t" indicate tables and "b" indicate boxes.